Delirium

Christopher G. Hughes • Pratik P. Pandharipande
E. Wesley Ely
Editors

Delirium

Acute Brain Dysfunction in the Critically Ill

Springer

Editors
Christopher G. Hughes
Critical Illness, Brain Dysfunction, and Survivorship Center and the Division of Anesthesiology Critical Care Medicine
Vanderbilt University Medical Center
Nashville, TN
USA

Pratik P. Pandharipande
Critical Illness, Brain Dysfunction, and Survivorship Center and the Division of Anesthesiology Critical Care Medicine
Vanderbilt University Medical Center
Nashville, TN
USA

E. Wesley Ely
Critical Illness, Brain Dysfunction, and Survivorship (CIBS) Center
Department of Medicine
Pulmonary and Critical Care
Vanderbilt University School of Medicine and the Tennessee Valley Veteran's Affairs Geriatric Research Education Clinical Center (GRECC)
Nashville, TN
USA

ISBN 978-3-030-25750-7 ISBN 978-3-030-25751-4 (eBook)
https://doi.org/10.1007/978-3-030-25751-4

This Springer imprint is published by the registered company Springer Nature Switzerland AG
The registered company address is: Gewerbestrasse 11, 6330 Cham, Switzerland

Preface

"A long habit of not thinking a thing wrong, gives it a superficial appearance of being right" was written by Thomas Paine in his pamphlet entitled *Common Sense* circa 1776. And while the context of this statement involved fighting for a democratic government and not fighting disease, the same philosophies hold true for much of our "practice" of medicine. Acute brain dysfunction during acute illness has, unfortunately, proven this concept time and time again throughout the history of medicine. It has long been associated with severe and critical illness, but for practitioners and even patients, it was typically considered an expected and often insignificant consequence – one that we now know is dangerous and costly in its own right and that should not be underestimated.

Patients with critical illness commonly demonstrate acute brain dysfunction secondary to their disease processes and as a consequence of the therapies required to treat their disease. This brain dysfunction and altered mental status can present in a wide collection of signs and symptoms, ranging from coma to hyperactivity and psychosis. Though this brain dysfunction has historically been described in many terms, the medical community has converged on "delirium" as the construct to advance clinical care, communication, and research.

Evidence over recent years from numerous disciplines has pointed us not only to the importance of diagnosing, preventing, and treating delirium during critical illness but also to the need to educate clinical care providers, patients, and families about its significance and bearing. Delirium in and of itself is unpleasant, unsettling, frightening, and often dangerous. Further, it is independently associated with worse patient-centered outcomes both in the short term and years after its presentation, including cognitive impairment and dementia. In order to improve both survival and survivorship of our patients with critical illness, we need to limit the prevalence and impact of delirium. As expected from its complicated origins and clinical presentations, this is not a simple task.

With the contents of this book, we summarize current knowledge, provide valuable clinical insights and strategies, emphasize the importance of multidisciplinary efforts, and stimulate future patient care and research. Thus, this book provides a comprehensive, state-of-the-art overview of delirium and acute brain dysfunction in the critically ill. It covers the basic pathophysiology of delirium, epidemiology, risk factors, outcomes associated with delirium, prevention and treatment of delirium, and challenges and techniques for improving delirium awareness. The chapters of the book were written by experts in the field (to which we owe our gratitude, respect, and admiration) to provide one of the most in-depth resources on delirium in the critically ill.

GL Engel and J. Romano in their article "Delirium, a syndrome of cerebral insufficiency" in the *Journal of Chronic Disease* in 1959 wrote "The physician who is greatly concerned to protect the functional integrity of the heart, liver, and kidneys of his patient has not yet learned to have similar regard for the functional integrity of the brain. This is a serious and, perhaps, tragic omission." We, and the evidence, agree! Advancing awareness and knowledge of delirium is an individual and public health imperative. It is our conviction that empowering readers with this valuable resource on delirium will help guide patient management and stimulate investigative efforts.

Nashville, TN, USA

Christopher G. Hughes
Pratik P. Pandharipande
E. Wesley Ely

Contents

Contributors

Bret D. Alvis, MD Division of Anesthesiology Critical Care Medicine, Department of Anesthesiology, Vanderbilt University Medical Center, Nashville, TN, USA

Elizabeth Archambault, LICSW Center of Innovation in Long Term Services and Supports, Providence VAMC, Providence, RI, USA

Rakesh C. Arora, MD, PhD Max Rady College of Medicine, Rady Faculty of Health Sciences, University of Manitoba, Winnipeg, MB, Canada

Cardiac Sciences Program, St. Boniface Hospital, Winnipeg, MB, Canada

Michele C. Balas, PhD, RN, CCRN-K, FCCM, FAAN The Ohio State University, College of Nursing, Columbus, OH, USA

Mary Ann Barnes-Daly, MS, RN, CCRN-K, DC Sutter Health, Sacramento, CA, USA

Sean S. Barnes, MD, MBA Department of Anesthesiology and Critical Care Medicine, Johns Hopkins Charlotte R. Bloomberg Children's Center, Baltimore, MD, USA

Leanne M. Boehm, RN, PhD, ACNS-BC Critical Illness, Brain Dysfunction, and Survivorship Center and the Vanderbilt University School of Nursing, Nashville, TN, USA

Malaz Boustani, MD Center for Brain Care Innovation, Regenstrief Institute, Indiana University School of Medicine, Indianapolis, IN, USA

Noll L. Campbell, PharmD, MS Department of Pharmacy Practice, Purdue University College of Pharmacy, West Lafayette, IN, USA

Center for Health Innovation and Implementation Science, Regenstrief Institute, Indianapolis, IN, USA

Indiana University Center for Aging Research, Regenstrief Institute, Indianapolis, IN, USA

John W. Devlin, PharmD School of Pharmacy Northeastern University, Boston, MA, USA

E. Wesley Ely, MD, MPH, FCCM Critical Illness, Brain Dysfunction, and Survivorship (CIBS) Center, Department of Medicine, Pulmonary and Critical Care, Vanderbilt University School of Medicine and the Tennessee Valley Veteran's Affairs Geriatric Research Education Clinical Center (GRECC), Nashville, TN, USA

Christopher Gabor, MSc Department of Emergency & Community Medicine, Hamilton Health Sciences, Hamilton, ON, Canada

Timothy D. Girard, MS, MSCI Department of Critical Care Medicine, University of Pittsburgh School of Medicine, Pittsburgh, PA, USA

Caroline L. Greene, PhD Geriatric Research Education and Clinical Center, Tennessee Valley Veterans Affairs Healthcare System, Nashville, TN, USA

Diane N. Haddad, MD Critical Illness, Brain Dysfunction, and Survivorship Center, Vanderbilt University Medical Center, Nashville, TN, USA

Division of Trauma, Surgical Critical Care, and Emergency General Surgery, Section of Surgical Sciences, Department of Surgery, Nashville, TN, USA

Christina J. Hayhurst, MD Division of Anesthesiology Critical Care Medicine, Department of Anesthesiology, Vanderbilt University Medical Center, Nashville, TN, USA

Christopher G. Hughes, MD, MS, FCCM Critical Illness, Brain Dysfunction, and Survivorship Center and the Division of Anesthesiology Critical Care Medicine, Vanderbilt University Medical Center, Nashville, TN, USA

Suzanne C. A. Hut, PhD Department of Intensive Care Medicine, University Medical Center Utrecht, Utrecht University, Utrecht, The Netherlands

UMC Utrecht Brain Center, Utrecht, The Netherlands

James C. Jackson, PsyD Geriatric Research Education and Clinical Center, Tennessee Valley Veterans Affairs Healthcare System, Nashville, TN, USA

Critical Illness, Brain Dysfunction, and Survivorship Center, Vanderbilt University Medical Center, Nashville, TN, USA

Laura Beth Kalvas, BSN, RN, PCCN The Ohio State University, College of Nursing, Columbus, OH, USA

Dustin Scott Kehler, MSc, PhD Department of Medicine, Division of Geriatric Medicine, Dalhousie University, Halifax, NS, Canada

Babar A. Khan, MD, MS Center for Health Innovation and Implementation Science, Regenstrief Institute, Indianapolis, IN, USA

Indiana University Center for Aging Research, Regenstrief Institute, Indianapolis, IN, USA

Department of Medicine, Indiana University School of Medicine, Indianapolis, IN, USA

Katarzyna Kotfis, MD, PhD, DESA Department of Anesthesiology, Intensive Therapy and Acute Intoxications, Pomeranian Medical University, Szczecin, Poland

Sapna R. Kudchadkar, MD, PhD Department of Anesthesiology and Critical Care Medicine, Pediatrics and Physical Medicine and Rehabilitation, Johns Hopkins Charlotte R. Bloomberg Children's Center, Baltimore, MD, USA

Frans S. Leijten, MD, PhD UMC Utrecht Brain Center, Utrecht, The Netherlands

Department of Neurology and Neurosurgery, University Medical Center Utrecht, Utrecht University, Utrecht, The Netherlands

Marcos G. Lopez, MD, MS Division of Anesthesiology Critical Care Medicine, Department of Anesthesiology, Vanderbilt University Medical Center, Nashville, TN, USA

José R. Maldonado, MD, FAPM, FACFE Division of Psychosomatic Medicine, Emergency Psychiatry Service, Stanford University School of Medicine, Stanford, CA, USA

Annachiara Marra, MD, PhD Department of Neurosciences, Reproductive and Odontostomatological Sciences, University of Naples, Federico II, Naples, Italy

Karin J. Neufeld, MD, MPH Johns Hopkins University School of Medicine, Baltimore, MD, USA

Mina F. Nordness, MD Critical Illness, Brain Dysfunction, and Survivorship Center, Vanderbilt University Medical Center, Nashville, TN, USA

Division of Trauma, Surgical Critical Care, and Emergency General Surgery, Section of Surgical Sciences, Department of Surgery, Vanderbilt University Medical Center, Nashville, TN, USA

Mayur B. Patel, MD, MPH, FACS, FCCM Critical Illness, Brain Dysfunction, and Survivorship Center, Vanderbilt University Medical Center, Nashville, TN, USA

Division of Trauma, Surgical Critical Care, and Emergency General Surgery, Section of Surgical Sciences, Department of Surgery, Nashville, TN, USA

Vanderbilt University Medical Center, Nashville, TN, USA

Geriatric Research Education and Clinical Center, Tennessee Valley Veterans Affairs Healthcare System, Nashville, TN, USA

Departments of Neurosurgery, and Hearing & Speech Sciences, Vanderbilt Brain Institute, Nashville, TN, USA

Surgical Service, Department of Veterans Affairs Medical Center, Tennessee Valley Healthcare System, Nashville, TN, USA

Brenda T. Pun, RN, DNP Division of Allergy, Pulmonary, and Critical Care Medicine, Department of Medicine, Vanderbilt University Medical Center, Nashville, TN, USA

Critical Illness, Brain Dysfunction, and Survivorship Center, Vanderbilt University Medical Center, Nashville, TN, USA

Shayan Rakhit, MD(c) Critical Illness, Brain Dysfunction, and Survivorship Center, Vanderbilt University Medical Center, Nashville, TN, USA

Division of Trauma, Surgical Critical Care, and Emergency General Surgery, Section of Surgical Sciences, Department of Surgery, Nashville, TN, USA

Vanderbilt University School of Medicine, Nashville, TN, USA

Paul Rowley, BS Department of Anesthesiology, University of Wisconsin School of Medicine and Public Health, Madison, WI, USA

James L. Rudolph, MD, SM Center of Innovation in Long Term Services and Supports, Providence VAMC, Providence, RI, USA

Robert Sanders, MBBS, PhD Department of Anesthesiology, University of Wisconsin School of Medicine and Public Health, Madison, WI, USA

Rohan M. Sanjanwala, MD, MPH Max Rady College of Medicine, Rady Faculty of Health Sciences, University of Manitoba, Winnipeg, MB, Canada

Marianne Shaughnessy, GNP, PhD Office of Geriatrics and Extended Care, Veterans Health Administration, Washington, DC, USA

Arjen J. C. Slooter, PhD Department of Intensive Care Medicine, University Medical Center Utrecht, Utrecht University, Utrecht, The Netherlands

UMC Utrecht Brain Center, Utrecht, The Netherlands

Heidi A. B. Smith, MD, MSCI Department of Anesthesiology and Pediatrics, Vanderbilt University Medical Center, Nashville, TN, USA

Kristina Stepanovic, BA Department of Medicine, Division of Allergy, Pulmonary and Critical Care Medicine, Vanderbilt University School of Medicine, Nashville, TN, USA

Mark van den Boogaard, PhD Department Intensive Care Medicine, Radboud University Medical Center, Radboud Institute for Health Sciences, IQ Healthcare, Nijmegen, The Netherlands

Stacey R. Williams, NP Department of Pediatrics, Nurse Practitioner, Division of Pediatric Critical Care, Vanderbilt University Medical Center, Nashville, TN, USA

Jo Ellen Wilson, MD, MPH Critical Illness, Brain Dysfunction, and Survivorship Center and the Department of Psychiatry and Behavioral Sciences, Vanderbilt University Medical Center, Nashville, TN, USA

Chapter 1
Delirium Definitions and Subtypes

Christina J. Hayhurst, Bret D. Alvis, and Timothy D. Girard

Introduction

Delirium has long been recognized as a pathologic syndrome, but as our understanding of it continues to evolve, so does the way we define it. In ancient Greece, Hippocrates used the term "phrenitis" when describing patients with cognitive and behavioral disturbances, agitation, and restlessness and used the term "lethargus" to describe those with memory impairment, somnolence, and listlessness. The term "delirium" was first used by the Roman physician Celsus, who described patients' delusions and perceptual disturbances in association with fever as delirium (the root word "delirare" means to go out of the furrow). In the nineteenth century, a French psychiatrist, Philippe Chaslin, coined the term "confusion mentale primitive" to indicate "an acute brain disorder, consecutive to a significant organic disease, with cognitive impairment associated with delusions, hallucinations, psychomotor agitation, or reciprocally, with psychomotor retardation and inertia" [1]. Thus the complex and changing nature of delirium has been long recognized, and the inconsistency of symptoms and variable clinical presentations have led to multiple attempts to define delirium throughout the modern era. Such changes in definition and terminology are one of the multiple reasons delirium can be difficult to diagnose, study, and treat. Prior to the *Diagnostic and Statistical Manual of Mental Disorders* (DSM-III, 1980) introduction of the term delirium, there were multiple terms used to describe acute generalized brain dysfunction. These terms included "acute confusional state, encephalopathy, acute brain failure, ICU psychosis, and even subacute

---

C. J. Hayhurst (✉) · B. D. Alvis
Division of Anesthesiology Critical Care Medicine, Department of Anesthesiology, Vanderbilt University Medical Center, Nashville, TN, USA
e-mail: christina.j.hayhurst@vumc.org

T. D. Girard
Department of Critical Care Medicine, University of Pittsburgh School of Medicine, Pittsburgh, PA, USA

C. G. Hughes et al. (eds.), *Delirium*, https://doi.org/10.1007/978-3-030-25751-4_1

befuddlement." These terms referred to delirium resulting from acute illness or intoxications and presenting in different treatment settings or patient populations (e.g., intensive care unit [ICU] vs hospital ward). Combining all of these clinical constructs under the unifying term *delirium* has resulted in a more coherent approach to clinical practice and research but leads to further questions about specific definitions and subtypes commonly encountered in the critically ill. Even among medical professionals, there remains scientific "confusion" around the topic, and only 54% of the healthcare professionals surveyed used the term accurately [2]. This chapter will review the current definitions and clinical subtypes of delirium most often encountered in the ICU.

Current Definition

Though controversy over how to define delirium persists in some circles, most experts and authoritative bodies consider the American Psychological Association's definition of delirium to be the reference standard (Table 1.1). In the DSM-V, delirium is defined by the following criteria: "A. Disturbance in *attention* (i.e., reduced ability to direct, focus, sustain, and shift attention) and awareness (reduced *orientation to the environment*). B. The disturbance develops over a short period of time (usually hours to a few days), *represents an acute change from baseline attention and awareness*, and tends to fluctuate in severity during the course of a day. C. An additional disturbance in cognition (e.g., memory deficit, disorientation, language, visuospatial ability, or perception). *D. The disturbances in Criteria A and C* are not better explained by a pre-existing, established or evolving neurocognitive disorder and *do not occur in the context of a severely reduced level of arousal such as coma* [3]. Though these criteria are an important reference standard and are used by psychiatrists in their daily practice, non-psychiatrist providers frequently rely on delirium assessment tools that have been validated against the DSM criteria. These tools facilitate rapid and reliable diagnosis of delirium in multiple settings, including the ICU.

Table 1.1 DSM-V diagnostic criteria

A. Disturbance in attention (i.e., reduced ability to direct, focus, sustain, and shift attention) and awareness (reduced orientation to the environment)
B. The disturbance develops over a short period of time (usually hours to a few days), represents a change from baseline attention and awareness, and tends to fluctuate in severity during the course of a day
C. An additional disturbance in cognition (e.g., memory deficit, disorientation, language, visuospatial ability, or perception)
D. The disturbances in Criteria A and C are not better explained by another pre-existing, established, or evolving neurocognitive disorder and do not occur in the context of a severely reduced level of arousal, such as coma
E. There is evidence from the history, physical examination, or laboratory findings that the disturbance is a direct physiological consequence of another medical condition, substance intoxication or withdrawal (i.e., due to a drug of abuse or to a medication), or exposure to a toxin or is due to multiple etiologies

Diagnosis of Delirium in the ICU

Delirium is highly prevalent in the ICU, with some studies reporting occurrence in up to 80% of patients [4, 5]. Unfortunately, delirium is often underdiagnosed in the ICU without regular screening using a validated assessment tool [6]. Several factors likely contribute to failure to recognize delirium in the ICU, including lack of awareness that delirium during critical illness is often the hypoactive subtype and misattribution of delirium signs and symptoms to sedation and/or sleep.

A reliable yet more easily administered tool than the DSM definition was needed to help care for ICU patients and detect delirium efficiently. Several tools have been developed to rapidly diagnose delirium in the ICU; the most studied and best validated include the Confusion Assessment Method for the ICU (CAM-ICU) and Intensive Care Delirium Screening Checklist (ICDSC) [7, 8]. Details about delirium monitoring using these tools are provided in the following chapter.

Based on assessment of psychometric properties and performance in the ICU clinical setting, the CAM-ICU and ICDSC are the screening tools recommended by the Society of Critical Care Medicine guidelines on pain, sedation, and agitation from 2018 [9]. Delirium diagnosis is now being expanded upon to consider severity, motoric subtypes, and clinical phenotypes (Fig. 1.1).

Unlike the Delirium Rating Scale-Revised-98, which was validated as a measure of delirium severity in non-ICU patients, the CAM-ICU and the ICDSC were originally validated to assess delirium presence but not measure delirium severity. Both tools, however, have subsequently been used in this way, and recent studies found severity of delirium to be correlated with outcomes. The ICDSC is scored from 0 to 8, with a score 4 or above indicating clinical delirium. However any score above zero has been associated with an increase in mortality. When a diagnosis of clinical delirium does not exist, patients can still demonstrate subsyndromal delirium (SSD). This classification is typically made when the subject demonstrates cognitive and attentional deficits without meeting all the diagnostic criteria for delirium [10]. There is still not a clear definition in the literature of SSD, but it is often considered if the ICDSC score is between 1 and 3 or if 1–2 of the features on the CAM-ICU are positive [11]. In one

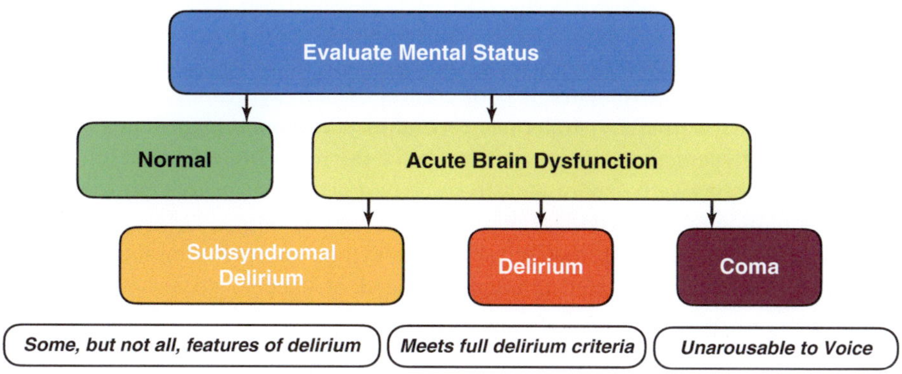

Fig. 1.1 Severity of delirium

study, ICU mortality rates were 2.4% for those patients with a ICDSC score of 0, 10.6% with a score of 1–3 (SSD), and 15.9% in those with a score between 4 and 8 (delirium) [12]. There are conflicting data regarding the outcomes of SSD compared with delirium. One study showed increased ICU mortality in those with SSD compared with those without any delirium symptoms [12], while another found no differences in outcomes [13]. SSD was associated in several studies with increased length of stay [11]. The distinction between SSD and no delirium is sometimes difficult, and more studies are required to explore neuropsychological tools that will help identify SSD and to determine whether it has important outcome consequences.

Due to interest in severity of delirium and not only a positive/negative assessment value, the CAM-ICU was adapted to include a numbered scale (0–2) for each delirium feature. This severity scale, known as the CAM-ICU-7, was found in one study to correlate with an increase in mortality [14]. More research is needed, however, before the CAM-ICU-7 or any delirium severity measure can be recommended for routine use in clinical practice.

Motoric Subtypes

Delirium, according to the DSM-V, must involve disturbances in both attention and cognition with an acute onset and organic etiology. As recognized by the ancient Greeks, these symptoms can be accompanied by a variety of psychomotor presentations. Importantly, several studies have found that the expression of these motoric subtypes of delirium is associated with differing outcomes [15–18]. In prior medical literature, hyperactive delirium was often termed "ICU psychosis," while the neurology literature called the hyperactive presentation "delirium" and termed hypoactive delirium "acute encephalopathy." There is suggestion to classify all delirium into clinical subtypes based on motoric symptoms and level of arousal [19, 20]. Lipowski first suggested categorizing delirium based on psychomotor presentation, using the terms hyperalert-hyperactive and hypoalert-hypoactive, and later added a mixed phenotype [21, 22].

The definitions of hyperactive and hypoactive delirium have traditionally included a listing of associated symptoms to distinguish the two subtypes. Hyperactive delirium is typically identified by increased activity levels, increased speed of actions or speech, involuntary movements, loss of control of activity, restlessness, abnormal content of verbal output, hyperalertness, irritability, and/or combativeness [22–25]. Patients with hyperactive delirium often receive the most clinical focus in the ICU due to their disruptive behavior and, in some cases, the danger they pose to themselves by pulling at intravascular lines, catheters, and monitors.

Hypoactive delirium, alternatively, involves symptoms such as reduced activity, apathy, listlessness, decreased amount or speed of speech, decreased alertness, withdrawal, unawareness, or hypersomnolence [22–25]. Patients with hypoactive delirium are less likely to draw attention to themselves, and the diagnosis of delirium may be missed entirely unless they are actively screened, as they do not exhibit overtly disruptive behavior.

A mixed subtype, wherein a patient fluctuates and exhibits both motoric features at different times, may be the most common motoric subtype in the ICU. It is difficult to precisely quantify its frequency, however, due to the often rapidly changing nature of the symptoms. Some studies have determined hypoactive to be the most common form of delirium and mixed to be the second most common. One thing is clear—pure hyperactive delirium is rare in the ICU—and as described later in the chapter, is generally associated with better outcomes than the other two motoric subtypes. What is not clear, however, is whether the association between hyperactive delirium and better outcomes reflects a biological difference in the mechanisms underlying the motoric subtypes of delirium or the effects of the sedative medications that are frequently given to ICU patients which can heavily influence the motor features exhibited during delirium.

In the ICU, a patient's level of arousal is often determined using a validated sedation scale, such as the Richmond Agitation and Sedation Scale (RASS) [26]. Originally developed by Sessler and colleagues [26], the RASS was initially designed as a monitoring tool for sedation related to medications given in the ICU. It was further validated for use in goal-directed sedation protocols [27]. It can, however, also be applied to patients who are not pharmacologically sedated as an assessment of their level of arousal. The RASS includes the following criteria, numbered between −5 and +4: unarousable, deep sedation, moderate sedation, light sedation, drowsy, alert and calm, restless, agitated, very agitated, and combative (Fig. 1.2).

+4	COMBATIVE	Combative, violent, immediate danger to staff	
+3	VERY AGITATED	Pulls to remove tubes or catheters; aggressive	
+2	AGITATED	Frequent non-purposeful movement, fights ventilator	
+1	RESTLESS	Anxious, apprehensive, movements not aggressive	
0	ALERT & CALM	Spontaneously pays attention to caregiver	
−1	DROWSY	Not fully alert, but has sustained awakening to voice (eye opening & contact >10 sec)	Verbal Stimulation
−2	LIGHT SEDATION	Briefly awakens to voice (eyes open & contact <10 sec)	
−3	MODERATE SEDATION	Movement or eye opening to voice (no eye contact)	
−4	DEEP SEDATION	No response to voice, but movement or eye opening to physical stimulation	Physical Stimulation
−5	UNAROUSEABLE	No response to voice or physical stimulation	

Procedure for RASS Assessment

1. Observe patient
   a. Patient is alert, restless, or agitated. **(score 0 to +4)**

2. If not alert, state patient's name and ***say*** to open eyes and look at speaker.
   b. Patient awakens with sustained eye opening and eye contact. **(score −1)**
   c. Patient awakens with eye opening and eye contact, but not sustained. **(score −2)**
   d. Patient has any movement in response to voice but no eye contact. **(score −3)**

3. When no response to verbal stimulation, physically stimulate patient by shaking shoulder and/or rubbing sternum.
   e. Patient has any movement to physical stimulation. **(score −4)**
   f. Patient has no response to any stimulation. **(score −5)**

Fig. 1.2 Richmond Agitation-Sedation Scale (RASS)

In many studies of ICU delirium, patients with delirium and a concomitant RASS >0 (which would include restless, agitated, and combative patients) were considered hyperactive. Patients with RASS ≤ -1, which described drowsy, light, or moderate sedation, were considered hypoactive, and patients with RASS ≤ -4, deep sedation or unarousable, were considered coma [28]. Patients with a RASS 0, indicating normal arousal level, at time of positive delirium assessment have most commonly been classified as hypoactive delirium due to the lack of hyperactive symptomatology. Other methods of determining the motoric subtype include motor subtyping from delirium checklists and visual analogue scales. However, the RASS is already commonly used in the ICU, making it a more accessible option.

In recent studies, it has been shown that the outcomes of hypoactive delirium compared to hyperactive delirium are generally worse. Liptzin and Levkoff suggest this might indicate the severity of the underlying illness. Healthier patients might be the ones who are physically able to become agitated or combative [29]. However, more recent work that has adjusted for severity of illness has still found hypoactive delirium as an independent risk factor for worse outcomes [30]. Hypoactive delirium is associated with increased short- and long-term mortality after critical illness. A prospective study of 1613 patients found in-hospital mortality to be the highest for patients with hypoactive or mixed subtypes [30]. In a study of 1292 ICU survivors, those with hypoactive delirium had a higher mortality rate at 18 months [31]. Interestingly, compared to the group with mixed or hyperactive phenotypes, they scored better on their healthcare-related quality of life questionnaires, which may be due to survivor bias. Patients with hypoactive delirium after surgery had a higher 6-month mortality compared to those with mixed delirium [15]. Patients in a palliative care ward were noted to have increased mortality at 1 month if their predominant motoric subtype was hypoactive [32]. Patients with hypoactive delirium are also at increased risk for pressure ulcers and hospital-acquired infections [15]. In patients with intracerebral hemorrhage, hypoactive delirium was associated with longer length of stay and worse functional outcomes and quality of life than hyperactive delirium [33]. Further study is needed to elucidate whether the hypoactive phenotype is merely representative of a more severe critical illness or whether it is a causative factor in outcomes.

Clinical Phenotypes

Most studies on subtypes of delirium in the ICU have focused on motoric subtypes, but delirium can also be examined according to clinical phenotypes in an effort to identify clinical risk factors and potential underlying causes of delirium that may be useful to guide therapy or predict outcomes. To date, only one study has taken this approach in the ICU, identifying five clinical phenotypes in a large multicenter cohort: metabolic, hypoxic, septic, sedative-associated, and unclassified [34]. Notably, these phenotypes were not considered mutually exclusive and, in fact, were found to frequently coexist [34] (Fig. 1.3). Girard et al. evaluated 1040

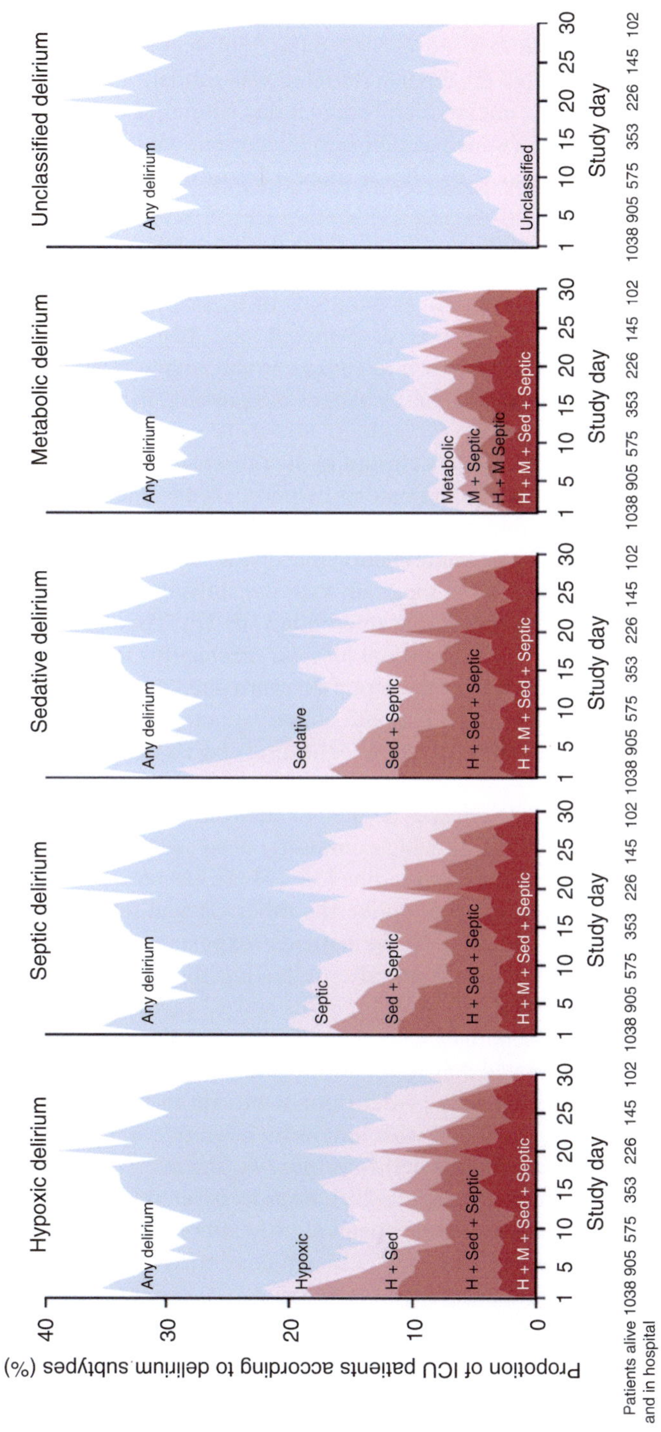

Fig. 1.3 Prevalence of delirium phenotype per study day

subjects and found rates of hypoxic, septic, sedative-associated, metabolic, and unclassified delirium to be 71%, 56%, 51%, 64%, 25%, and 22%, respectively [34]. They also demonstrated that the median duration was similar (3 days) no matter the phenotype, with only the "unclassified" being 1 day shorter [34].

Hypoxic delirium was defined as delirium concurrent with hypoxemia or shock [34]. Hypoxemia was defined as two or more 15-min intervals during which the lowest blood oxygen saturation level was <90%, and shock was defined as a lactate >4.4 mmol/L or two or more 15-min intervals during which lowest mean arterial pressure was <65 mmHg [34]. The duration of hypoxic delirium was found to predict long-term outcomes, with longer durations of hypoxic delirium being associated with worse cognitive deficits at 3-month and 12-month follow-up [34]. Intermittent hypoxia has been shown to cause cortical, subcortical, and hippocampal injury to rodent brains [35]. These changes are possible mechanisms to explain the long-term cognitive effects.

Septic delirium was defined as delirium in the presence of a known or suspected infection and ≥2 systemic inflammatory response syndrome criteria [34]. The effects of sepsis on the brain have only recently begun to be elucidated in animal models [34, 36]. The systemic inflammation that characterizes sepsis leads to monocyte and neutrophil infiltration in the brain with the activation of pro-inflammatory cytokines and chemokines within the microglia [36, 37]. This has been shown to lead to cortical and subcortical neuronal loss—a mechanism for cognitive impairment [34, 38]. Longer duration of the septic delirium phenotype, like hypoxic delirium, was associated with worse 12-month cognitive outcomes [34]. Much like the other phenotypes, the treatment of septic delirium is based on the general management of sepsis [36].

Sedative-associated delirium was defined as delirium in the setting of administration of at least one of the following commonly used sedatives: benzodiazepine, propofol, opioid, and/or dexmedetomidine [34]. There has been a strong interest in this particular phenotype because, unlike the other clinical delirium phenotypes, the clinician has direct control over the patients' exposure [34]. Prolonged durations of sedative-associated delirium, after adjusting for covariates, were associated with worse cognitive function at 3 months and 12 months [34]. Additionally, when specific classes of sedatives were examined (e.g., benzodiazepine-associated delirium, propofol-associated delirium), no specific class was more or less likely to predict long-term cognitive decline—delirium in the setting of any sedative, regardless of drug class, was associated with long-term cognitive impairment [34]. One study divided sedative-associated delirium into two forms: rapidly reversible and persistent sedative-associated delirium [39]. Rapidly reversible sedative-associated delirium was defined as delirium that abates shortly after sedative interruption [39], whereas persistent sedative-associated delirium continued after cessation of sedatives [39]. Patel et al. found that patients with rapidly reversible sedative-associated delirium had fewer ventilator, ICU, and hospital days than those with persistent delirium, but rapidly reversible sedative-associated delirium was much less common (only 12% of patients compared to 77% with persistent delirium) [39]. Persistent delirium was also associated with an increased 1-year mortality, whereas rapidly reversible delirium was not [39]. Whether sedative exposure, which can have effects that last longer than 2 h after discontinuation, played a role in persistent delirium could not be determined, and no evidence exists regarding the relationship between these two subsets of sedative-associated delirium and long-term cognition.

Metabolic delirium was defined as delirium concurrent with any of the following metabolic derangements that represent renal or hepatic dysfunction: blood urea nitrogen greater than 17.85 mmol/L, glucose <2.5 mmol/L, international normalized ratio >2.5, aspartate transaminase or alanine transaminase >200 U/L, sodium <120 mmol/L, and sodium >160 mmol/L [34]. The pathophysiology of metabolic delirium is poorly understood and could differ significantly from that of the other phenotypes. Recent experimental data indicate that acute kidney injury can lead to inflammation in the brain and other remote organs and a reduction in the clearance of medications, metabolites, and/or other potential neurotoxins—any or all of these conditions may explain the findings of a recent study showing that acute kidney injury is a risk factor for delirium during critical illness [40]. Mechanisms of delirium in the setting of liver failure have not been defined but similar conclusions have been drawn with regard to a reduction in the clearance of medications and metabolites with hepatic failure [41]. In the study of 1040 ICU patients, duration of metabolic phenotype was not associated with cognitive outcomes assessed at 3-month and 12-month follow-up [34]. This may indicate that the mechanisms of delirium during acute kidney and liver dysfunction do not cause lasting brain injury, but additional research is needed to test this hypothesis.

In their study of clinical phenotypes of delirium, Girard et al. labeled a fifth phenotype as "unclassified"—delirium in the absence of hypoxia, sepsis, sedation, and metabolic dysfunction [34]. Regarding cognitive deficits at 3 months and 12 months, the unclassified phenotype behaves similar to the sedative-associated phenotype [34]. Longer durations of unclassified delirium predicted worse cognitive function at 3 and 12 months [34]. In fact, a prolonged period of this phenotype was one of the strongest predictors for worse long-term cognitive impairment [34]. Given the generic nature of this phenotype, characterizing this further into more detailed subsets could prove prudent. One example of this would be to separate out surgical phenotypes. Cavallari et al. demonstrated that microstructural brain abnormalities predispose subjects to delirium under the stress of surgery [42, 43]. This study identified a significant relationship between brain abnormalities and postoperative delirium incidence and severity independent of age, vascular comorbidities, gender, and preoperative cognition [44]. These findings support that surgery alone, in some patients, could be a separate phenotype for delirium. Significantly more research needs to be performed to identify the utility of making this a separate phenotype and whether or not there are cognitive deficits associated with surgical delirium.

Conclusions

As our understanding of delirium during critical illness continues to evolve, our definitions must as well. The current practice of using validated tools in the ICU to diagnose delirium has provided an easy framework for clinical care and research. These tools have also led to an increase in delirium diagnoses, leaving fewer patients unrecognized. Delirium diagnosis must be expanded upon in the future to consider severity, motoric subtypes, and clinical phenotypes. These additional classification systems have demonstrated important outcome differences between the subtypes and may guide treatment options for them.

References

1. Camus V. Phenomenology of acute confusional states. Br J Psychiatry. 2002;181:256–7.
2. Morandi A, Pandharipande P, Trabucchi M, et al. Understanding international differences in terminology for delirium and other types of acute brain dysfunction in critically ill patients. Intensive Care Med. 2008;34(10):1907–15.
3. European Delirium A, American Delirium S. The DSM-5 criteria, level of arousal and delirium diagnosis: inclusiveness is safer. BMC Med. 2014;12:141.
4. Ely EW, Shintani A, Truman B, et al. Delirium as a predictor of mortality in mechanically ventilated patients in the intensive care unit. JAMA. 2004;291(14):1753–62.
5. McNicoll L, Pisani MA, Zhang Y, Ely EW, Siegel MD, Inouye SK. Delirium in the intensive care unit: occurrence and clinical course in older patients. J Am Geriatr Soc. 2003;51(5):591–8.
6. Spronk PE, Riekerk B, Hofhuis J, Rommes JH. Occurrence of delirium is severely underestimated in the ICU during daily care. Intensive Care Med. 2009;35(7):1276–80.
7. Ely EW, Inouye SK, Bernard GR, et al. Delirium in mechanically ventilated patients: validity and reliability of the confusion assessment method for the intensive care unit (CAM-ICU). JAMA. 2001;286(21):2703–10.
8. Bergeron N, Dubois MJ, Dumont M, Dial S, Skrobik Y. Intensive care Delirium screening checklist: evaluation of a new screening tool. Intensive Care Med. 2001;27(5):859–64.
9. Devlin JW, Skrobik Y, Gelinas C, et al. Clinical practice guidelines for the prevention and Management of Pain, agitation/sedation, Delirium, immobility, and sleep disruption in adult patients in the ICU. Crit Care Med. 2018;46(9):e825–73.
10. Lowery DP, Wesnes K, Brewster N, Ballard C. Subtle deficits of attention after surgery: quantifying indicators of sub syndrome delirium. Int J Geriatr Psychiatry. 2010;25(10):945–52.
11. Serafim RB, Soares M, Bozza FA, et al. Outcomes of subsyndromal delirium in ICU: a systematic review and meta-analysis. Crit Care. 2017;21(1):179.
12. Ouimet S, Riker R, Bergeron N, Cossette M, Kavanagh B, Skrobik Y. Subsyndromal delirium in the ICU: evidence for a disease spectrum. Intensive Care Med. 2007;33(6):1007–13.
13. Breu A, Stransky M, Metterlein T, Werner T, Trabold B. Subsyndromal delirium after cardiac surgery. Scand Cardiovasc J. 2015;49(4):207–12.
14. Khan BA, Perkins AJ, Gao S, et al. The confusion assessment method for the ICU-7 Delirium severity scale: a novel Delirium severity instrument for use in the ICU. Crit Care Med. 2017;45(5):851–7.
15. Robinson TN, Raeburn CD, Tran ZV, Brenner LA, Moss M. Motor subtypes of postoperative delirium in older adults. Arch Surg. 2011;146(3):295–300.

16. Avelino-Silva TJ, Campora F, Curiati JAE, Jacob-Filho W. Prognostic effects of delirium motor subtypes in hospitalized older adults: a prospective cohort study. PLoS One. 2018;13(1):e0191092.
17. Kiely DK, Jones RN, Bergmann MA, Marcantonio ER. Association between psychomotor activity delirium subtypes and mortality among newly admitted post-acute facility patients. J Gerontol A Biol Sci Med Sci. 2007;62(2):174–9.
18. Kim SY, Kim SW, Kim JM, et al. Differential associations between delirium and mortality according to delirium subtype and age: a prospective cohort study. Psychosom Med. 2015;77(8):903–10.
19. Milisen K, Foreman MD, Godderis J, Abraham IL, Broos PL. Delirium in the hospitalized elderly: nursing assessment and management. Nurs Clin North Am. 1998;33(3):417–39.
20. Trzepacz PT. Update on the neuropathogenesis of delirium. Dement Geriatr Cogn Disord. 1999;10(5):330–4.
21. Lipowski ZJ. Transient cognitive disorders (delirium, acute confusional states) in the elderly. Am J Psychiatry. 1983;140(11):1426–36.
22. Lipowski ZJ. Delirium in the elderly patient. N Engl J Med. 1989;320(9):578–82.
23. Stagno D, Gibson C, Breitbart W. The delirium subtypes: a review of prevalence, phenomenology, pathophysiology, and treatment response. Palliat Support Care. 2004;2(2):171–9.
24. O'Keeffe ST, Lavan JN. Clinical significance of delirium subtypes in older people. Age Ageing. 1999;28(2):115–9.
25. Meagher DJ, Moran M, Raju B, et al. Motor symptoms in 100 patients with delirium versus control subjects: comparison of subtyping methods. Psychosomatics. 2008;49(4):300–8.
26. Sessler CN, Gosnell MS, Grap MJ, et al. The Richmond agitation-sedation scale: validity and reliability in adult intensive care unit patients. Am J Respir Crit Care Med. 2002;166(10):1338–44.
27. Ely EW, Truman B, Shintani A, et al. Monitoring sedation status over time in ICU patients: reliability and validity of the Richmond Agitation-Sedation Scale (RASS). JAMA. 2003;289(22):2983–91.
28. Pandharipande PP, Pun BT, Herr DL, et al. Effect of sedation with dexmedetomidine vs lorazepam on acute brain dysfunction in mechanically ventilated patients: the MENDS randomized controlled trial. JAMA. 2007;298(22):2644–53.
29. Liptzin B, Levkoff SE. An empirical study of delirium subtypes. Br J Psychiatry. 1992;161:843–5.
30. van den Boogaard M, Schoonhoven L, van der Hoeven JG, van Achterberg T, Pickkers P. Incidence and short-term consequences of delirium in critically ill patients: a prospective observational cohort study. Int J Nurs Stud. 2012;49(7):775–83.
31. van den Boogaard M, Schoonhoven L, Evers AW, van der Hoeven JG, van Achterberg T, Pickkers P. Delirium in critically ill patients: impact on long-term health-related quality of life and cognitive functioning. Crit Care Med. 2012;40(1):112–8.
32. Meagher DJ, Leonard M, Donnelly S, Conroy M, Adamis D, Trzepacz PT. A longitudinal study of motor subtypes in delirium: relationship with other phenomenology, etiology, medication exposure and prognosis. J Psychosom Res. 2011;71(6):395–403.
33. Naidech AM, Beaumont JL, Rosenberg NF, et al. Intracerebral hemorrhage and delirium symptoms. Length of stay, function, and quality of life in a 114-patient cohort. Am J Respir Crit Care Med. 2013;188(11):1331–7.
34. Girard TD, Thompson JL, Pandharipande PP, et al. Clinical phenotypes of delirium during critical illness and severity of subsequent long-term cognitive impairment: a prospective cohort study. Lancet Respir Med. 2018;6(3):213–22.
35. Zhang SX, Wang Y, Gozal D. Pathological consequences of intermittent hypoxia in the central nervous system. Compr Physiol. 2012;2(3):1767–77.
36. Ebersoldt M, Sharshar T, Annane D. Sepsis-associated delirium. Intensive Care Med. 2007;33(6):941–50.

37. Singer BH, Newstead MW, Zeng X, et al. Cecal ligation and puncture results in long-term central nervous system myeloid inflammation. PLoS One. 2016;11(2):e0149136.
38. Semmler A, Hermann S, Mormann F, et al. Sepsis causes neuroinflammation and concomitant decrease of cerebral metabolism. J Neuroinflammation. 2008;5:38.
39. Patel SB, Poston JT, Pohlman A, Hall JB, Kress JP. Rapidly reversible, sedation-related delirium versus persistent delirium in the intensive care unit. Am J Respir Crit Care Med. 2014;189(6):658–65.
40. Siew ED, Fissell WH, Tripp CM, et al. Acute kidney injury as a risk factor for delirium and coma during critical illness. Am J Respir Crit Care Med. 2017;195(12):1597–607.
41. Bhattacharya B, Maung A, Barre K, et al. Postoperative delirium is associated with increased intensive care unit and hospital length of stays after liver transplantation. J Surg Res. 2017;207:223–8.
42. Cavallari M, Guttmann CR, Jones RN, Inouye SK, Alsop DC, Group SS. Reply: neural substrates of vulnerability to post-surgical delirium with prospective diagnosis. Brain. 2016;139(Pt 10):e55.
43. Cavallari M, Dai W, Guttmann CR, et al. Neural substrates of vulnerability to postsurgical delirium as revealed by presurgical diffusion MRI. Brain. 2016;139(Pt 4):1282–94.
44. Lindroth H, Sanders RD. Neural substrates of vulnerability to post-surgical delirium with prospective diagnosis. Brain. 2016;139(Pt 10):e54.

Chapter 2
Monitoring for Delirium in Critically Ill Adults

Annachiara Marra, Leanne M. Boehm, Katarzyna Kotfis, and Brenda T. Pun

Introduction

Delirium is the most common manifestation of acute brain dysfunction and is increasingly understood as a serious medical event during hospitalization. It is most commonly precipitated by underlying medical conditions, iatrogenic causes (e.g., administration of deliriogenic medications), sensory impairment (e.g., removal of eye glasses or hearing aids), immobilization, and alterations of sleep cycle. It is a prevalent complication in people receiving care throughout the hospital, especially in older people, those with dementia, and patients admitted to intensive care, postoperative, geriatric, and palliative care units [1, 2]. Delirium during the ICU period is a strong predictor of increased length of mechanical ventilation, longer ICU and hospital stays, increased risk of falls, increased health care cost, mortality [3–7], and is linked to negative outcomes long after hospital discharge such as increased mortality and cognitive impairment [4, 8, 9]. The first step in managing ICU delirium is systematic monitoring with a validated delirium assessment tool. Current recommendations

A. Marra (✉)
Department of Neurosciences, Reproductive and Odontostomatological Sciences, University of Naples, Federico II, Naples, Italy

L. M. Boehm
Critical Illness, Brain Dysfunction, and Survivorship Center and the Vanderbilt University School of Nursing, Nashville, TN, USA

K. Kotfis
Department of Anesthesiology, Intensive Therapy and Acute Intoxications, Pomeranian Medical University, Szczecin, Poland

B. T. Pun
Division of Allergy, Pulmonary, and Critical Care Medicine, Department of Medicine, Vanderbilt University Medical Center, Nashville, TN, USA

Critical Illness, Brain Dysfunction, and Survivorship Center, Vanderbilt University Medical Center, Nashville, TN, USA

C. G. Hughes et al. (eds.), *Delirium*, https://doi.org/10.1007/978-3-030-25751-4_2

focus on valid assessment of pain, sedation, and delirium in tandem [10, 11]. This highlights the fundamental interconnectedness of delirium and other patient symptoms and interventions in the ICU. Delirium assessment is so fundamental to critical care management that it is now a core feature in the evidence-based organizational approach referred to as the "ABCDEF bundle" (awakening and breathing coordination, choice of sedatives, delirium monitoring, early mobility, and family engagement and empowerment) [10–14]. Currently, there are enormous variations in practice, with most patients not routinely monitored for delirium in hospital wards and ICUs around the world and with most delirium going undiagnosed [15].

This chapter describes the most common delirium assessment tools for the ICU and outlines how to use those tools to inform delirium prevention and management strategies.

Definition of Delirium

Delirium is an acute neuropsychiatric disorder that is characterized by a loss of attention and accompanied by cognitive change, perceptual disturbance, and/or change in level of consciousness (LOC). Delirium first appeared in medical writings over 2000 years ago [16], and today the term is widely used in medicine and in everyday language and pop culture. There are bands, movies, and beers that bear the name. As a result, there is widespread variation in defining the term [17]. In this era that demands ICU clinicians to practice in multiprofessional teams, it is important that each team member uses medical terms accurately and consistently in order to maximize the care and treatment for patients and families. The primary source for defining delirium has become the *Diagnostic and Statistical Manual of Mental Disorders* (DSM). The DSM details explicit diagnostic criteria for delirium and thus serves as the reference standard (see previous chapter for further details). The most recent revision, the DSM-5, outlines the core criteria for delirium providing more detailed descriptions of each feature and differentiates it from severe neurocognitive disorders and coma [18]. According to DSM-5 criteria, delirium is defined as an acutely developing deficit in attention (reduced ability to direct, focus, sustain, and shift attention) coupled with a change in cognition (memory deficit, disorientation, or perceptual disturbance) [18]. While no major criteria were changed in the revision, it did include some minor changes that prompted some to criticize that the new criteria could be interpreted too narrowly [19]. Meagher and colleagues compared the DSM-IV and two versions of the DSM-5, a strict version (all DSM-5 criteria in their most explicit forms) and a relaxed version (delirium features in all possible forms) with more general interpretation of the criteria. The strict application of DSM-5 criteria interpretation excluded cases with substantial delirium symptoms, but the relaxed version included these patients, thus leading the authors to recommend the relaxed interpretation [19]. The European Delirium Association and the American Delirium Society both endorse a relaxed approach to the criteria interpretation [20]. This debate underscores that, while the DSM-5 provided more detailed explanations of the delirium criteria, it still requires psychiatric training to navigate and interpret. This complexity does not lend itself to widespread application; thus, valid and reliable assessment tools are needed for general bedside practitioners.

Delirium Assessment Tools for the ICU

Despite the high prevalence of delirium, delirium goes undetected by bedside nurses and medical practitioners in up to three out of four patients when structured assessment tools are not used [21–23]. This is, in part, because symptoms of delirium are often "quiet" (hypoactive rather than hyperactive), challenging to recognize in patients who are sedated or nonverbal [24–27], and frequently fluctuate during the day. Bedside critical care clinicians need delirium assessment tools that, while validated against the DSM standards, are easy to use, are easy to communicate, and have good inter-rater reliability. While many tools have been developed over time, they do not all have strong psychometric properties. In 2013, the Clinical Practice Guidelines for the Management of Pain, Agitation, and Delirium (PAD) in Adult Patients in the ICU evaluated a myriad of ICU delirium assessment tools and identified two tools satisfying the threshold for recommendation: Confusion Assessment Method for the ICU (CAM-ICU) [28, 29] and Intensive Care Delirium Screening Checklist (ICDSC) [30]. Gelinas and colleagues reproduced the PAD guideline psychometric evaluation using updated data and again concluded only the CAM-ICU and ICDSC met the acceptable threshold for delirium monitoring [31]. Other tools evaluated for psychometric and feasibility properties that *did not* meet the acceptable threshold include the Cognitive Test for Delirium, the Delirium Detection Score, and the Nursing Delirium Screening Scale. In 2018, the updated version of the guidelines confirmed the role of validated screening tools, including CAM-ICU and ICDSC to improve delirium recognition [10].

There are a variety of other tools developed for use outside the ICU (e.g., Confusion Assessment Method [CAM], 4 A's Test [4AT] [32], Nursing Delirium Screening Scale [Nu-DESC] [33], Delirium Observation Screening Scale [34], Single Question in Delirium [SQiD] [35], Recognizing Acute Delirium As part of your Routine [RADAR] [36]). However, this chapter focuses on tools developed and validated for use in critically ill patients. The following sections provide an overview of the two guideline-recommended and validated ICU delirium monitoring tools.

CAM-ICU

The CAM-ICU scale (Fig. 2.1a) was designed as an adaptation of the original CAM [37] in order to evaluate delirium objectively in a largely nonverbal population due to mechanical ventilation [28, 29]. It is a point-in-time assessment tool. The CAM-ICU evaluates for delirium by assessing four diagnostic features: (1) sudden changes/fluctuations in mental status, (2) inattention, (3) altered levels of consciousness, and (4) disorganized thinking. The patient is considered CAM-ICU positive (i.e., delirious) if he/she manifests both features 1 and 2, plus either feature 3 or 4. The original

CAM-ICU validation study was conducted with 111 patients being evaluated by two independent observers. The observer CAM-ICU evaluations were compared with an assessment conducted by a psychiatrist employing the DSM-IV criteria for delirium diagnosis. Analysis revealed a specificity of 93% and 100% for both raters, respectively, and a sensitivity of 98% and 100% for both raters, respectively [28]. Further studies have demonstrated the usefulness of the CAM-ICU in routine clinical assessment of delirium in ICU patients in other critical care environments to include surgery,

a **CAM-ICU Worksheet**

Feature 1: Acute Onset or Fluctuating Course	Score	Check here if Present
Is the patient different than his/her baseline mental status? OR Has the patient had any fluctuation in mental status in the past 24 hours as evidenced by fluctuation on a sedation/level of consciousness scale (i.e., RASS/SAS), GCS, or previous delirium assessment?	Either question Yes →	☐
Feature 2: Inattention		
<u>**Letters Attention Test**</u> (See training manual for alternate **Pictures**) <u>Directions</u>: Say to the patient, *"I am going to read you a series of 10 letters. Whenever you hear the letter 'A,' indicate by squeezing my hand."* Read letters from the following letter list in a normal tone 3 seconds apart. **S A V E A H A A R T** or **C A S A B L A N C A** or **A B A D B A D A A Y** **Errors are counted when patient fails to squeeze on the letter "A" and when the patient squeezes on any letter other than "A."**	Number of Errors >2 →	☐
Feature 3: Altered Level of Consciousness		
Present if the Actual RASS score is anything other than alert and calm (zero)	RASS anything other than zero →	☐
Feature 4:Disorganized Thinking		
<u>**Yes/No Questions**</u> (See training manual for alternate set of questions) 1. Will a stone float on water? 2. Are there fish in the sea? 3. Does one pound weigh more than two pounds? 4. Can you use a hammer to pound a nail? **Errors are counted when the patient incorrectly answers a question.** <u>**Command**</u> Say to patient: "Hold up this many fingers" (Hold 2 fingers in front of patient) "Now do the same thing with the other hand" (Do not repeat number of fingers) *If the patientis unable to move both arms, for 2nd part of command ask patient to "Add one more finger" **An error is counted if patient is unable to complete the entire command.**	Combined number of errors >1→	☐

Overall CAM-ICU **Feature 1 <u>plus</u> 2 <u>and</u> either 3 <u>or</u> 4 present = CAM-ICU positive**	**Criteria Met →**	☐ **CAM-ICU Positive** **(Delirium Present)**
	Criteria Not Met →	☐ **CAM-ICU Negative** **(No Delirium)**

Fig. 2.1 Assessment of the content of consciousness: (**a**) Confusion Assessment Method for the ICU (CAM-ICU) (Ely et al. [28, 53]); (**b**) Intensive Care Delirium Screening checklist (ICDSC). (Used with permission from John Devlin. Sessler et al. [54], Ely et al. [55])

b **Intensive Care Delirium Screening Checklist Worksheet (ICDSC)**

- Score your patient over the entire shif. Components don't all need to be present at the same tme.
- Components #1 through #4 require a focused bedside patient assessrnent. This cannot be completed when the patient is deeply sedated or comatose (ie. SAS = 1 or 2; RASS = -4 or -5).
- Components #5 through #8 are based on observations throughout the entire shift. information from the prior 24 hrs (ie, from prior 1-2 nursing shifts) should be obtained for components #7 and #8.

1. **Altered Level of Consciousness** — **NO 0 1 Yes**
   Deep sedation/coma over entire shift (SAS= 1, 2; RASS = -4,-5] = Not assessable
   Agitation [SAS = 5,6, or 7; RASS= 1-4] at any point = 1 point
   Normal wakefulness [SAS = 4: RASS = 0] over the entire shift = 0 points
   Light sedation [SAS = 3; RASS= -1, -2, -3]: = 1 point (if no recent sedatives)
   = 0 points (if recent sedatives)
2. **Inattention** — **NO 0 1 Yes**
   Difficulty following instructions conversation, patient easily distracted by external stimuli.
   Will not reliably squeeze hands to spoken letter A: **S A V E A H A A R T**
3. **Disorientation** — **NO 0 1 Yes**
   In addition to name, place, and date, does the patient recognize ICU caregivers?
   Does patient know what kind of place they are in?
   (list examples: dentist's office, home, work, hospital)
4. **Hallucination, delusion, or psychosis** — **NO 0 1 Yes**
   Ask patient if they are having hallucinations or delusions.
   (e.g. trying to catch an object that isn't there
   Are they afraid of the people or things around them?
5. **Psychomotor agitation or retardation** — **NO 0 1 Yes**
   Either: a) Hyperactivity requiring the use of sedative drugs or restraints in order to control potentially dangerous behavior (e.g. pulling IV lines cut or hitting staff)
   OR b) Hypoactive or clinically noticeable psychomotor slowing or retardation
6. **Inappropriate speech or mood** — **NO 0 1 Yes**
   Patient displays; inappropriate emotion; disorganized or incoherent speech; sexual or inappropriate interactions; is either apathetic or overty demanding
7. **Sleep-wake cycle disturbance** — **NO 0 1 Yes**
   Either; frequent awakening/< 4 hours sleep at night OR sleeping during much of the day
8. **Symptom Fluctuation** — **NO 0 1 Yes**
   Fluctuation of any of the above symptoms over a 24 hr period.

TOTAL SHIFT SCORE: ______ **(0 – 8)**

Score	Classification
0	Normal
1-3	Subsyndromal Delirium
4-8	Delirium

Fig. 2.1 (continued)

trauma, burn, cardiovascular, and neurological ICU settings [38]. A meta-analysis performed by Gusmao-Flores et al. demonstrated excellent accuracy of the CAM-ICU with pooled sensitivity of 80% (95% confidence intervals (CI): 77.1–82.6%) and specificity of 95.9% (95% CI: 94.8–96.8%) for detecting delirium [39]. Evaluation of CAM-ICU features is conducted through objective evaluation. The CAM-ICU has been translated in over 30 languages which can be found at www.icudelirium.org/cibs-center along with training materials and videos.

There is one recent adaptation of the CAM-ICU to highlight [10]. The *CAM-ICU-7* is a severity rating scale based on the CAM-ICU assessment. Specific points are assigned for each feature. The CAM-ICU-7 scores are categorized as 0–2, no delirium; 3–5, mild to moderate delirium; and 6–7, severe delirium [40] (Table 2.1). A recent observational study using the CAM-ICU-7 suggests an association between delirium severity and worse outcomes (i.e., ICU and hospital length of stay and the probability of returning home) [40].

Table 2.1 The confusion assessment method for the ICU-7 delirium severity scale

Items (assessed using CAM-ICU criteria)	Grading
1. Acute onset or fluctuation of mental status	0 for absent
	1 for present
2. Inattention	0 for absent (correct: ≥8)
	1 for inattention (correct: 4–7)
	2 for severe inattention (correct: 0–3)
3. Altered LOC	0 for absent (RASS: 0)
	1 for altered level (RASS: 1, −1)
	2 for severe altered level (RASS: >1, <−1)
4. Disorganized thinking	0 for absent (correct: ≥4)
	1 for disorganized thinking (correct: 2, 3)
	2 for severe disorganized thinking (correct: 0, 1)
Score	0–2: no delirium
	3–5: mild to moderate delirium
	6–7: severe delirium

Adapted from: Khan et al. [40]

ICDSC

Intensive Care Delirium Screening Checklist (ICDSC) is an 8-item checklist (Fig. 2.1b) validated in 2001 by Bergeron et al. [30]. The ICDSC incorporates both a point-of-care focused evaluation by the bedside clinician and evaluation of other delirium features manifesting during the remainder of a specified time period (e.g., 12-h nursing shift). The eight predefined diagnostic criteria as per DSM-IV include altered LOC, inattention, disorientation, hallucination or delusion, changes in psychomotor activity (agitation and retardation), inappropriate mood or speech, sleep/wake cycle disturbances, and symptom fluctuation [30]. Patients are given one point for each delirium symptom manifesting over the course of a shift. The ICDSC is positive for delirium when at least four out of eight criteria are present. The validation study performed by Bergeron et al. compared ICDSC to a psychiatric evaluation and reported sensitivity of 99% and specificity of 64% in detecting ICU delirium. According to the meta-analysis by Gusmao-Flores et al., the ICDSC has good accuracy (area under ROC 0.89) with pooled sensitivity of 74% (95% CI: 65.3–81.5%) and pooled specificity of 81.9% (95% CI: 76.7–86.4%) [39].

Incorporating Delirium Assessment into Clinical Practice

Regular monitoring of delirium with a valid and reliable tool allows for enhanced detection of delirium and facilitates a coherent clinical plan in which specific management of the patient's delirium is planned alongside other aspects of care, thus coordinating care and optimizing therapeutic interventions [41–46]. Moreover, delirium monitoring can reveal early signs of acute and serious physiologic problems (e.g., acute disruption to homeostasis, adverse drug effects, organ dysfunction) and stimulate rapid and responsive medical care. Routine delirium monitoring can help overcome delirium miscommunications between the multidisciplinary team [47] and improve precision of diagnostic understanding and language. This enhanced communication is achieved by counteracting the numerous misnomers for delirium (*ICU psychosis, confusion, and terminal agitation*) which downplay the significance and severity of delirium and contribute to its under-recognition, poor assessment, and inadequate follow-up care [48].

Assessment Recommendations

Delirium assessment should be performed serially in order to obtain the best picture of the patient's mental status. Delirium assessment can be performed by any healthcare professional, although nurses most commonly perform the assessment and should be included as part of standard care. The role of nurses in this process is critically important due to the nurse's consistent close patient contact and interaction. Since a key feature of delirium is fluctuation, the guidelines recommend delirium evaluation be performed at least every shift (e.g., every 8 or 12 h) and each time a change in mental status is noted [10, 49]. Delirium assessment can most often be completed in <1 min. The result of delirium assessments should be recorded in patient medical record documents to enable its use for members of the multidisciplinary team.

The assessment of delirium is an important element of general assessment of the state of consciousness and is conducted in two stages. The first step is to assess the LOC, via either the Richmond Agitation-Sedation Scale (RASS) (see previous chapter for figure) or Sedation Agitation Scale (SAS) (Fig. 2.2). The next step is to assess the content of consciousness (i.e., delirium). In cases of coma (e.g., RASS −4, RASS −5 or SAS 1, SAS 2), it is impossible to assess for delirium because the patient is unresponsive to external stimuli. Coma disqualifies the patient from delirium evaluation. However, a patient can be assessed for delirium if there is any responsiveness to verbal stimulation (e.g., RASS −3 to +4 or SAS 3–7). When it is possible to obtain at least the beginnings of meaningful reactions (e.g., any response to voice), the content of consciousness should be evaluated, and delirium can be assessed.

Implementation Recommendations

Implementation of routine delirium monitoring requires not only appropriate practical training (e.g., expert lectures, workshops, case-based scenarios, visual aids, mnemonics, bedside teaching) in the ICU environment but also institutional support and acknowledgment of the necessity for delirium screening [50]. Implementation trials have shown that great importance must be put on follow-up teaching, reinforcement, and audits of delirium screening in order to maintain high levels of compliance and reliability many years after implementation [51].

Riker Sedation-Agitation Scale (SAS)

Score	Term	Descriptor
7	Dangerous Agitation	Pulling at ET tube, trying to remove catheters, climbing over bedrail, striking at staff, thrashing side-to-side
6	Very Agitated	Requiring restraint and frequent verbal reminding of limits, biting ETT
5	Agitated	Anxious or physically agitated, calms to verbal instructions
4	Calm and Cooperative	Calm, easily arousable, follows commands
3	Sedated	Difficult to arouse but awakens to verbal stimuli or gentle shaking, follows simple commands but drifts off again
2	Very Sedated	Arouses to physical stimuli but does not communicate or follow commands, may move spontaneously
1	Unarousable	Minimal or no response to noxious stimuli, does not communicate or follow commands

Fig. 2.2 Sedation Agitation Scale (SAS). Guidelines for SAS Assessment: (1) agitated patients are scored by their most severe degree of agitation as described. (2) If patient is awake or awakens easily to voice ("awaken" means responds with voice or head shaking to a question or follows commands), that's a SAS 4 (same as calm and appropriate – might even be napping). (3) If more stimuli such as shaking are required but patient eventually does awaken, that's SAS 3. (4) If patient arouses to stronger physical stimuli (may be noxious) but never awakens to the point of responding yes/no or following commands, that's a SAS 2. (5) Little or no response to noxious physical stimuli represents a SAS 1. This helps separate sedated patients into those you can eventually wake up (SAS 3), those you can't awaken but can arouse (SAS 2), and those you can't arouse (SAS 1)

A "delirium vigilance approach" can enhance implementation success by employing altered LOC as a trigger to perform delirium assessment [52], brain roadmaps for multiprofessional communication, mnemonics for risk identification, and structured documentation systems for quality improvement performance tracking [20, 47]. Clinical dashboards can trigger delirium assessment if a patient's LOC meets criteria for delirium assessment (i.e., RASS −3 to +4, SAS 3–7) but delirium status has not been documented. The brain roadmap (Fig. 2.3) provides the script for communicating delirium assessment results in addition to relevant information to guide delirium management discussion during interdisciplinary rounds. Components of the brain roadmap communication framework are pain assessment, target and actual LOC, delirium assessment, and sedative/analgesic/antipsychotic medications received in the previous 24 h [50]. Mnemonics (Table 2.2) [e.g., Dr. DRE, THINK, DELIRIUM(S)] can then be applied to guide discussion of predisposing and precipitating factors contributing to delirium and, thus, determine a patient-centered therapeutic management approach. Finally, quality improvement feedback can be

Brain Road Map for Rounds
(Script for Interdisciplinary Communication)

Skipping any of these steps could leave the clinical team wanting more information!

Investigate (Ask these questions)	Report (only takes 10 seconds)
Where is the patient going?	Target level of consciousness (RASS, SAS)
Where is the patient now?	Actual level of consciousness (RASS, SAS) Delirium assessment (CAM-ICU, ICDSC) Pain assessment (NRS, CPOT, BPS)
How did they get there?	Drug exposures

Fig. 2.3 The brain roadmap for rounds. (Adapted from www.icudelirium.org)

Table 2.2 Mnemonics for delirium

Dr. DRE Strategies to consider when delirium is present	**Dr** Diseases (sepsis, COPD, CHF)
	DR Drug removal (especially sedatives)
	E Environment (immobilization, sleep, day/night variation, hearing aids, glasses)
THINK What to THINK about when delirium is present	**T** Toxic situations (heart failure, shock, dehydration, deliriogenic meds [especially sedatives], new organ failure)
	H Hypoxemia
	I Infection/sepsis, immobilization
	N Nonpharmacological interventions (sensory aids, reorientation, sleep, music, noise control, ambulation)
	K+ or electrolyte problems
DELIRIUM (S) Differential diagnosis for patients with delirium (Remember: delirium usually has more than one cause)	**D** Drugs
	E Eyes, ears, other sensory deficits
	L Low O2 states (heart attack, stroke, pulmonary embolism)
	I Infection
	R Retention (urine or stool)
	I Ictal state
	U Underhydration/undernutrition
	M Metabolic causes (diabetes, postoperative state, sodium abnormalities)

Used with permission from www.icudelirium.org

created using data from the medical record. Structured delirium documentation and recording delirium components in addition to only the overall assessment result can provide data for tracking process and outcome measures for quality improvement initiatives to reduce delirium prevalence in addition to monitoring assessment reliability.

Interprofessional Approach to Delirium Management

The PAD-IS guidelines recommend using a multidisciplinary ICU team approach to facilitate pain, agitation, and delirium management [10, 49]. The ABCDEF bundle, a group of evidence-based critical care practices, provides a framework for implementation of this recommendation. This bundle emphasizes essential routine patient assessments (i.e., pain, LOC, delirium) and prioritizes key interventions (e.g., sedation cessation, spontaneous breathing trials, early mobility). Implementation of the ABCDEF bundle maximizes the likelihood of successful patient engagement in each individual bundle component. Outcomes associated with ABCDEF bundle implementation include reduced duration of delirium and mechanical ventilation and a higher likelihood of early mobilization and hospital survival [11–14].

Conclusion

Delirium monitoring should become part of routine clinical care for every ICU patient. Validated simple and quick assessment tools are available for routine use by non-psychiatric personnel. The choice of which validated delirium assessment tool and implementation process to use is dependent on patient needs, goals of care, and organizational structure. Regular monitoring of delirium allows an enhanced detection of delirium that could facilitate the clinical management of the patient leading to improved patient outcomes and increased awareness of early signs of acute and serious physiological problems, thus stimulating rapid and responsive medical care.

References

1. Ryan DJ, O'Regan NA, Caoimh RÓ, Clare J, O'Connor M, Leonard M, et al. Delirium in an adult acute hospital population: predictors, prevalence and detection. BMJ Open. 2013;3(1). https://doi.org/10.1136/bmjopen-2012-001772.
2. Hosie A, Davidson PM, Agar M, Sanderson CR, Phillips J. Delirium prevalence, incidence, and implications for screening in specialist palliative care inpatient settings: a systematic review. Palliat Med. 2013;27(6):486–98.
3. Ely EW, Baker AM, Dunagan DP, Burke HL, Smith AC, Kelly PT, et al. Effect on the duration of mechanical ventilation of identifying patients capable of breathing spontaneously. N Engl J Med. 1996;335(25):1864–9.
4. Ely EW, Shintani A, Truman B, Speroff T, Gordon SM, Harrell FE Jr, et al. Delirium as a predictor of mortality in mechanically ventilated patients in the intensive care unit. JAMA. 2004;291(14):1753–62.
5. Salluh JI, Wang H, Schneider EB, Nagaraja N, Yenokyan G, Damluji A, et al. Outcome of delirium in critically ill patients: systematic review and meta-analysis. BMJ. 2015;350:h2538.
6. Klein Klouwenberg PMC, Zaal IJ, Spitoni C, Ong DSY, van der Kooi AW, Bonten MJM, et al. The attributable mortality of delirium in critically ill patients: prospective cohort study. BMJ. 2014;349:g6652.

7. Leslie DL, Marcantonio ER, Zhang Y, Leo-Summers L, Inouye SK. One-year health care costs associated with delirium in the elderly population. Arch Intern Med. 2008;168(1):27–32.
8. Pandharipande PP, Girard TD, Jackson JC, Morandi A, Thompson JL, Pun BT, et al. Long-term cognitive impairment after critical illness. N Engl J Med. 2013;369(14):1306–16.
9. Girard TD, Jackson JC, Pandharipande PP, Thompson JL, Shintani AK, Ely EW. Duration of delirium as a predictor of long-term cognitive impairment in survivors of critical illness. Am J Respir Crit Care Med. 2009;179:A5477.
10. Devlin JW, Skrobik Y, Gelinas C, Needham DM, Slooter AJC, Pandharipande PP, et al. Clinical practice guidelines for the prevention and management of pain, agitation/sedation, delirium, immobility, and sleep disruption in adult patients in the ICU. Crit Care Med. 2018;46(9):e825–e73.
11. Barnes-Daly M, Phillips G, Ely E. Improving hospital survival and reducing brain dysfunction at 7 California community hospitals: implementing PAD guidelines via the ABCDEF bundle in 6,064 patients. Crit Care Med. 2017;45(2):171–8.
12. Balas MC, Vasilevskis EE, Olsen KM, Schmid KK, Shostrom V, Cohen MZ, et al. Effectiveness and safety of the awakening and breathing coordination, delirium monitoring/management, and early exercise/mobility bundle. Crit Care Med. 2014;42(5):1024–36.
13. Ely EW. The ABCDEF bundle: science and philosophy of how ICU liberation serves patients and families. Crit Care Med. 2017;45(2):321–30.
14. Barnes-Daly MA, Pun BT, Harmon LA, Byrum DG, Kumar VK, Devlin JW, et al. Improving health care for critically ill patients using an evidence-based collaborative approach to ABCDEF bundle dissemination and implementation. Worldviews Evid-Based Nurs. 2018;15(3):206–16.
15. Morandi A, Piva S, Ely EW, Myatra SN, Salluh JIF, Amare D, et al. Worldwide survey of the "assessing pain, both spontaneous awakening and breathing trials, choice of drugs, delirium monitoring/management, early exercise/mobility, and family empowerment" (ABCDEF) bundle. Crit Care Med. 2017;45:e1111–22.
16. Deksnyte A, Aranauskas R, Budrys V, Kasiulevicius V, Sapoka V. Delirium: its historical evolution and current interpretation. Eur J Intern Med. 2012;23(6):483–6.
17. Morandi A, Pandharipande P, Trabucchi M, Rozzini R, Mistraletti G, Trompeo AC, et al. Understanding international differences in terminology for delirium and other types of acute brain dysfunction in critically ill patients. Intensive Care Med. 2008;34(10):1907–15.
18. Association. AP. Diagnostic and statistical manual of mental disorders: DSM-5. Washington, DC: American Psychiatric Association; 2013.
19. Meagher DJ, Morandi A, Inouye SK, Ely W, Adamis D, Maclullich AJ, et al. Concordance between DSM-IV and DSM-5 criteria for delirium diagnosis in a pooled database of 768 prospectively evaluated patients using the delirium rating scale-revised-98. BMC Med. 2014;12:164.
20. European Delirium A, American Delirium S. The DSM-5 criteria, level of arousal and delirium diagnosis: inclusiveness is safer. BMC Med. 2014;12:141.
21. Devlin JW, Fong JJ, Schumaker G, O'Connor H, Ruthazer R, Garpestad E. Use of a validated delirium assessment tool improves the ability of physicians to identify delirium in medical intensive care unit patients. Crit Care Med. 2007;35(12):2721–4.
22. Han JH, Eden S, Shintani A, Morandi A, Schnelle J, Dittus RS, et al. Delirium in older emergency department patients is an independent predictor of hospital length of stay. Acad Emerg Med. 2011;18(5):451–7.
23. Inouye SK, Foreman MD, Mion LC, Katz KH, Cooney LM Jr. Nurses' recognition of delirium and its symptoms: comparison of nurse and researcher ratings. Arch Intern Med. 2001;161(20):2467–73.
24. Patel SB, Kress JP. Accurate identification of delirium in the ICU: problems with translating the evidence in the real-life setting. Am J Respir Crit Care Med. 2011;184(3):287–8.
25. Spronk PE, Riekerk B, Hofhuis J, Rommes JH. Occurrence of delirium is severely underestimated in the ICU during daily care. Intensive Care Med. 2009;35(7):1276–80.
26. Devlin JW, Fong JJ, Howard EP, Skrobik Y, McCoy N, Yasuda C, et al. Assessment of delirium in the intensive care unit: nursing practices and perceptions. Am J Crit Care. 2008;17(6):555–65.. quiz 66

27. Pun BT, Devlin JW. Delirium monitoring in the ICU: strategies for initiating and sustaining screening efforts. Semin Respir Crit Care Med. 2013;34(2):179–88.
28. Ely EW, Margolin R, Francis J, May L, Truman B, Dittus R, et al. Evaluation of delirium in critically ill patients: validation of the Confusion Assessment Method for the Intensive Care Unit (CAM-ICU). Crit Care Med. 2001;29(7):1370–9.
29. Ely EW, Inouye SK, Bernard GR, Gordon S, Francis J, May L, et al. Delirium in mechanically ventilated patients: validity and reliability of the confusion assessment method for the intensive care unit (CAM-ICU). JAMA. 2001;286(21):2703–10.
30. Bergeron N, Dubois MJ, Dumont M, Dial S, Skrobik Y. Intensive care delirium screening checklist: evaluation of a new screening tool. Intensive Care Med. 2001;27(5):859–64.
31. Gelinas C, Berube M, Chevrier A, Pun BT, Ely EW, Skrobik Y, et al. Delirium assessment tools for use in critically ill adults: a psychometric analysis and systematic review. Crit Care Nurse. 2018;38(1):38–49.
32. McLullich A. The 4AT – a rapid assessment test for delirium 2014. Available from: http://www.the4at.com/.
33. Gaudreau JD, Gagnon P, Harel F, Tremblay A, Roy MA. Fast, systematic, and continuous delirium assessment in hospitalized patients: the nursing delirium screening scale. J Pain Symptom Manag. 2005;29(4):368–75.
34. Schuurmans MJ, Shortridge-Baggett LM, Duursma SA. The delirium observation screening scale: a screening instrument for delirium. Res Theory Nurs Pract. 2003;17(1):31–50.
35. Sands MB, Dantoc BP, Hartshorn A, Ryan CJ, Lujic S. Single Question in Delirium (SQiD): testing its efficacy against psychiatrist interview, the confusion assessment method and the memorial delirium assessment scale. Palliat Med. 2010;26(6):561–5.
36. Voyer P, Champoux N, Desrosiers J, Landreville P, McCusker J, Monette J, et al. Recognizing acute delirium as part of your routine [RADAR]: a validation study. BMC Nurs. 2015;14:19.
37. Inouye SK, van Dyck CH, Alessi CA, Balkin S, Siegal AP, Horwitz RI. Clarifying confusion: the confusion assessment method. A new method for detection of delirium. Ann Intern Med. 1990;113(12):941–8.
38. Soja SL, Pandharipande PP, Fleming SB, Cotton BA, Miller LR, Weaver SG, et al. Implementation, reliability testing, and compliance monitoring of the confusion assessment method for the intensive care unit in trauma patients. Intensive Care Med. 2008;34(7):1263–8.
39. Gusmao-Flores D, Salluh JI, Chalhub RA, Quarantini LC. The Confusion Assessment Method for the Intensive Care Unit (CAM-ICU) and Intensive Care Delirium Screening Checklist (ICDSC) for the diagnosis of delirium: a systematic review and meta-analysis of clinical studies. Crit Care. 2012;16(4):R115.
40. Khan BA, Perkins AJ, Gao S, Hui SL, Campbell NL, Farber MO, et al. The confusion assessment method for the ICU-7 delirium severity scale: a novel delirium severity instrument for use in the ICU. Crit Care Med. 2017;45(5):851–7.
41. Hshieh TT, Yue J, Oh E, Puelle M, Dowal S, Travison T, et al. Effectiveness of multicomponent nonpharmacological delirium interventions: a meta-analysis. JAMA Intern Med. 2015;175(4):512–20.
42. Lakatos BE, Capasso V, Mitchell MT, Kilroy SM, Lussier-Cushing M, Sumner L, et al. Falls in the general hospital: association with delirium, advanced age, and specific surgical procedures. Psychosomatics. 2009;50(3):218–26.
43. Mudge AM, Maussen C, Duncan J, Denaro CP. Improving quality of delirium care in a general medical service with established interdisciplinary care: a controlled trial. Intern Med J. 2013;43(3):270–7.
44. van den BM, Pickkers P, van der HH, Roodbol G, van AT, Schoonhoven L. Implementation of a delirium assessment tool in the ICU can influence haloperidol use. Crit Care. 2009;13(4):R131.
45. Inouye SK, Westendorp RG, Saczynski JS. Delirium in elderly people. Lancet. 2014;383(9920):911–22.
46. Luetz A, Weiss B, Boettcher S, Burmeister J, Wernecke KD, Spies C. Routine delirium monitoring is independently associated with a reduction of hospital mortality in critically ill surgical patients: a prospective, observational cohort study. J Crit Care. 2016;35:168–73.

47. Brummel NE, Vasilevskis EE, Han JH, Boehm L, Pun BT, Ely EW. Implementing delirium screening in the intensive care unit: secrets to success. Crit Care Med. 2013;41(9):2196.
48. Morandi A, Solberg LM, Habermann R, Cleeton P, Peterson E, Ely EW, et al. Documentation and management of words associated with delirium among elderly patients in postacute care: a pilot investigation. J Am Med Dir Assoc. 2009;10(5):330–4.
49. Barr J, Fraser GL, Puntillo K, Ely EW, Gelinas C, Dasta JF, et al. Clinical practice guidelines for the management of pain, agitation, and delirium in adult patients in the intensive care unit. Crit Care Med. 2013;41(1):263–306.
50. Brummel NE, Vasilevskis EE, Han JH, Boehm L, Pun BT, Ely EW. Implementing delirium screening in the ICU: secrets to success. Crit Care Med. 2013;41(9):2196–208.
51. Vasilevskis EE, Morandi A, Boehm L, Pandharipande PP, Girard TD, Jackson JC, et al. Delirium and sedation recognition using validated instruments: reliability of bedside intensive care unit nursing assessments from 2007 to 2010. J Am Geriatr Soc. 2011;59(Suppl 2):S249–55.
52. Chester JG, Beth Harrington M, Rudolph JL, Group VADW. Serial administration of a modified Richmond agitation and sedation scale for delirium screening. J Hosp Med. 2012;7(5):450–3.
53. Ely EW, et al. Delirium in mechanically ventilated patients: validity and reliability of the confusion assessment method for the intensive care unit. JAMA. 2003;289:2983–91.
54. Sessler CN, Gosnell M, Grap MJ, Brophy GT, O'Neal PV, Keane KA, et al. The Richmond Agitation-Sedation Scale: validity and reliability in adult intensive care patients. Am J Respir Crit Care Med. 2002;166:1338–44.
55. Ely EW, Truman B, Shintani A, Thomason JWW, Wheeler AP, Gordon S, et al. Monitoring sedation status over time in ICU patients: the reliability and validity of the Richmond Agitation Sedation Scale (RASS). JAMA. 2003;289:2983–91.

Chapter 3
Epidemiology of Delirium in Critically Ill Adults: Prevalence, Risk Factors, and Outcomes

Dustin Scott Kehler, Rohan M. Sanjanwala, and Rakesh C. Arora

Abbreviations

ADL	Activities of daily living
APACHE II	Acute Physiology and Chronic Health Evaluation II
CAM-ICU	Confusion Assessment Method for the ICU
DECCA	Delirium Epidemiology in Critical Care
IADL	Instrumental activities of daily living
ICDSC	Intensive Care Delirium Screening Checklist
ICU	Intensive care unit
IQCODE	Informant Questionnaire on Cognitive Decline in the Elderly
PICS	Post-intensive care syndrome
PTSD	Post-traumatic stress disorder
RASS	Richmond Agitation-Sedation Scale

D. S. Kehler
Department of Medicine, Division of Geriatric Medicine, Dalhousie University, Halifax, NS, Canada

R. M. Sanjanwala
Max Rady College of Medicine, Rady Faculty of Health Sciences, University of Manitoba, Winnipeg, MB, Canada

R. C. Arora (✉)
Max Rady College of Medicine, Rady Faculty of Health Sciences, University of Manitoba, Winnipeg, MB, Canada

Cardiac Sciences Program, St. Boniface Hospital, Winnipeg, MB, Canada

C. G. Hughes et al. (eds.), *Delirium*, https://doi.org/10.1007/978-3-030-25751-4_3

Introduction

Delirium is common in critically ill patients. It is characterized by a transient, fluctuating, altered mental state and thought to be a manifestation of acute brain dysfunction [1]. Symptoms of delirium include disturbances or disruptions in consciousness, attention, and thinking [2]. Delirium has multiple interacting etiologies, resulting in a multitude of risk factors that predispose or precipitate delirium in vulnerable patients. While this clinical syndrome may resolve in the hospital, patients who develop delirium are at a significantly higher risk for adverse events during hospitalization and following hospital discharge [3]. This chapter provides an overview of the prevalence, incidence, risk factors, and outcomes of delirium in critically ill adult patients.

Prevalence

Patients admitted to the intensive care unit (ICU) experience acute brain dysfunction which can manifest as the clinical syndrome of delirium. The overall prevalence of delirium in critically ill patients varies across different populations studied and ranges from 16% to 89% a [4, 5]. The clinical presentation of delirium is varied from patient to patient or often in the same patient on different days. Motoric and other delirium subtypes are described in more detail in Chap. 1; however, the most common motoric subtypes of delirium are hypoactive (symptoms of drowsiness, inactivity [~40% of cases]) and mixed (~50%); sole hyperactive (e.g., symptoms of restlessness, agitation) delirium is the least common. [3] Major contributing factors for differences in delirium prevalence include patient precipitating factors (e.g., baseline vulnerability, severity of disease), the ICU case mix (patient type: medical, surgical, trauma), and severity of ICU stressors (e.g., mechanical ventilation duration, sedation/analgesia), which are described later in this chapter. Prevalence and incidence estimates are also affected by the delirium screening tool used, frequency of screening, and administrator competence. The delirium screening and assessment tools recommended for use in critically ill patients are described in more detail in Chap. 2.

As the North American population continues to **age**, increasingly older (age >65 years) and vulnerable adults are admitted to the ICU, constituting more than half of all ICU admissions and ICU days [6, 7]. By extension, there are more patients being admitted to the ICU with multiple, interacting, chronic conditions. **Pre-existing cognitive decline** is common among older ICU patients which may result in a higher prevalence of delirium among this age group. In a study of 304 patients admitted to a medical ICU who were at least 60 years old, patients were considered to have dementia if they scored >3.3 with the Short Form of Informant Questionnaire on Cognitive Decline in the Elderly (IQCODE) by a patient proxy [8]. The authors found that 86 of 92 patients (93%) with dementia experienced delirium within the first 48 h of their admission. However, another study demonstrated that only 41% of patients with dementia (n = 36) experienced delirium, while 26% of patients without dementia had delirium (n = 83) [9]. The small sample sizes of the studies could account for these differences. Even so, it appears that significant cognitive vulnerability at baseline results in a higher delirium prevalence when critical illness develops.

Delirium is common in **mechanically ventilated** patients, although accurate delirium diagnosis is hindered by limited communication between the patient and healthcare provider or the researcher. The Confusion Assessment Method for the ICU (CAM-ICU) [10] and Intensive Care Delirium Screening Checklist (ICDSC) [11] are the two best studied and most widely utilized scales in clinical practice (described in more detail in Chap. 2) [1]. Earlier studies have reported a higher prevalence of delirium in mechanically ventilated patients (80%) [12–14] compared to those not requiring mechanical ventilation (20–50%) [1]. In a study that assessed delirium using the CAM-ICU, the prevalence of delirium was over 80% among mechanically ventilated patients (N = 111). However, delirium was detected in approximately 40% of nonventilated, alert patients, who were initially considered cognitively intact [10]. Other reports have observed slightly higher estimates of patients who were not mechanically ventilated, approximately half of medical ICU patients [15]. The need for mechanical ventilation could be a surrogate of severity of illness such that delirium is a consequence of higher morbidity. The multicenter Delirium Epidemiology in Critical Care (DECCA) study is a large cohort of patients who evaluated ICU patients using the CAM-ICU screening test [1]. The study population (N = 975,497) consisted of 64% of patients with a medical condition, 22% with an elective surgical procedure, and 14% with an emergent diagnosis [1]. After excluding the deeply sedated and unarousable patients with a Richmond Agitation-Sedation Scale (RASS) score of −3 to −5, 75 of 232 (32%) patients were diagnosed to have delirium [1]. This finding is in agreement with the results from a previous systematic review and meta-analysis, which included studies evaluating ICU, non-cardiac surgical patients who were assessed with a validated delirium screening tool. A meta-analysis of 16,595 patients (n = 42 studies) identified that the prevalence of delirium was 32% [16]. These large-scale studies provide a real-world picture of delirium prevalence across different critical care settings.

Risk Factors

Risk factors for delirium are typically separated into predisposing factors, (which increases a patients' risk for developing delirium (e.g., older age, disease burden, functional status) and precipitating factors (e.g., surgery, mechanical ventilation, sleep disturbances). Risk factors described in this chapter are provided in Table 3.1 and Fig. 3.2.

Table 3.1 Associations between risk factors and delirium

Risk factor	Deleterious association	Protective association	No association
Predisposing risk factors			
Older age	[3, 17, 18][a]		
Sex (male)	[20][b]		[17][b]
Severity of illness	[19][a]		
Hypertension	[17, 18][b]		
Hypercholesterolemia		[20][b]	
Alcohol consumption	[18][b]		[23]
Smoking			[17, 18][b]
Hypoalbuminuria	[24]		
Frailty	[25, 26, 27]		
Dementia/cognitive impairment	[3, 17, 19][a]		
Depression	[28]		
Psychotropic drug use	[28]		
Precipitating risk factors			
Emergent event	[3, 17, 19][a, b]		
Length of surgical operation			[20][b]
ICU length of stay	[20][b]		
APACHE II score	[18][b]		
Sedatives/analgesics			
Benzodiazepine use	[30, 33]		
Long-term drug exposure	[23]		
↑Nighttime sedatives	[31, 32]		
Sedative-induced coma	[17][b]		
Short-action sedatives (e.g., dexmedetomidine)		[3, 17, 36, 37][a, b]	
Statins		[21][a]	[22][b]
ICU sleep quality		[3, 19][a]	[29]
Sleep aids		[29]	
Physical restraint use	[19][a]		
Pain	[3][a]		

[a]Indicates non-systematic review
[b]Indicates systematic review and/or meta-analysis

Predisposing Factors

Older age of critically ill adults (>65 years old) is associated with an inflection point of an increase in incidence of delirium [3, 17, 18]. Indeed, hospitalized patients who are 65 years or older have more than twice the risk of developing delirium compared to their younger counterparts [18]. This finding is not necessarily surprising as comorbidity burden, which also contributes to delirium risk, increases with older age. In fact, overall comorbidity and severity of illness are shown to increase the risk of delirium by 1.3 to 5.6-fold in the non-cardiac critically ill population [19]. Hypertension has been associated with a risk of delirium in the ICU, with almost a doubling in the observed incidence of delirium [17, 18]. Conversely, hypercholesterolemia was previously shown to reduce the risk of delirium in vascular surgery patients [20]. This counterintuitive finding could be due to the proposed delirium-protective effect of statin use among vascular surgical patients having higher atherosclerotic burden in the vascular surgical patients, rather than the burden of high cholesterol [21], although this hypothesis is controversial [21, 22].

The evidence is conflicting whether there are differences in delirium risk between males and females among critically ill patients. This may be related to specific patient populations (e.g., older medical patients vs. younger trauma patients) and subtypes of delirium. A systematic review examining non-cardiac surgical, critically ill adults found no differences in the risk of delirium between males and females [17], whereas a meta-analysis of 11 studies ($n = 2777$ patients) admitted for vascular surgery revealed a 30% increased odds of developing delirium for males [20].

There are limited data regarding the impact of behavioral factors prior to hospital admission on delirium risk. Alcohol abuse and/or dependence is associated with a more than twofold increased risk of delirium in the critically ill patients [18]. A multicenter observational study of patients admitted to medical, surgical, cardiac, neurologic, and trauma ICUs, however, did not confirm this association [23]. Similarly, while low brain oxygen saturation is thought to be a plausible mechanism that leads to delirium, smoking has not been consistently associated with increased delirium risk [17, 18].

Severe hypoalbuminemia, defined as serum albumin of ≤30.0 g/L, a surrogate measure of a poor nutritional state, was significantly associated with a threefold higher odds of delirium risk compared to patients admitted to the ICU after non-cardiac surgery [24]. While there are limited data on what mechanisms drive the delirium risk among patients having a poor nutritional state, it is thought that malnutrition negatively impacts cerebral function [24].

Low physiologic (e.g., functional and cognitive) reserve is associated with an increased risk of delirium in patients with a critical illness. Frailty, depending on the measurement tool used, resulted in a three-(measured by a frailty index) to eightfold (measured by the Short Performance Physical Battery) increased risk of delirium in the ICU among patients who underwent elective cardiac surgery [25, 26]. Single markers of frailty including slow gait speed and weak grip strength were also shown to be associated with a higher delirium risk independent of age, activities of daily living (ADL), and previous cardiovascular disease among patients admitted to an acute geriatric unit [27]. Clinical diagnosis of dementia and cognitive impairment prior to hospitalization increase the risk of delirium in the older general medicine and surgical (cardiac and non-cardiac) population [3, 17, 19]. There is also emerging evidence that depression or use of psychotropic drugs is linked with a higher delirium risk in the ICU [28]. The pathophysiological link between low functional and cognitive reserve, as well as psychopathology (i.e., depression and psychotropic drug use), is likely due to the interference of neurotransmission through a systematic activation of pro-inflammatory cytokines, at least indirectly, that may already be impaired at baseline [19].

Precipitating Risk Factors

There are a multitude of contributing factors that precipitate delirium in acutely ill hospitalized adults [17]. Generally speaking, more significant insults such as invasive surgery compared to elective procedures or events requiring mechanical ventilation are associated with a higher risk of developing delirium [3, 19].

Severity of Illness

Factors relating to severity of illness and medical and surgical treatment requirements impact delirium risk. A meta-analysis revealed that every additional point in the Acute Physiology and Chronic Health Evaluation II (APACHE II) score was associated with a 1.13 (95% CI 1.06–1.21) increased odds of developing delirium among patients admitted to the ICU [18]. The length of operation for vascular surgical patients was not associated with delirium; however, the length of time spent in the ICU was significantly associated with delirium, and each additional day increase in ICU length of stay was associated with a higher delirium risk (mean difference of 1.06 [95% CI 0.39–1.73]) [20].

Pharmacological Agents

Sedation and analgesic agents impact the risk of delirium in the ICU. Continuous benzodiazepine and opioid infusions in critically ill patients are significantly associated with a higher odds of delirium transition (OR 4.02 [95% CI 2.19–7.38]) [29]. Further, higher doses of benzodiazepines increased the risk of transitioning to either delirium or a coma by 1.2-fold, independent of demographics, comorbidity, and severity of illness [30]. Prolonged drug exposure ($\geq$48 h) to benzodiazepines (HR 1.08 [95% CI 1.04–1.12]) per 5 mg midazolam-equivalent increment) and anticholinergic drugs (HR 2.45 [95%CI 1.08–5.54]) has been shown to increase delirium risk [23]. Increasing the dose of benzodiazepine during nighttime may also be hazardous (2.5-fold increased odds of delirium), and this practice is estimated to occur in 40% of patients (23.3 mg higher than daytime doses) receiving mechanical ventilation [31, 32]. Delirium risk is increased while in the ICU by the number of days spent in a sedative-induced coma [17], and early deep sedation within the first 48 h was significantly associated with increased risk [33–35]. A plausible mechanism for increased delirium risk is prolonged drug exposure leading to drug accumulation due to changing volumes of distribution and renal or hepatic insufficiency commonly seen in critically ill patients.

Other non-benzodiazepine and opioid agents such as dexmedetomidine have been associated with a lower risk of developing delirium in surgical and in general medical conditions [3, 17], with a strong relative risk reduction among cardiac surgery patients (0.35 [95% CI 0.20–0.62]) [36]. A multicenter randomized trial found that mechanically ventilated patients receiving dexmedetomidine had a significantly lower prevalence of delirium compared to patients receiving midazolam (54% vs. 77%) [37]. Another randomized trial found that dexmedetomidine led to a decreased incidence and duration of postoperative delirium compared to propofol in patients after cardiac surgery [38]. The protective effects of dexmedetomidine on delirium risk are thought to be due to decreased sympathetic tone, decreased inflammation, and less disturbed sleep [36], although it has been suggested that dexmedetomidine administration simply attenuates delirium risk because of a reduction in exposure to gamma-aminobutyric acid (GABA) agonist agents (i.e., benzodiazepines, propofol) [17, 39].

The evidence is less clear regarding the role of HMG-CoA reductase agents (a.k.a. statins) and their association with delirium risk. Previous reports have suggested that statins may have a protective effect through reductions in oxidative stress and apoptosis [21]. In a study by Mather and colleagues, patients admitted to a medical ICU who were propensity matched for comorbidities determined that statin users had a significant decreased odds of developing delirium (OR 0.47 [95% CI 0.38–0.56]) compared to those who did not use statins [21]. Two additional prospective cohort studies also found benefit with statin administration [40, 41]. However, this protective association is not consistently demonstrated in critically ill patients. Three randomized controlled trials found no difference in delirium between statin and placebo [42–44]. A meta-analysis ($n = 4382$ patients) demonstrated no association of delirium risk with exposure to statins in cardiac surgery patients and in otherwise critically ill patients ($n = 289{,}773$ patients) [22]. The authors of that meta-analysis also discuss that the doses of statins administered in the included studies were significantly lower than what is recommended for the prevention of cardiovascular disease events [22]. Therefore, it is plausible that statins have a dose-dependent effect on delirium risk reduction, but this has not been fully established in the extant literature.

Sleep Deprivation

Other factors related to the care of critically ill patients may impact delirium risk. There is some evidence to suggest that sleep quality in the ICU has an effect on delirium risk [3, 19]. However, patient-perceived sleep quality in the 24 h preceding delirium was not associated with risk for developing delirium in hospital. [29] Rather, the use of pharmacological sleep aids at home prior to hospital admission were shown to be independently associated with a reduced risk of delirium development.

Outcomes

Delirium in critically ill patients has been associated with adverse outcomes, which are described below and displayed in Fig. 3.1. The exact pathophysiology surrounding delirium occurrence and its impact on in-hospital and post-discharge outcomes has yet to be determined [45, 46].

Mortality

The impact of delirium on inhospital mortality is unclear. A meta-analysis of 28 studies found that critically ill patients presenting with delirium were twice as likely to die in the hospital compared to patients without delirium (risk ratio 2.19 [95% CI, 1.78–2.70]) [16]. These findings were consistent even after adjusting for confounders such as age, baseline severity of illness (APACHE II score), and female sex. In contrast, a prospective study of 1112 patients admitted to the ICU (50% had at least one episode of delirium) revealed no association between delirium occurrence and inhospital mortality after adjusting for disease severity before the onset of delirium [47]. Nonetheless, a sensitivity analysis in that study demonstrated a strong association between persistent delirium (>2 days) and inhospital mortality risk [2], suggesting that persistent delirium lasting at least 48 h increases the risk of inhospital

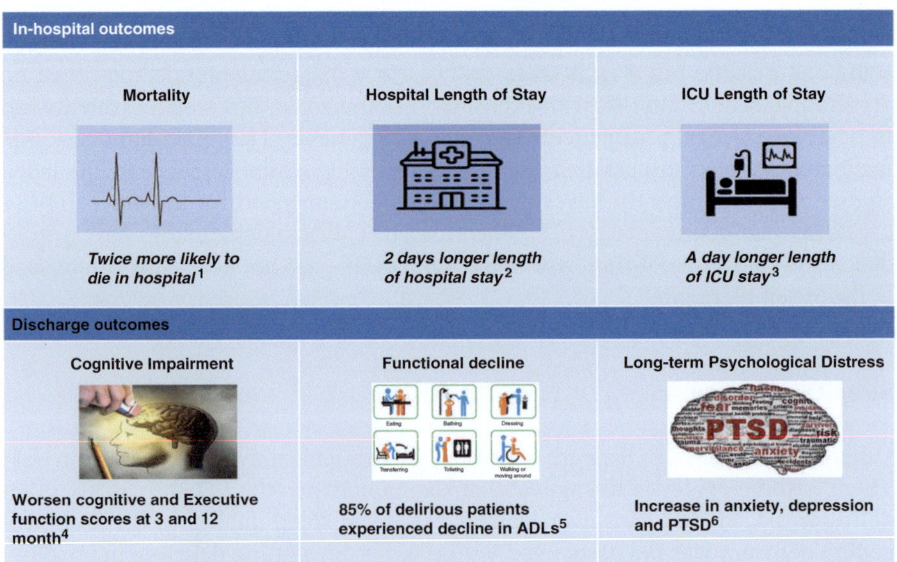

Fig. 3.1 Adverse in- hospital and post discharge among critically ill patients experiencing delirium (Salluh et al. [16], Thomason et al. [15]. Salluh et al. [1]. Pandharipande et al. [60]. Khan [65]. Marra et al. [75])

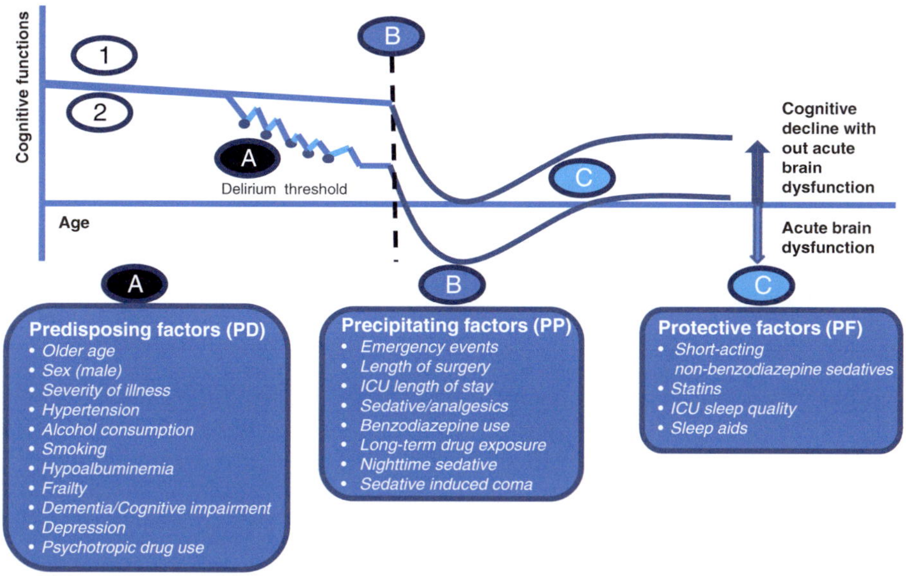

Fig. 3.2 The trajectory of cognitive decline secondary to acute insults (precipitating factors) among patients with/without preexisting vulnerability (predisposing factors): There is age-associated cognitive decline among older adult patients. The acute stressor events in such patients will result in further decline in cognitive functioning (patient 1). However, among patients with higher vulnerability (i.e., multiple predisposing factors), there is a preexisting cumulative cognitive decline. Such patients experiencing acute insult are at higher risk of developing acute brain dysfunction (i.e., delirium) (patient 2)

mortality. Interestingly, one study showed that rapidly reversible delirium resulting from sedation was not associated with a higher inhospital mortality risk [48]. However, while randomized controlled trials using pharmacological (e.g., dexmedetomidine, antipsychotic, rivastigmine, clonidine) and non-pharmacological (e.g., spontaneous awakening, early mobilization, increased perfusion) interventions reduces delirium duration, they were not shown to reduce mortality rates compared to placebo or control group participants [49]. It is possible that such interventions which result in shorter delirium duration do not completely alleviate acute brain or associated multi-organ dysfunction [49]. Even so, persistent delirium is significantly associated with worse inhospital outcomes.

Delirium has a negative health impact that continues beyond hospital discharge among patients with a critical illness [6]. In fact, after controlling for age, illness severity, cognition, and functional status, delirium has been shown to increase 1 year mortality risk following hospital discharge [6]. That study also reported that the duration of delirium contributed to a higher mortality risk following hospitalization, in so much that each additional day with delirium was associated with a 10% increased risk of mortality (HR 1.10 [95% CI 1.02–1.18]). A prospective study of ICU survivors found a nonsignificant increase in post-discharge mortality in those with delirium during the hospital stay (HR 1.26 [95% CI 0.93–1.71]) [50].

A meta-analysis of older adults (>65 years old) experiencing delirium (7 studies, n = 2957) demonstrated that patients experiencing delirium in the ICU had an increased risk of death at 2-year post-discharge (HR 1.95 [95% CI 1.51–2.52]) [51]. The risk of mortality appears to be at its highest in the short term. In an analysis of 26,245 delirious and 262,450 randomly selected controls who were discharged from the emergency department, adjusted 30-day mortality was significantly higher (HR 4.82 [95% CI 4.60–5.04]) compared to 12-month mortality (HR 2.07 [95% CI 2.01–2.13)]) [52]. The mitigated long-term mortality risk at 1 year following hospital discharge may suggest that patients who recover successfully from their previous critical illness have a more favorable long-term prognosis, although more required data are needed to confirm this hypothesis.

ICU and Hospital Length of Stay

Delirium in critical care patients independently predicts a longer ICU and hospital length of stay [12]. A meta-analysis of 42 studies showed that patients with delirium have a longer ICU (standard mean difference 1.38 [0.99–1.77]) and hospital stay (0.97 [0.61–1.33]) compared to patients without delirium [16]. Patients who experienced delirium at any time during their hospital stay were in the hospital for 2 days longer and a day longer in the ICU compared to those who never experienced delirium [15]. The duration of delirium may also contribute to a longer hospital stay in so much that each additional day with delirium was associated with an additional 1.18 days in the hospital. [12] In turn, delirium is associated with a higher cost related to longer ICU and hospital stay, approximately a 1.4-fold and 1.3-fold higher, respectively [53].

Psychological Burden in Patients and Family Caregiver

The critical care patient and their family caregivers experience extreme levels of acute psychological distress. However, the emotional consequence for the delirious patients and their caregiver has not been studied extensively, partly because of the lack of sufficient instrumentation which can adequately assess subjective perception of stress while also quantifying the emotional burden among delirious patients and their caregivers. A previous study evaluating the experiences of patients who had a delirium episode reported that only 28% remembered the episode and recollected being confused, fearful, and anxious. In addition, patients reported experiencing visual hallucinations [54]. A recent prospective study of medical and surgical hospitalized patients who were at least 70 years old also demonstrated that both the patient with delirium and their caregiver reported significantly higher emotional burden [55].

Post-intensive Care Syndrome

Post-intensive care syndrome (PICS) is an umbrella term for acute onset (or aggravation of preexisting) cognitive, physical, and psychological impairment that persists among ICU survivors following critical illness [56, 57]. Although the precise prevalence of PICS is still a source of significant investigative interest, current estimates suggest that more than 50% of the ICU survivors will experience some component of PICS [58–61]. Delirium occurrence has been associated with an increased incidence of different domains of PICS, including higher burden of cognitive and functional impairment as well as psychological distress among patients and their family caregiver [62].

PICS-Cognitive Dysfunction

Critically ill patients experiencing delirium frequently have prolonged cognitive impairment following hospital discharge [16, 63]. The resulting cognitive impairment may not resolve for an extended period of time, and it is possible that the patient may not achieve prehospital cognitive status [63]. Indeed, a study found that longer delirium duration was associated with worse cognitive function, including global cognition and executive function, at 3 and 12 months following hospital discharge [60]. Another study of mechanically ventilated medical ICU survivors ($n = 77$) experiencing delirium aligns with these findings which demonstrated that 79% and 71% of patients with delirium had cognitive impairment on neuropsychological testing at 3 and 12 months following hospitalization, respectively [63]. A large ($n = 1101$) 12-month follow-up study revealed that delirious ($n = 412$) patients had a higher odds of mild (OR 2.41 [95% CI 1.57–3.69]) and severe (OR 3.10 95% CI [1.10–8.74]) cognitive dysfunction compared to the non-delirious critical care survivors ($n = 689$) [50]. As a result of a new cognitive impairment, the critically ill patient may experience additional negative outcomes that impact socialization with others and their overall quality of life [64].

PICS: Functional Impairment

The occurrence of delirium has been associated with an increased risk of long-term limitations in activities of daily living (ADL) in critical illness survivors. In a small study ($n = 27$) of adults 65 years or older who were delirious during their hospital stay, ADLs were evaluated 3 months post-discharge. The study revealed that 85% of patients experienced a decline in their ADLs and 52% experienced worse instrumental ADLs (IADLs) compared to their prehospital status with a mean difference of 1.1 for ADLs and a 3.0 for IADLs based on the Katz and Lawton ADL scale [65]. Evidence also suggests that the prolonged delirium (>5 days) linearly increases the probability of having a disability in ADLs at 12 months from hospital discharge

[58]. The milieu of inhospital complications which result in delirium (e.g., longer ICU and hospital stay, sleep disturbances, use of physical restraints) and overlap in potential inflammatory pathophysiologic mechanisms may explain why delirium is associated with worse ADLs [66, 67].

PICS: Psychological Distress

The neuropsychological sequelae that occur following a critical care admission are numerous and can be highly distressing for patients and their families. Depression, anxiety, and post-traumatic stress disorder (PTSD) are common among critical care survivors. A study of patients with community acquired pneumonia and acute respiratory distress syndrome demonstrated that longer duration of delirium was associated with a higher risk of developing PTSD. Moreover, a series of studies have revealed that patients developing PTSD following critical illness had significantly lower mental health scores [68–70]. However, symptoms of PTSD for patients who experience delirium may not persist 1 year following hospital discharge [71].

Discharge Health-Related Quality of Life

To understand the long-term implications of delirium in critically ill patients, health-related quality of life (HRQoL) needs to be elucidated. A number of studies have not found an association between developing delirium in the hospital and poor quality of life following hospital discharge [50, 64, 72, 73]. However, patients with different subtypes of delirium reported disparate levels of quality of life following hospital discharge. Participants with hyperactive and mixed delirium were more likely to have poor health-related quality of life compared to patients with hypoactive delirium after adjusting for urgency and severity of illness, as well as ICU and hospital length of stay [64]. The small number of investigations to date drive the need for further study to elucidate the impact of delirium on health-related quality of life following hospital discharge. Furthermore, the studies here have excluded the most severely ill who would have likely had the worst health-related quality of life compared to the analyzed sample.

Institutionalization After Discharge

Delirium in the critically ill patient is associated with diminished independence following hospital discharge and necessity for placement in a long-term care facility. In a study of 700 older adults (>65 years old) admitted to the emergency department requiring ICU care, only 9% (56/613) of patients who were not delirious were discharged to a chronic care facility compared to 37% (23/63) of delirious patients, representing a fourfold increased (unadjusted) odds in the delirious patient requiring additional care [74]. A meta-analysis of 7 studies ($n = 2579$ patients) with an average 14-month follow-up supports this finding that delirium increases the risk of institutionalization [51]. The analyses revealed that patients that experience delirium are more likely to be placed in a long-term care facility (OR 2.41 [95% CI 1.77–3.29]) compared to those who did not experience delirium in hospital. Indeed, the patients who experience delirium should be considered at an especially higher likelihood to require institutional care following hospital discharge, and, consequently, requiring additional healthcare resources compared to their non-delirious peers.

Conclusion

Delirium is common in the critically ill patient, but the reported prevalence estimates vary significantly (16–89%) across conditions, the type of screening and assessment tool used, and the number of predisposing and precipitating risk factors present. Delirium has a negative impact on health outcomes in the hospital and following hospital discharge, although more evidence is needed to confirm the long-term consequences of ICU delirium. The early identification of risk, therefore, is essential to facilitate the healthcare team in developing prevention and management strategies for this syndrome.

References

1. Salluh JI, et al. Delirium epidemiology in critical care (DECCA): an international study. Crit Care. 2010;14:R210. https://doi.org/10.1186/cc9333.
2. Wong CL, Holroyd-Leduc J, Simel DL, Straus SE. Does this patient have delirium?: value of bedside instruments. JAMA. 2010;304:779–86. https://doi.org/10.1001/jama.2010.1182.
3. Hayhurst CJ, Pandharipande PP, Hughes CG. Intensive care unit delirium: a review of diagnosis, prevention, and treatment. Anesthesiology. 2016;125:1229–41. https://doi.org/10.1097/aln.0000000000001378.
4. Brigola AG, et al. Relationship between cognition and frailty in elderly: a systematic review. Dement Neuropsychologia. 2015;9:110–9. https://doi.org/10.1590/1980-57642015dn92000005.
5. van Eijk MM, Slooter AJ. Delirium in intensive care unit patients. Semin Cardiothorac Vasc Anesth. 2010;14:141–7. https://doi.org/10.1177/1089253210371495.
6. Pisani MA, et al. Days of delirium are associated with 1-year mortality in an older intensive care unit population. Am J Respir Crit Care Med. 2009;180:1092–7. https://doi.org/10.1164/rccm.200904-0537OC.
7. Pisani MA, Redlich C, McNicoll L, Ely EW, Inouye SK. Underrecognition of preexisting cognitive impairment by physicians in older ICU patients. Chest. 2003;124:2267–74.
8. Pisani MA, Murphy TE, Van Ness PH, Araujo KL, Inouye SK. Characteristics associated with delirium in older patients in a medical intensive care unit. Arch Intern Med. 2007;167:1629–34. https://doi.org/10.1001/archinte.167.15.1629.
9. McNicoll L, et al. Delirium in the intensive care unit: occurrence and clinical course in older patients. J Am Geriatr Soc. 2003;51:591–8.

10. Ely EW, et al. Delirium in mechanically ventilated patients: validity and reliability of the confusion assessment method for the intensive care unit (CAM-ICU). JAMA. 2001;286:2703–10.
11. Bergeron N, Dubois MJ, Dumont M, Dial S, Skrobik Y. Intensive care delirium screening checklist: evaluation of a new screening tool. Intensive Care Med. 2001;27:859–64.
12. Ely EW, et al. The impact of delirium in the intensive care unit on hospital length of stay. Intensive Care Med. 2001;27:1892–900. https://doi.org/10.1007/s00134-001-1132-2.
13. Ely EW, et al. Delirium as a predictor of mortality in mechanically ventilated patients in the intensive care unit. JAMA. 2004;291:1753–62. https://doi.org/10.1001/jama.291.14.1753.
14. Pandharipande P, et al. Prevalence and risk factors for development of delirium in surgical and trauma intensive care unit patients. J Trauma. 2008;65:34–41. https://doi.org/10.1097/TA.0b013e31814b2c4d.
15. Thomason JW, et al. Intensive care unit delirium is an independent predictor of longer hospital stay: a prospective analysis of 261 non-ventilated patients. Crit Care. 2005;9:R375–81. https://doi.org/10.1186/cc3729.
16. Salluh JI, et al. Outcome of delirium in critically ill patients: systematic review and meta-analysis. BMJ. 2015;350:h2538. https://doi.org/10.1136/bmj.h2538.
17. Zaal IJ, Devlin JW, Peelen LM, Slooter AJ. A systematic review of risk factors for delirium in the ICU. Crit Care Med. 2015;43:40–7. https://doi.org/10.1097/ccm.0000000000000625.
18. Huai J, Ye X. A meta-analysis of critically ill patients reveals several potential risk factors for delirium. Gen Hosp Psychiatry. 2014;36:488–96. https://doi.org/10.1016/j.genhosppsych.2014.05.002.
19. Inouye SK, Westendorp RG, Saczynski JS. Delirium in elderly people. Lancet. 2014;383:911–22. https://doi.org/10.1016/s0140-6736(13)60688-1.
20. Oldroyd C, et al. A systematic review and meta-analysis of factors for delirium in vascular surgical patients. J Vasc Surg. 2017;66:1269–1279.e1269. https://doi.org/10.1016/j.jvs.2017.04.077.
21. Mather JF, et al. Statin and its association with delirium in the medical ICU. Crit Care Med. 2017;45:1515–22. https://doi.org/10.1097/ccm.0000000000002530.
22. Vallabhajosyula S, Kanmanthareddy A, Erwin PJ, Esterbrooks DJ, Morrow LE. Role of statins in delirium prevention in critical ill and cardiac surgery patients: a systematic review and meta-analysis. J Crit Care. 2017;37:189–96. https://doi.org/10.1016/j.jcrc.2016.09.025.
23. Burry LD, et al. Delirium and exposure to psychoactive medications in critically ill adults: a multi-Centre observational study. J Crit Care. 2017;42:268–74. https://doi.org/10.1016/j.jcrc.2017.08.003.
24. Zhang DF, et al. Preoperative severe hypoalbuminemia is associated with an increased risk of postoperative delirium in elderly patients: results of a secondary analysis. J Crit Care. 2018;44:45–50. https://doi.org/10.1016/j.jcrc.2017.09.182.
25. Jung P, et al. The impact of frailty on postoperative delirium in cardiac surgery patients. J Thorac Cardiovasc Surg. 2015;149:869.
26. Brown CH t, et al. The association between preoperative frailty and postoperative delirium after cardiac surgery. Anesth Analg. 2016;123:430–5. https://doi.org/10.1213/ane.0000000000001271.
27. Bellelli G, et al. The association between delirium and sarcopenia in older adult patients admitted to acute geriatrics units: results from the GLISTEN multicenter observational study. Clin Nutr. 2017; https://doi.org/10.1016/j.clnu.2017.08.027.
28. Sajjad A, et al. Psychopathology prior to critical illness and the risk of delirium onset during intensive care unit stay. Intensive Care Med. 2018; https://doi.org/10.1007/s00134-018-5195-8.
29. Kamdar BB, et al. Delirium transitions in the medical ICU: exploring the role of sleep quality and other factors. Crit Care Med. 2015;43:135–41. https://doi.org/10.1097/ccm.0000000000000610.
30. Pandharipande P, et al. Lorazepam is an independent risk factor for transitioning to delirium in intensive care unit patients. Anesthesiology. 2006;104:21–6.

31. Seymour CW, et al. Diurnal sedative changes during intensive care: impact on liberation from mechanical ventilation and delirium. Crit Care Med. 2012;40:2788–96. https://doi.org/10.1097/CCM.0b013e31825b8ade.
32. Mehta S, et al. Variation in diurnal sedation in mechanically ventilated patients who are managed with a sedation protocol alone or a sedation protocol and daily interruption. Crit Care. 2016;20:233. https://doi.org/10.1186/s13054-016-1405-3.
33. Shehabi Y, et al. Sedation depth and long-term mortality in mechanically ventilated critically ill adults: a prospective longitudinal multicentre cohort study. Intensive Care Med. 2013;39: 910–8. https://doi.org/10.1007/s00134-013-2830-2.
34. Stephens RJ, et al. Practice patterns and outcomes associated with early sedation depth in mechanically ventilated patients: a systematic review and meta-analysis. Crit Care Med. 2018;46:471–9. https://doi.org/10.1097/ccm.0000000000002885.
35. Shehabi Y, et al. Sedation intensity in the first 48 hours of mechanical ventilation and 180-day mortality: a multinational prospective longitudinal cohort study. Crit Care Med. 2018;46:850–9. https://doi.org/10.1097/ccm.0000000000003071.
36. Geng J, Qian J, Cheng H, Ji F, Liu H. The influence of perioperative dexmedetomidine on patients undergoing cardiac surgery: a meta-analysis. PLoS One. 2016;11:e0152829. https://doi.org/10.1371/journal.pone.0152829.
37. Riker RR, et al. Dexmedetomidine vs midazolam for sedation of critically ill patients: a randomized trial. JAMA. 2009;301:489–99. https://doi.org/10.1001/jama.2009.56.
38. Djaiani G, et al. Dexmedetomidine versus propofol sedation reduces delirium after cardiac surgery: a randomized controlled trial. Anesthesiology. 2016;124:362–8. https://doi.org/10.1097/aln.0000000000000951.
39. Subramaniam B, et al. Effect of intravenous acetaminophen vs placebo combined with propofol or dexmedetomidine on postoperative delirium among older patients following cardiac surgery: the DEXACET randomized clinical trial. JAMA. 2019;321:686–96. https://doi.org/10.1001/jama.2019.0234.
40. Page VJ, et al. Statin use and risk of delirium in the critically ill. Am J Respir Crit Care Med. 2014;189:666–73. https://doi.org/10.1164/rccm.201306-1150OC.
41. Morandi A, et al. Statins and delirium during critical illness: a multicenter, prospective cohort study. Crit Care Med. 2014;42:1899–909. https://doi.org/10.1097/ccm.0000000000000398.
42. Needham DM, et al. Rosuvastatin versus placebo for delirium in intensive care and subsequent cognitive impairment in patients with sepsis-associated acute respiratory distress syndrome: an ancillary study to a randomised controlled trial. Lancet Respir Med. 2016;4:203–12. https://doi.org/10.1016/s2213-2600(16)00005-9.
43. Page VJ, et al. Evaluation of early administration of simvastatin in the prevention and treatment of delirium in critically ill patients undergoing mechanical ventilation (MoDUS): a randomised, double-blind, placebo-controlled trial. Lancet Respir Med. 2017;5:727–37. https://doi.org/10.1016/s2213-2600(17)30234-5.
44. Billings FT t, et al. High-dose perioperative atorvastatin and acute kidney injury following cardiac surgery: a randomized clinical trial. JAMA. 2016;315:877–88. https://doi.org/10.1001/jama.2016.0548.
45. Smith M, Meyfroidt G. Critical illness: the brain is always in the line of fire. Intensive Care Med. 2017;43:870–3. https://doi.org/10.1007/s00134-017-4791-3.
46. Maldonado JR. Delirium pathophysiology: an updated hypothesis of the etiology of acute brain failure. Int J Geriatr Psychiatry. 2017; https://doi.org/10.1002/gps.4823.
47. Klein Klouwenberg PM, et al. The attributable mortality of delirium in critically ill patients: prospective cohort study. BMJ. 2014;349:g6652. https://doi.org/10.1136/bmj.g6652.
48. Patel SB, Poston JT, Pohlman A, Hall JB, Kress JP. Rapidly reversible, sedation-related delirium versus persistent delirium in the intensive care unit. Am J Respir Crit Care Med. 2014;189:658–65. https://doi.org/10.1164/rccm.201310-1815OC.

49. Al-Qadheeb NS, et al. Randomized ICU trials do not demonstrate an association between interventions that reduce delirium duration and short-term mortality: a systematic review and meta-analysis. Crit Care Med. 2014;42:1442–54. https://doi.org/10.1097/ccm.0000000000000224.
50. Wolters AE, et al. Long-term outcome of delirium during intensive care unit stay in survivors of critical illness: a prospective cohort study. Crit Care. 2014;18:R125. https://doi.org/10.1186/cc13929.
51. Witlox J, et al. Delirium in elderly patients and the risk of postdischarge mortality, institutionalization, and dementia: a meta-analysis. JAMA. 2010;304:443–51. https://doi.org/10.1001/jama.2010.1013.
52. Israni J, Lesser A, Kent T, Ko K. Delirium as a predictor of mortality in US Medicare beneficiaries discharged from the emergency department: a national claims-level analysis up to 12 months. BMJ Open. 2018;8:e021258. https://doi.org/10.1136/bmjopen-2017-021258.
53. Milbrandt EB, et al. Costs associated with delirium in mechanically ventilated patients. Crit Care Med. 2004;32:955–62.
54. Grover S, Ghosh A, Ghormode D. Experience in delirium: is it distressing? J Neuropsychiatr Clin Neurosci. 2015;27:139–46. https://doi.org/10.1176/appi.neuropsych.13110329.
55. Racine AM, et al. Delirium burden in patients and family caregivers: development and testing of new instruments. Gerontologist. 2018; https://doi.org/10.1093/geront/gny041.
56. Rawal G, Yadav S, Kumar R. Post-intensive care syndrome: an overview. J Transl Intern Med. 2017;5:90–2. https://doi.org/10.1515/jtim-2016-0016.
57. Needham DM, et al. Improving long-term outcomes after discharge from intensive care unit: report from a stakeholders' conference. Crit Care Med. 2012;40:502–9. https://doi.org/10.1097/CCM.0b013e318232da75.
58. Brummel NE, et al. Delirium in the ICU and subsequent long-term disability among survivors of mechanical ventilation. Crit Care Med. 2014;42:369–77. https://doi.org/10.1097/CCM.0b013e3182a645bd.
59. Griffiths J, et al. An exploration of social and economic outcome and associated health-related quality of life after critical illness in general intensive care unit survivors: a 12-month follow-up study. Crit Care. 2013;17:R100. https://doi.org/10.1186/cc12745.
60. Pandharipande PP, et al. Long-term cognitive impairment after critical illness. N Engl J Med. 2013;369:1306–16. https://doi.org/10.1056/NEJMoa1301372.
61. Jackson JC, et al. Depression, post-traumatic stress disorder, and functional disability in survivors of critical illness in the BRAIN-ICU study: a longitudinal cohort study. Lancet Respir Med. 2014;2:369–79. https://doi.org/10.1016/s2213-2600(14)70051-7.
62. McPeake J, Mikkelsen ME. The evolution of post intensive care syndrome. Crit Care Med. 2018;46:1551–2. https://doi.org/10.1097/ccm.0000000000003232.
63. Girard TD, et al. Delirium as a predictor of long-term cognitive impairment in survivors of critical illness. Crit Care Med. 2010;38:1513–20. https://doi.org/10.1097/CCM.0b013e3181e47be1.
64. van den Boogaard M, et al. Delirium in critically ill patients: impact on long-term health-related quality of life and cognitive functioning. Crit Care Med. 2012;40:112–8. https://doi.org/10.1097/CCM.0b013e31822e9fc9.
65. Khan B in C50. Critical care: delirium and sedation in the ICU A5273-A5273.
66. Altman MT, et al. Association of intensive care unit delirium with sleep disturbance and functional disability after critical illness: an observational cohort study. Ann Intensive Care. 2018;8:63. https://doi.org/10.1186/s13613-018-0408-4.
67. Rengel KF, Hayhurst CJ, Pandharipande PP, Hughes CG. Long-term cognitive and functional impairments after critical illness. Anesth Analg. 2019;128:772–80. https://doi.org/10.1213/ane.0000000000004066.
68. Denke C, et al. Long-term sequelae of acute respiratory distress syndrome caused by severe community-acquired pneumonia: delirium-associated cognitive impairment and post-traumatic stress disorder. J Int Med Res. 2018;46:2265–83. https://doi.org/10.1177/0300060518762040.
69. Svenningsen H, et al. Symptoms of posttraumatic stress after intensive care delirium. Biomed Res Int. 2015;2015:876947. https://doi.org/10.1155/2015/876947.

70. Marra A, Pandharipande PP, Patel MB. Intensive care unit delirium and intensive care unit-related posttraumatic stress disorder. Surg Clin North Am. 2017;97:1215–35. https://doi.org/10.1016/j.suc.2017.07.008.
71. Wolters AE, et al. Long-term mental health problems after delirium in the ICU. Crit Care Med. 2016;44:1808–13. https://doi.org/10.1097/ccm.0000000000001861.
72. Abraham CM, et al. Hospital delirium and psychological distress at 1 year and health-related quality of life after moderate-to-severe traumatic injury without intracranial hemorrhage. Arch Phys Med Rehabil. 2014;95:2382–9. https://doi.org/10.1016/j.apmr.2014.08.005.
73. Svenningsen H, et al. Intensive care delirium – effect on memories and health-related quality of life – a follow-up study. J Clin Nurs. 2014;23:634–44. https://doi.org/10.1111/jocn.12250.
74. Kennedy M, et al. Delirium risk prediction, healthcare use and mortality of elderly adults in the emergency department. J Am Geriatr Soc. 2014;62:462–9. https://doi.org/10.1111/jgs.12692.
75. Marra A, et al. Intensive care unit delirium and Intensive Care Unit –related posttraumatic stress disorder. J Crit Care. 2018;43:88–94. https://doi.org/10.1016/j.jcrc.2017.08.034.. Epub 2017 Aug 24

Chapter 4
The Relationship Between Delirium and Mental Health Outcomes: Current Insights and Future Directions

Kristina Stepanovic, Caroline L. Greene, James C. Jackson, and Jo Ellen Wilson

Learning Objectives
After reading the chapter, individuals will be able to:

- Describe the epidemiology of common psychiatric conditions after critical illness
- Articulate the relationship between delirium and depression and PTSD
- Explain the clinical relevance of an association between delirium and mental health conditions
- Recognize the need for more focused research delirium and psychiatric outcomes

K. Stepanovic
Department of Medicine, Division of Allergy, Pulmonary and Critical Care Medicine, Vanderbilt University School of Medicine, Nashville, TN, USA

C. L. Greene
Geriatric Research Education and Clinical Center, Tennessee Valley Veterans Affairs Healthcare System, Nashville, TN, USA

J. C. Jackson (✉)
Geriatric Research Education and Clinical Center, Tennessee Valley Veterans Affairs Healthcare System, Nashville, TN, USA

Critical Illness, Brain Dysfunction, and Survivorship Center, Vanderbilt University Medical Center, Nashville, TN, USA
e-mail: james.c.jackson@vanderbilt.edu; https://www.icudelirium.org

J. E. Wilson
Critical Illness, Brain Dysfunction, and Survivorship Center and the Department of Psychiatry and Behavioral Sciences, Vanderbilt University Medical Center, Nashville, TN, USA

C. G. Hughes et al. (eds.), *Delirium*, https://doi.org/10.1007/978-3-030-25751-4_4

Introduction

Delirium is a neurological syndrome marked by an acute disturbance of consciousness with inattention and a change in cognition or perceptual disturbance that fluctuates over time. Delirium affects up to 80% of elderly patients and the risk of delirium increases consistently with increased age [1]. Delirium is associated with a wide array of adverse outcomes such as longer hospital lengths of stay, greater length of mechanical ventilation, and increased mortality in the ICU and hospital. Delirium has long been associated with negative consequences even after hospital discharge including discharge to a nursing home, increased risk of death over 2 years, as well as incident dementia [2]. While delirium has consistently been shown to be related to deficits in cognition [3] (with questions persisting related to whether it is simply a marker of injury or fundamentally injurious), less is known regarding the association between delirium and a wide array of mental health difficulties (the three conditions typically studied in ICU survivors are anxiety, depression, and PTSD [post-traumatic stress disorder], not necessarily in that order) [4]. Figure 4.1 describes the overlap of symptoms of PTSD, major depressive disorder (MDD), and delirium. However, early evidence suggests the possibility of linkages of various kinds between delirium and psychiatric phenomena, and this notion

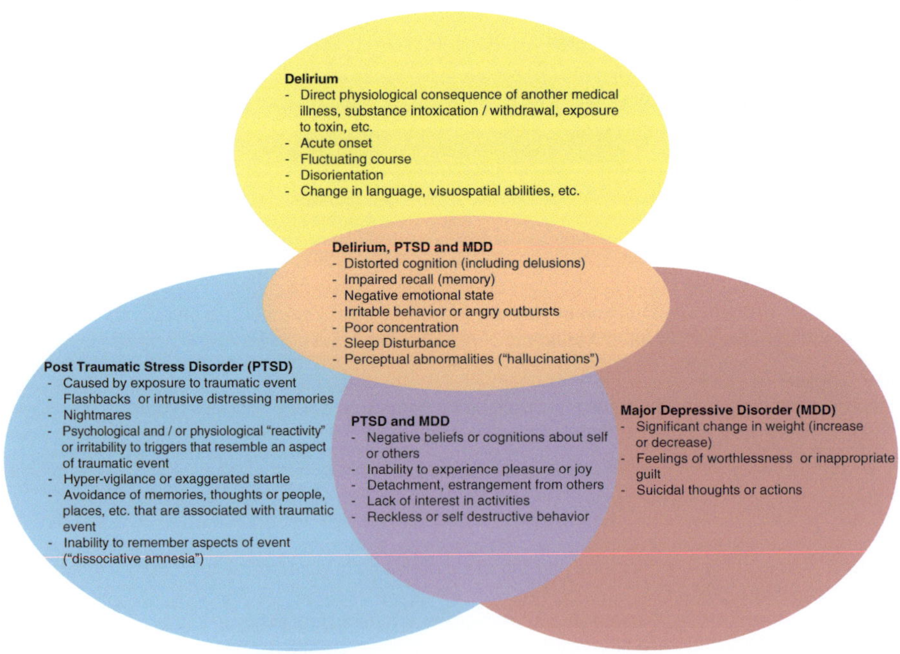

Fig. 4.1 Overlap of signs and symptoms of delirium, post-traumatic stress disorder, and major depressive disorder. During an episode of delirium, patients may experience significant anxiety and mood disturbances, and following an episode of delirium, they remain at an elevated risk to develop symptoms of PTSD or MDD

certainly fits with the experience of seasoned clinicians working with patients following critical illness and other settings in which delirium is a central problem [5]. While a clear imperative exists to treat delirium as a major public health concern, if it is the case that delirium contributes to sequelae of a psychiatric nature, this urgently underscores the importance of finding solutions to prevent and reduce this condition, as doing so may greatly reduce the burden of emotional distress in individuals after the ICU. In the pages that follow, we will describe the epidemiology of common psychiatric conditions in survivors of critical illness, engage issues related to their intersection with delirium, and offer practical solutions for clinicians and recommendations for researchers related to delirium and mental health conditions.

General Anxiety

General anxiety symptoms are exceedingly common among survivors of critical illness, with approximately half of all ICU survivors reporting marked and clinically meaningful symptoms of anxiety up to a year after discharge – a number much higher than the general population's prevalence [6–7]. Although anxiety is often quite a normal reaction in the context of stress, it can interfere with and impede recovery in multitudinous ways. Symptoms of anxiety during critical illness can have a negative impact on post-ICU psychological functioning and are associated with longer-term PTSD and worse quality of life. While relatively little is known regarding risk factors for ICU-related anxiety, published risk factors to date include demographic and historical variables (e.g., younger age, female gender, premorbid history of anxiety); in-ICU medical and physiological variables (e.g., length of mechanical ventilation, illness severity, sedation management); and environmental variables (e.g., stressful/noisy/chaotic ICU environment) as increasing the likelihood of anxiety [8]. Somewhat surprisingly, no investigations to date have formally explored the relationship between anxiety as a predisposing risk factor for delirium and, alternatively, whether delirium in the ICU is associated with a greater likelihood of anxiety after discharge, perhaps because anxiety, itself, has been studied less than PTSD and depression after critical illness, in particular. As such, we will devote little attention to issues related to delirium and anxiety, focusing instead on issues related to PTSD and depression.

Acute and Post-traumatic Stress

PTSD is a syndrome that develops, by definition, in response to exposure to a trauma or highly stressful event (in this chapter, we will refer to this "trauma" as the experience of critical illness and intensive care treatment). Although it was long characterized as an anxiety disorder, this is no longer the case. Critical illness survivors can develop acute stress symptoms during the course of hospitalization (acute stress disorder is distinct from PTSD with regard to duration of symptoms) and post-traumatic stress (PTS) symptoms afterward [9, 10]. PTS symptoms are described as symptoms of PTSD without meeting full criteria for PTSD and may include symptoms such as flashbacks, nightmares, unwanted upsetting memories, negative affect, inability to recall key features of the trauma, insomnia, irritability, etc. It has been estimated that at least 20% of ICU survivors experience clinically significant symptoms of PTS during the 1st year after ICU discharge, which is substantially higher than the overall prevalence of these symptoms among individuals in North America and the world [9, 11]. Although these symptoms are often expressed following combat, sexual assault, or a traumatic injury, they also can be a reaction to exposure to critical illness and/or the ICU environment. They may be related to disturbing memories of events that appear "real" to patients but which did not, in fact, actually happen in the way they are recalled (these have been termed "delusional memories") or, potentially, to delirious states experienced during hospitalization. See below for a more detailed list of risk factors [9, 12]. PTS symptoms after critical illness often include fear of recurrence of the medical condition and/or functional decline that could result in another fear-invoking hospitalization. Avoidant symptoms tend to predominate and manifest as denial of difficulties, apprehension about discussing any signs or symptoms of a possible medical condition with providers, and reluctance to seek help in the first place. Patients often avoid medical appointments and, as a result, may experience greater severity of chronic conditions that have gone untreated.

To meet diagnostic criteria for a formal diagnosis of PTSD, individuals must report complaints across a range of dimensions including intrusion, avoidance, negative changes in cognition or mood, and arousal/avoidance. These symptoms must be present for at least 1 month after exposure to trauma, and they must contribute to some degree of meaningful clinical impairment [13]. As a brief aside, although PTSD is often thought of in "all-or-nothing" terms, symptoms of PTSD fall at points on a spectrum [14]. To be sure, the *Diagnostic and Statistical Manual of Mental Disorders* 5th Edition (DSM-V) provides a very specific definition of PTSD which must be met for individuals to have a formal "PTSD" diagnosis. However, even isolated PTSD symptoms can have a profound impact on individuals and, in some cases, can be disabling.

To provide a clinical example of such cases, one of us (JCJ) worked with a patient many years ago who had classic avoidant features in the absence of other significant symptoms. Mr. Smith (not his real name) had undergone a particularly stressful emergency surgery in which he almost died. In the year after this surgery, he developed a bunion on his foot that made it difficult to walk and was beginning to contribute to problems at his job (which involved walking up to 5 miles a day). After an evaluation with a podiatrist, he was advised that his bunion could be easily removed via a "bunionectomy" – a simple, same-day, office procedure – and that he would quickly be "as good as new." Despite the probable ease and simplicity of this procedure, he ultimately chose not to undergo surgery due to extreme anxiety about "going under" and to a desire to avoid any situations that might potentially provoke reminders of his previous experience. Sadly, his pain and problems walking persisted until he eventually lost his job.

Risk Factors for PTSD in ICU Survivors: What About Delirium?

As noted, risk factors for PTSD in ICU survivors have been a source of high interest among both researchers and clinicians, and certain variables such as younger age, female sex, and pre-existing mental health diagnoses appear to consistently confer increased risk of PTSD both in survivors of critical illness and more generally [8]. Memories of frightening psychotic experiences during ICU hospitalization – as we mentioned, these are commonly referred to as "delusional memories" – have been linked with later PTS, though findings in this regard are unequivocal. While perhaps it is the case that most researchers believe delusional memories are particularly likely to form the basis for PTSD in ICU survivors, not all investigations have supported this finding. For example, in an investigation of Swedish ICU patients – 41% of whom reported having delusional memories – no signification associations were observed between delusional memories and anxiety or PTSD [15]. In our clinical experience with ICU survivors, this finding resonates, as some patients seem largely unphased by the presence of bizarre and terrifying "delusional" memories developed in the context of delirium even as others are profoundly traumatized.

As it relates to delirium, the connection between this neurologic syndrome and PTSD is controversial and complicated to unpack. While the notion that delirium – frequently, but not always, described by our patients as deeply disturbing – is a reliable contributor to PTSD seems logical, relatively little *empirical* data support this assertion. Weinert and colleagues, for example, determined that memories of a delirious nature were associated with greater symptoms of PTSD and observed that individuals who were the most alert and awake during critical illness had the lowest risk of PTSD [16]. More generally, however, no clear patterns reflecting specific associations between delirium and PTSD have been found. One recent case series ($N = 2$) of veterans with pre-existing PTSD suggested the possibility that those already suffering from PTSD might be at risk of what is known as "emergence delirium" or "ED" after anesthesia, but this idea, while interesting, has yet to be explored or demonstrated in a larger cohort [17].

Reducing Delirium as a Method of Decreasing PTSD?

To the extent that delirium and delusional memories are possible contributors to PTSD, it appears reasonable to consider carefully exploring sedation strategies as a target for intervention. This has been done in the context of ICU care recently, as certain approaches to sedation and pain management, for example, are widely known to be deliriogenic. In particular, researchers have focused on the role of benzodiazepines such as midazolam and lorazepam as well as opiates, as all of these have been found in at least some studies to be potentially related to post-ICU PTSD [18]. While the thoughtful use and reduction of medications of various kinds in the ICU should be heralded as progress, and while a clear "sea change" has occurred in recent years (resulting in patients being more active and alert and probably less delirious as a result), the impact of this paradigm shift on PTSD is unclear. Regardless, the other benefits of sedation reduction are substantial despite the mental effects of such an approach being unclear. Data from several sources indicates that factual memories of ICU-related experiences – presumably more likely to occur within the context of sedation – may be protective against future psychiatric distress [19–20]. Lighter sedation may in fact be protective of neuropsychiatric disorders after discharge, and amnesia of the ICU stay has been associated with increased neurocognitive sequelae [21, 22]. Briefly, the notion here is that factual memories of medical or ICU-related events – even if quite upsetting – have the effect of grounding patients in "reality" which may be preferable to the presence of psychotic or delusional memories.

Depression

Depression and depressive symptoms also are prevalent in the context of critical illness and ICU hospitalization. It appears that the point prevalence of clinically significant depressive symptoms may be as high as 30% after discharge, much higher than the US population's 7% for major depressive disorder or 10% for any mood disorder (which includes major depressive disorder, dysthymia, and bipolar I and II) [23]. Depression includes cognitive-affective and somatic symptoms (believed to be particularly prominent in the context of critical illness), and it has been posited that cognitive-affective symptoms in particular (feelings of hopelessness, affective symptoms, etc.) may underlie the relationship between depression and chronic diseases through mechanisms which may include dysregulated cortisol and nonadherence to medical regimens [24]. Alternatively, in survivors of medical and surgical critical illness, somatic symptoms that largely involve such things as fatigue, problems sleeping, deficits in initiation, etc. appear to be primary [25]. In general, symptoms of depression may increase vulnerability to critical illness as individuals with significant symptoms of depression may be likely to succumb to unhelpful health-related behaviors such as smoking, inactivity, excessive alcohol use, poor dietary choices, and non-compliance with recommended treatment regimens [26]. It appears that patients with serious depression tend to die up to a decade earlier than their non-depressed counterparts, often from chronic health conditions such as cardiac disease, chronic obstructive pulmonary disease (COPD), and diabetes, among many others [27–28].

Exploring the Association Between Delirium and Depression

Nearly 30 studies have explored the complex relationship between depression and delirium, with most of them evaluating depression as a risk factor for delirium and a few of them focusing on whether delirium drives the development of depression [29–32]. In general, it appears that depression reliably heightens the likelihood of experiencing delirium, and this finding is generally consistent across a wide array of patient populations, including those with critical illness. While the strength of the relationship between depression and delirium varies, the increased risk of delirium in individuals with depression is often very high [29–30]. Less is known about whether delirium contributes to poorer psychiatric outcomes, perhaps because most researchers have focused on the cognitive sequelae of delirium to the exclusion of a focus on psychiatric outcomes (not surprising, as delirium is widely conceived of as a neurologic and not a psychiatric condition) [33]. Despite the widely varying methodology and rigor of the studies in question, a majority have identified an association between delirium and subsequent depression, reflected in outcomes such as higher scores on depression measures at distal timepoints [34].

Common Processes Underlying Delirium and Depression

As depression is the primary psychiatric condition to be associated with delirium, we will briefly unpack issues related to physiology that may potentially undergird both of these conditions, recognizing that few if any investigations have explored these relationships as such. While questions exist regarding the mechanisms that contribute to the development of delirium, one of the most prominent theories involves imbalances in dopaminergic and cholinergic pathways as well as disruptions pertaining to inflammation [34]. Importantly, these are the same mechanisms widely implicated in the emergence and maintenance of depression, along, perhaps, with altered cytokine expression, itself, a major risk factor for depression. Also fundamental to both delirium and depression are various pathologies related to sleep, reflecting potential issues in circadian regulation [35].

Treatment of Delirium and Depression

If it is the case that delirium and depression potentially are influenced by common mechanisms, this insight may have practical pharmacologic implications. One key implication, certainly, involves exploration of whether the mood-related difficulties potentially present in delirium are simply reflective of this neurologic syndrome or whether, alternatively, they are reflective of an actual disorder of mood [36]. If depression is indeed present, then treatment should likely avoid agents with prominent anticholinergic properties as there is some evidence that these may be deliriogenic [37–38]. Yet another clinical insight pertains, as we've discussed, to the centrality of circadian rhythm disruption in those with both delirium and depression. It may be that sleep-related interventions, among them melatonin, might be effective in the management of both these conditions, although evidence for the effectiveness of melatonin in delirium is extremely preliminary [39, 40]. Finally, if it is the case that depression is a major risk factor for the development of delirium, the integration of mental health strategies in the ICU in an effort to prevent the development of delirium may be crucial as a reduction in incident depression may translate into a reduction in incident delirium.

A Research Agenda Related to Delirium and Mental Health

Individuals who have been hospitalized in the ICU and experience delirium tend to experience longer hospital duration and higher mortality rates than those who did not experience delirium. There are many risk factors for development of delirium including genetic (e.g., APOE-4 allele), pathophysiological (e.g., infection), medical (e.g., sedating medications), environmental (e.g., chaotic ICU environment, dysregulation of sleep/wake cycle), or mental health (e.g., depression). A prior history of depressive symptoms and depressive disorders is common among individuals who experience delirium, and depression also is a common consequence of delirium. The exact mechanisms by which delirium and mental health are correlated in a bi-directional manner following critical illness remain largely unknown. There can be noted disruptions to cognition during both delirium and depressive episodes. Throughout the extant literature, there is indication of a similar pathophysiological pathway for development of both depression and delirium, a pathway involving stress and inflammatory responses as well as monoaminergic and melatonergic functions. Exposure to various medications also has been associated with onset and duration of delirium (e.g., benzodiazepine and opioid medications) as well as environmental culprits such as physical restraint or immobilization.

Among all the various psychological, behavioral, and environmental interventions thought to prevent delirium, early mobilization (e.g., ambulation, exercise, and range of motion implemented within the first days of ICU hospitalization) may be key. Mobilization, or physical activity, also has been associated with prevention of a depressive episode as well as enhanced management of depressive symptoms, regardless of any other intervention employed (e.g., psychotherapy or antidepressant medication). All of this evidence for a common etiology and common pathophysiological pathway highlights the promising possibility for common modes of prevention and intervention. At this point, however, the field of critical care psychology lacks animal models and basic science research that can further enhance our understanding of the pathophysiological mechanisms, as well as the intersection between delirium and mental health outcomes. As a field, we also are lacking studies designed to enhance our understanding of the various phenotypes of delirium that may present and how those phenotypes may be associated with a mental health history or mental health outcomes. We also are desperately in need of better tools of assessment – both for delirium and depressive symptoms/depressive disorders – for enhanced sensitivity and specificity of diagnosis to guide treatment efforts.

Conclusions

Delirium continues to be pervasive in critically ill populations and in medical and geriatric populations more generally. While commonly linked to cognitive problems, this neurologic syndrome is also associated with mental health difficulties and, more specifically, with depression. Evidence of an association between delirium and PTSD is so far inconsistent. Indeed, the presence of delirium increases vulnerability to the development of mental health-related difficulties. Interventions to decrease delirium in a variety of populations may in turn prevent the emergence of incident depression or even PTSD, but this remains a question in need of future study. Although little attention continues to be paid to the dynamic interplay between delirium and psychiatric conditions, clinicians and patients should be aware of the relevance of delirium not only to outcomes such as mortality, hospital length of stay, and cognition but also to conditions such as depression.

Take-Home Messages

- The nature of the association between delirium and mental health difficulties has been relatively little studied and remains somewhat unclear.
- While research on the link between delirium and PTSD has been somewhat contradictory, evidence consistently supports a relationship between delirium and depression, and this relationship exists in both directions.
- Interventions that reduce delirium may also decrease the incidence of prevalence of ICU-associated psychiatric syndromes, although this requires further study.
- Dedicated research programs – marked by increasingly sophisticated multidisciplinary approaches – should continue to elucidate the fundamental underpinnings of the relationships between delirium, anxiety, depression, and PTSD.

References

1. Pandharipande P, Shintani A, Peterson J, et al. Lorazepam is an independent risk factor for transitioning to delirium in intensive care unit patients. Anesthesiology. 2006;104:21–6.
2. Witlox J, Eurelings LS, De Jonghe JF, et al. Delirium in elderly patients and the risk of postdischarge mortality, institutionalization, and dementia: a meta-analysis. JAMA. 2010;304:443–51.
3. Pandharipande P, Girad TD, Jackson JC, et al. Long-term cognitive impairment after critical illness. New England Journal of Medicine. 2013;369:1306–16.

4. Girard TD, Jackson JC, Pandharipande PP, et al. Delirium as a predictor of long-term cognitive impairment in survivors of critical illness. Crit Care Med. 2010;38:1513–20.
5. Minden SL, Carbone LA, Barsky A, et al. Predictors and outcomes of delirium. Gen Hosp Psychiatry. 2005;27:209–14.
6. Davydow DS, Desai SV, Needham DM, et al. Psychiatric morbidity in survivors of the acute respiratory distress syndrome: a systematic review. Psychosom Med. 2008;70:512–9.
7. Nikayin S, Rabiee A, Hashem MD, et al. Anxiety symptoms in survivors of critical illness: a systematic review and meta-analysis. Gen Hosp Psychiatry. 2016;43:23–9.
8. Marra A, Pandharipande P, Patel M. Intensive care unit delirium and intensive care unit-related posttraumatic stress disorder. Surg Clin North Am. 2017;97:1215–35.
9. Jackson JC, Hart RP, Gordon SM, Hopkins RO, et al. Post-traumatic stress disorder and post-traumatic stress symptoms following critical illness in medical intensive care unit patients: assessing the magnitude of the problem. Crit Care. 2007;11:R27.
10. Patel MB, Jackson JC, Morandi A, et al. Incidence and risk factors for intensive care unit-related post-traumatic stress disorder in veterans and civilians. Am J Respir Crit Care Med. 2016;93:1373–81.
11. Cuthbertson BH, Hull A, Strachan M, et al. Post-traumatic stress disorder after critical illness requiring general intensive care. Intensive Care Med. 2004;30:450–5.
12. Jones C, Griffiths RD, Humphries G, et al. Memory, delusions, and the development of acute posttraumatic stress disorder-related symptoms after intensive care. Crit Care Med. 2001;29:573–80.
13. American Psychiatric Association. Diagnostic and statistical manual of mental disorders. 5th ed. Washington, DC: American Psychiatric Association; 2013.
14. Moreau C, Zisook S. Rationale for a posttraumatic stress spectrum disorder. Pyschiatr Clin North Am. 2002;25:775–90.
15. Sackey PV, et al. Short- and long-term follow-up of intensive care unit patients after sedation with isoflurane and midazolam – a pilot study. Crit Care Med. 2008;36:801–6.
16. Weinert CR, Sprenkle M. Post-ICU consequences of patient wakefulness and sedative exposure during mechanical ventilation. Intensive Care Med. 2008;34:82–90.
17. Muacevic A, Adler JR, Nguyen S, et al. Emergence delirium with post-traumatic stress disorder among military veterans. Cureus. 2016;8:e921.
18. Bienvenu OJ, Gellar J, Althouse BM, et al. Post-traumatic stress disorder symptoms after acute lung injury: a 2-year prospective longitudinal study. Psychol Med. 2013;43:2657–71.
19. Kress JP, Pohlman AS, O'Connor MF, et al. Daily interruption of sedative infusions in critically ill patients undergoing mechanical ventilation. N Engl J Med. 2000;342:1471–7.
20. Girard TD, Kress JP, Fuchs BD, et al. Efficacy and safety of a paired sedation and ventilator weaning protocol for mechanically ventilated patients in intensive care (Awakening and Breathing Controlled trial): a randomised controlled trial. Lancet. 2008;371:126–34.
21. Larson MJ, Weaver LK, Hopkins RO. Cognitive sequelae in acute respiratory distress syndrome patients with and without recall of the intensive care unit. J Int Neuropsychol Soc. 2007;13(4):595–605. https://doi.org/10.1017/S1355617707070749.
22. Treggiari MM, Romand JA, Yanez ND, Deem SA, Goldberg J, Hudson L, et al. Randomized trial of light versus deep sedation on mental health after critical illness. Crit Care Med. 2009;37(9):2527–34. https://doi.org/10.1097/CCM.0b013e3181a5689f.
23. Davydow DS, Zatzick D, Hough CL, et al. A longitudinal investigation of posttraumatic stress and depressive symptoms over the course of the year following medical–surgical intensive care unit admission. Gen Hosp Psychiatry. 2013;35:226–32.
24. Cheng HT, Ho MC, Hung KY. Affective and cognitive rather than somatic symptoms of depression predict 3-year mortality in patients on chronic hemodialysis. Sci Rep. 2018;8:5868.
25. Jackson JC, Pandharipande PP, Girard TD, et al. Depression, post-traumatic stress disorder, and functional disability in survivors of critical illness in the BRAIN-ICU study: a longitudinal cohort study. Lancet Respir Med. 2014;2:369–79.

26. DiMatteo MR, Lepper HS, Croghan TW. Depression is a risk factor for noncompliance with medical treatment – meta-analysis of the effects of anxiety and depression on patient adherence. Arch Intern Med. 2000;160:2010–107.
27. Burg M. Depression prior to CABG predicts 6-month and 2-year morbidity and mortality. Psychosom Med. 2001;63:103.
28. Zhang X, Norris SL, Gregg EW, et al. Depressive symptoms and mortality among persons with and without diabetes. Am J Epidemiol. 2005;161:652–60.
29. Smith PJ, Attix DK, Craig Weldon B, et al. Executive function and depression as independent risk factors for postoperative delirium. Anesthesiology. 2009;110:781–7.
30. Wilson K, Broadhurst C, Diver M, et al. Plasma insulin growth factor-1 and incident delirium in older people. Int J Geriatr Psychiatry. 2005;20:154–9.
31. Slor CJ, Witlox J, Jansen RW, et al. Affective functioning after delirium in elderly hip fracture patients. Int Psychogeriatr. 2013;25:445–55.
32. Fann JR, Alfano CM, Roth-Roemer S, et al. Impact of delirium on cognition, distress, and health-related quality of life after haematopoietic stem-cell transplantation. J Clin Oncol. 2007;25:1223–31.
33. Pandharipande PP, Girard TD, Jackson JC. Long-term Cognitive Impairment after Critical Illness. N Engl J Med. 2013;369:1306–16.
34. O'Sullivan R, Inouye SK, Meagher D. Delirium and depression: inter-relationship and overlap in elderly people. Lancet Psychiatry. 2014;1:303–11.
35. Figueroa-Ramos MI, Arroyo-Novoa CM, Lee KA, et al. Sleep and delirium in ICU patients: a review of mechanisms and manifestations. Intensive Care Med. 2009;35:781–95.
36. Gagliardi JP. Virtual mentor. Clinical pearl: differentiating among depression, delirium and dementia in elderly patients. Am Med Assoc J Ethics. 2010;10:383–8.
37. Zimmerman KM, Salow M, Skarf LM, et al. Increasing anticholinergic burden and delirium in palliative care inpatients. Palliat Med. 2014;28:335–41.
38. Wolters AE, Zaal IJ, Veldhuijzen DS, et al. Anticholinergic medication use and transition to delirium in critically ill patients: a prospective cohort study. Crit Care Med. 2015;43:1846–52.
39. Balan S, Leibovitz A, Zila SO, et al. The relation between the clinical subtypes of delirium and the urinary level of 6-SMT. J Neuropsychiatr Clin Neurosci. 2003;15:363–6.
40. Sultan SS. Assessment of role of perioperative melatonin in prevention and treatment of postoperative delirium after hip arthroplasty under spinal anesthesia in the elderly. Saudi J Anaesth. 2010;4:169–73.

Chapter 5
Prediction Models for Delirium in Critically Ill Adults

Mark van den Boogaard and John W. Devlin

Background

Delirium in critically ill adults is associated with deleterious short-term and long-term effects. Patients are frequently bothered by its symptoms; its occurrence is associated with increased stress among families. While delirium occurs, on average, in 30% of adults admitted to the ICU [1], its prevalence ranges widely depending on the number and types of predisposing and precipitating risk factors for delirium, which differ substantially between patients. For example, a middle-aged patient transitioning quickly through the ICU after elective, major surgery will have a far lower risk for developing delirium during their ICU stay than a very old patient with baseline cognitive dysfunction who is emergently admitted to the ICU with septic shock, requires mechanical ventilation and sedation, and ends up having a prolonged ICU stay. The average ICU patient who develops delirium has 11 different risk factors for delirium prior to its occurrence [2]. Daily recognition and removal of modifiable delirium risk factors, and the use of proven non-pharmacologic and pharmacologic prevention strategies, represent the hallmark of delirium prevention approaches that should be used in all critically ill adults.

The complex interplay between predisposing and precipitating risk factors, and the variability by which these factors occur in critically ill adults, makes accurate delirium prediction a challenge for most ICU clinicians. While one might assume that all effective delirium prevention strategies [3] are routinely provided to every patient every day, this approach is usually not feasible in most ICUs. Moreover, among patients at a low predicted risk for developing delirium in the ICU, the costs

M. van den Boogaard (✉)
Department Intensive Care Medicine, Radboud University Medical Center, Radboud Institute for Health Sciences, IQ Healthcare, Nijmegen, The Netherlands
e-mail: Mark.vandenBoogaard@Radboudumc.nl

J. W. Devlin
School of Pharmacy Northeastern University, Boston, MA, USA

C. G. Hughes et al. (eds.), *Delirium*, https://doi.org/10.1007/978-3-030-25751-4_5

and/or risks associated with delirium prevention strategies may exceed their potential benefit. ICU clinicians therefore require guidance regarding which of their patients are at greatest risk for delirium so that they can tailor delirium reduction efforts to those patients who will benefit most from these interventions [4].

To determine a patient's delirium risk, or even better, calculate a delirium risk score, one needs an ICU delirium prediction model that has been developed and validated in a heterogeneous cohort of ICU patients at varying risks for developing delirium and preferably in different ICU settings [5, 6]. Ideally, information regarding a patient's risk for delirium should be discussed with both the patient and their family [7]. Importantly, the use of delirium risk scores derived from a prediction model has been shown to be far better at predicting ICU delirium risk compared to clinician judgment alone [8]. This chapter seeks to review current ICU delirium prediction models, describe the steps used to develop, validate, and calibrate them, and provide guidance to ICU clinicians on how they can adopt a delirium prediction model into their practice.

Risk Factors Versus Predictors

A delirium risk factor is any substance, characteristic, condition, or exposure associated with delirium; in many cases a causal relationship with delirium may not yet have been proven. A delirium predictor is a delirium risk factor shown to be able to predict delirium. Many delirium risk factors are not necessarily delirium predictors. In general, the strength of the measured association between a risk factor and the clinical outcome (or event) of interest and both the distribution (across the patient population) and frequency by which it occurs will influence whether a risk factor can be considered a predictor.

Over the past decade, many risk factors for delirium have been identified [9, 10]. Although ICU delirium risk factors are extensively described in Chap. 3 of this book, additional comments about these risk factors in the context of delirium prediction are important to highlight. As noted in Chap. 3, risk factors can be categorized as being either predisposing (i.e., risk factor exists prior to critical illness) or precipitating (i.e., risk factor is attributable to critical illness and thus occurrence is just before or during ICU admission). Increasing age and preexisting cognitive decline are important predisposing factors. Precipitating factors are either modifiable (e.g., the administration of a benzodiazepine) or non-modifiable (e.g., a worsening severity of illness over the course of the ICU stay). ICU clinicians should focus their delirium reduction efforts on those variables that are modifiable. Therefore, any modifiable risk factors included in an ICU delirium prediction model provide the clinician with guidance on where to intervene to reduce delirium (over and above predicting its occurrence).

Development and Validation of an ICU Delirium Prediction Model

How a delirium prediction model will be used in clinical practice is an important consideration during its development. For example, if a delirium risk score is desired for a set period of time (e.g., the duration of ICU admission), then a once-only (e.g., risk factors evaluated once around the time of ICU admission) static prediction model is usually ideal. However, if one is seeking to know the predicted risk of delirium over a time unit (e.g., ICU shift, day or week), then a so-called dynamic prediction model is preferred. While data for time-dependent, dynamic models are more time consuming to collect and the models are more complex to design and run, they are also more accurate. Consideration of time-varying predictors (e.g., a medication associated with delirium whose use could vary from day to day) will result in less residual confounding. Another advantage of time-dependent, dynamic models is that unlike a static model, it accounts for a potential deterioration in patient health after the baseline delirium prediction is calculated (another source of residual confounding).

Basic rules exist when developing and validating prediction models. The most important methodological considerations when ICU delirium prediction models are developed include risk factor identification, sample size calculation, and model validation. More detailed information on prediction model development methods are described in the book: *Clinical Prediction Models: A Practical Approach to Development, Validation, and Updating* [6]. During delirium prediction model development, it is important that all patients are free of delirium at the time data collection is initiated, that data collection is prospective (vs. retrospective), and that all patients meeting model criteria are consecutively enrolled. Retrospective data collection is fraught with misclassification bias (given the inability to proactively identify the true presence of a risk factor and the outcome), and a lack of consecutive enrollment is fraught with selection bias [e.g., only patients at perceived greater delirium risk are included (or vice versa)].

The primary aim of any prediction model or prediction rule is to estimate the chance that a certain outcome, in this case ICU delirium, will occur. Importantly, this calculated risk should be considered an estimation and not an absolute rate. The larger the population used to develop the model, the more "stable" the prediction model/rule will be. For each risk factor (i.e., potential predictor) included in the model regression analysis, among the patients with the risk factor, at least 10–15 patients with delirium (i.e., cases) and 10–15 patients without delirium (i.e., non-cases) are required [11]. So the optimal sample size of any prediction model is predicated by the number of risk factors where a rationale to include exists. Therefore, prediction models with a larger sample size are generally more robust; the smaller the 95% confidence interval around each regression coefficient, the greater the robustness. An "unstable" delirium prediction model, reflected by a wide

95% confidence interval around one or more regression coefficients, will be more affected by a small change in the number of patients who develop delirium. In this situation, the misclassification of delirium in even a handful of patients could have important limitations on the ability to correctly consider all desired risk factors as predictors in the model. Lastly, the way by which missing values (e.g., delirium not evaluated or the presence of risk factor not recorded) are imputed in the model can also affect the end model result.

During the development of a delirium prediction model with good performance, both variables with a well-established association to delirium (e.g., age) and newer variables purported by experts to be associated with delirium (e.g., vascular disease, diabetes), where association is not well-established, should be included. Importantly, risk factors should only be considered for models if they can be readily collected during routine patient care. For example, although the presence of the APOE-4 allele [12] has been associated with delirium occurrence, the routine measurement of a genetic marker like this is not feasible in most ICU clinical settings. Once the prediction model has been developed, the model will generate an estimated predicted risk score for delirium occurrence for any ICU patient between 0% and 100%; this risk % can be categorized into risk groups (e.g., low, moderate, and high).

After development, a delirium prediction model needs to be validated in another independent patient dataset to demonstrate it works for patients with a different mix of delirium predictors than those patients used in the original development dataset. Both internal and external validity need to be determined. Internal validation evaluates model reproducibility. Given that a prediction model often overestimates delirium occurrence in the development cohort, it is important to confirm that model estimation is accurate (i.e., the model is not over-fitted) in a new patient cohort. Available internal validation techniques include apparent validation, split-sample validation, cross validation, and bootstrap validation. After the internal validation, the models need to be externally validated; this supports the generalizability of the model. When the new dataset includes patients from the same ICUs used for model development, but admitted in a period soon after the initial model validation period, then this validation is called temporal validation. If the new dataset consists of patients from ICUs not involved in the original validation, then this validation is called external validation. External validation is preferred over temporal validation as it results in a prediction model with greater generalizability (i.e., clinical applicability). This last step of validation is of importance for the use of an ICU delirium prediction model in daily practice.

Epidemiological Definitions and Rules

When evaluating the performance of an ICU prediction model, it is important to evaluate both model discrimination and calibration.

Discrimination refers to the ability of the model to differentiate between patients who will develop delirium with those who will not. The ability to adequately differentiate between these two patient groups in relation to their predicted risk for developing delirium is often presented in an "area under the receiver operating characteristic" (AUROC), (Fig. 5.1a, b). With the reported AUROC in this figure being 0.84, one can conclude that the model is a good predictor for delirium occurrence during the ICU admission (i.e., 84% of the time, this model will correctly predict delirium will occur when it actually does occur).

Discrimination can be evaluated by calculating model sensitivity and specificity and thus estimating the likelihood ratio for delirium occurrence (also known as pretest probability). The post-test probability of delirium occurrence can be determined after calculating the positive and negative predictive values of the delirium prediction model. *Sensitivity* is expressed in proportions ranging from 0% to 100% and is the proportion of actual patients who develop delirium that were correctly predicted as developing delirium, while *specificity* reflects the proportion of patients who did not develop delirium and who were correctly predicted not to develop it (Fig. 5.2).

Interpretation: At a predicted delirium risk of 25.1%, model sensitivity is 76.3% and model specificity is 80.4% (1–0.196). This indicates that 76.3% of the time this

Fig. 5.1 (**a**) Example of an AUROC of a delirium prediction model. (**b**) AUROC with 95% confidence interval for an ICU delirium prediction model

a

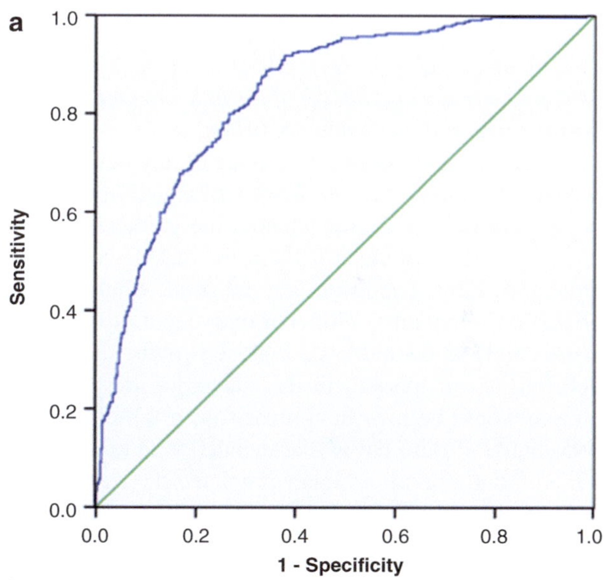

b

Test Result Variable(s):predicted_probability

Area	Std. Error[a]	Asymptotic Sig.[b]	Asymptotic 95% Confidence interval: Lower Bound	Asymptotic 95% Confidence interval: Upper Bound
.843	.013	.000	.817	.868

Fig. 5.2 Sensitivity and specificity for an ICU delirium prediction model

Positive if Greater Than or Equal To[a]	Sensitivity	1 - Specificity
,25073440	,764	,197
,25089471	,764	,197
,25096929	,763	,197
,25106898	,763	,196
,25122578	,763	,196
,25145288	,762	,196
,25180301	,762	,195
,25199835	,762	,195
,25203817	,762	,194
,25218872	,762	,194
,25291821	,762	,193
,25377146	,761	,193

prediction model will correctly predict delirium will occur for patients who do develop delirium and 80.3% of the time correctly predict delirium will not occur for patients who do not develop delirium.

When the statistical performance of any delirium prediction model is evaluated, model sensitivity and specificity will usually be provided (Fig. 5.2) given that this helps a clinician to decide whether the predicted delirium risk score the model provides is robust enough for them to trust it when making care decisions for their patient(s). For a condition like delirium, where its occurrence can have profound effects on a patient, a clinician may decide to choose to a predicted delirium risk score cutoff value that has a high sensitivity so that a patient at risk for developing delirium is not missed. In this scenario, the predicted delirium risk score cutoff chosen would be low. In comparison, if a medication existed that very effectively prevented delirium but was associated with undesirable safety concerns, then a clinician might choose a higher predicted delirium risk score as a cutoff (that would have higher specificity and lower sensitivity) given concerns about administering the medication to patient that was not actually going to develop delirium. Choosing the best delirium prediction model cutoff value is based solely on a clinician's assessment of their patient and the perceived risk/benefit for any intervention(s) that might prevent delirium occurrence.

The sensitivity and specificity of a delirium prediction model can be used to calculate a *likelihood ratio.* A *positive likelihood ratio (LR^+= sensitivity/1-specificity)* refers to the chance a patient with a high-risk classification for developing delirium will develop delirium in relation to patients with a high risk classification for developing delirium that do not develop delirium. A *negative likelihood ratio (LR^- = 1-sensitivity/specificity)* refers to the opposite scenario. In Fig. 5.2, the calculated LR^+ = 3.89 (0.763/0.196) means that a high-risk delirium prediction result is 3.89 more likely in a patient who goes on to develop delirium than the one who does not. A LR^- = 0.05 (1–0.763/0.804) means that for a patient with a low prediction score for delirium, there is only a 5% chance the patient goes on to develop delirium than in the patient who does not.

The *positive predictive value* defines the proportion of patients who develop delirium and who had a high predicted delirium risk score from the prediction model. This value is calculated by taking the number of delirium patients over the total of both the delirium and non-delirium patients in the high predicted delirium risk group. The *negative predicted value* is the proportion of patients who never developed delirium and had a low predicted delirium risk score over the total of both non-delirium patients and delirium patients in the total group of patients with a low predicted delirium risk score.

For each of these pre-test and post-test probabilities, the matrix for calculating these values is shown in Fig. 5.3: *Estimation of accuracy.*

Calibration of the model refers to the accuracy of the model predictions in relation to the observed events. This can be tested using the Hosmer-Lemeshow (HL) test, or more frequently used, calibration is estimated using a calibration plot (Fig. 5.4, *Calibration plot*) where the calculated predicted risk scores (x-axis) are plotted against the observed events (y-axis) (i.e., the percentage of patients where delirium occurs).

Interpretation of this calibration plot: At 20% predicted delirium risk (x-axis), the actual or observed delirium percentage is 20%. At an 80% predicted delirium

	Delirium patient	*Non-delirium patient*	
High predicted delirium risk	True predicted high risk (TP) = 150	False predicted high risk (TP) = 20	Positive predictive value =TP/(TP+FP) =150/(150+20)=0.88
Low predicted delirium risk	False predicted low risk (FN) = 10	True predicted low risk (TN) = 15	Negative predictive value =TN/(FN+TN) =15/(10+15)=0.60
	Sensitivity =TP/(TP+FN) =150/(150+10)=0.94	Specificity =TN/(FP+TN) =15/(10+15)=0.60	

Fig. 5.3 Estimation of accuracy for an ICU delirium prediction model

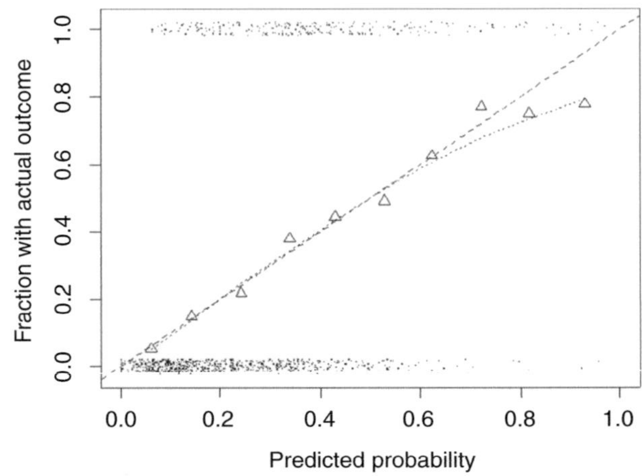

Fig. 5.4 Example of a calibration plot for an ICU delirium prediction model

risk, the observed delirium percentage is 75%. This suggests that prediction model is overestimating actual delirium occurrence for a predicted delirium risk ≥60%.

Existing ICU Delirium Prediction Models

Although the first delirium prediction model for elderly hospitalized patients was developed in the mid-1990s by Prof. Inouye [13], it took more than a decade before the first ICU delirium prediction model was developed [8]. Since then, a total of four ICU prediction models have been developed and published [8, 14–18]. The different prediction models, their development/validation, discriminating performance, and prediction rules are described as follows:

PRE-DELIRIC

The PREdiction DELIRium IC, PRE-DELIRIC model, was first developed in 2012 in a group of 1613 ICU patients, temporarily validated in cohort of 549 different ICU patients (from the same ICUs) and then subsequently validated in 894 ICU patients from multiple institutions [8]. The ICU patients in each cohort were a mixed population of surgical, medical, trauma, and neurology patients. The 25 different potential delirium predictors evaluated were derived from a systematic review [19] and collected within the first 24 h of ICU admission; the occurrence of delirium over the course of the ICU stay was the primary outcome variable. Patients with delirium at the time of ICU admission were excluded. A logistic regression analysis that used backward selection procedure was used to develop a prediction model that contained ten different delirium predictors: age, severity of illness (APACHE-II score), presence of coma, ICU admission category (e.g., medical, surgical),

Table 5.1 Prediction rules for the PRE-DELIRIC model

Risk of delirium = 1/(1+exp-(-4.0369))
+ 0.02 × age (year)
+ 0.03 × APACHE-II score (point)
+ 0 for non-coma/0.26 for drug induced coma/1.07 for miscellaneous coma/1.34 for combination coma
+ 0 for surgical patients/0.15 for medical patients/0.53 for trauma patients/0.65 for neurology or neurosurgical patients
+ 0.50 for infection
+ 0.14 for metabolic acidosis
+ 0 for no morphine use/0.19 for 0.01–7.1 mg per 24 h morphine use per 0.06 for 7.2–18.6 mg per 24 h morphine use/0.24 for >18.6 mg per 24 h morphine use
+ 0.66 for use of sedatives
+ 0.01 × urea concentration (mmol/L)
+ 0.19 for urgent admission

The scoring system's intercept is expressed as –4.0369; the other numbers represent the recalibrated regression coefficients (weight) of each predictor

presence of infection, presence of metabolic acidosis, use of morphine, use of a sedative, the serum urea level, and whether the ICU admission was urgent or elective. The model was well calibrated, and the discriminative power was 0.85 (95% CI 0.84–0.87) (see the prediction rule in Table 5.1). When considering a PRE-DELIRIC score of 35% or higher as a cutoff value for patient at high risk for developing delirium in the ICU, the sensitivity and specificity of the model were 67.1% and 86.5%, respectively. The positive likelihood ratio (LR^+) was 4.97, and the negative likelihood ratio (LR^-) was 0.41.

The ability of ICU nurses and physicians to predict ICU delirium occurrence was found to be significantly lower [0.59 (95% CI 0.49–0.70)] than that of the PRE-DELIRIC model. In a second, multinational study of 1824 ICU patients without delirium at the time of ICU admission, the calibration of PRE-DELIRIC was found to be poorer than in the original study, and therefore the PRE-DELIRIC model was recalibrated [14]. In a third, multinational study, the recalibrated PRE-DELIRIC model was used to predict delirium using either the CAM-ICU or the ICDSC; its predictive value for ICU delirium was comparable between CAM-ICU [0.75 (95% CI 0.72–0.78)] and ICDSC [0.71 (95% CI 0.67–0.75)] [15]. Furthermore, it was found that the PRE-DELIRIC model can also reliably predict subsyndromal delirium using the ICDSC [20].

Despite PRE-DELIRIC's static character (i.e., each predictor needs to be collected just once per ICU admission) and therefore increased risk for residual confounding, its predictive value is fairly good. Another potential drawback of the PRE-DELIRIC model (given that the APACHE-II score is calculated based on clinical values in the first 24 h after ICU admission) is that it can only be used to predict delirium occurrence 24 h after ICU admission. PRE-DELIRIC will therefore fail to predict those patients who will develop in the first 24 h of ICU admission – nearly 25% of the ICU patients who develop delirium after admission to the ICU [21, 22].

E-PRE-DELIRIC

In an effort to address the limitations of PRE-DELIRIC and be able to predict ICU delirium occurrence as quickly as possible after ICU admission, the Early PREdiction DELIRium ICu (E-PRE-DELIRIC) model was developed and validated. In a multinational study cohort of 2914 mixed ICU patients (derived from 13 ICUs in 7 countries), 16 potential delirium predictors, based on the PRE-DELIRIC model and a consensus of international delirium experts, were collected at the time of ICU admission; the occurrence of delirium over the course of the ICU stay (as assessed by the CAM-ICU) was again the primary clinical outcome. The dataset was split into a development set of 1962 patients and a validation set of 952 patients. The final model, developed using logistic regression analysis with a backward selection procedure, consisted of nine different predictors each evaluated at the time of ICU admission: age, history of cognitive impairment, history of alcohol abuse, ICU admission category, urgent admission, mean arterial blood pressure, use of corticosteroids, presence of respiratory failure, and serum urea concentration. Validation using the second dataset revealed the model to be well calibrated with a discriminative power of 0.75 (95% CI 0.71–0.79). The E-PRE-DELIRIC prediction rule is depicted in Table 5.2.

Using an E-PRE-DELIRIC score of ≥35% as a cutoff value for patients at high risk for developing delirium in the ICU, the model sensitivity was 50%, specificity 83%, LR^+ 2.9, and LR^- 0.6. In a subsequent multinational study where data was collected for both the PRE-DELIRIC and E-PRE-DELIRIC models, the statistical performance of the PRE-DELIRIC model [AUROC 0.74 (95% CI 0.71–0.76)] was significantly better than the E-PRE-DELIRIC model [0.68 (95% CI 0.66–0.71)] [15]. However, the clinicians in the study ICUs deemed the E-PRE-DELIRIC model to be more feasible for use in daily clinical practice. To accommodate these somewhat divergent results, a two-step approach is now recommended to predict delirium in the ICU. The E-PRE-DELIRIC model should be used first. When it generates

Table 5.2 Prediction rule of the E-PRE-DELIRIC model

Risk of delirium = 1/(1+exp – (-3.907))
+ 0.025 × age (year)
+ 0.878 for history of cognitive impairment
+ 0.505 for history of alcohol abuse
+ 0 for surgical patients/0.370 for medical patients /1.219 for trauma patients/ 0.504 for neurology or neurosurgical patients
+ 0.612 for urgent admission
–0.006 mean arterial blood pressure at the time of ICU admission (mmHg)
+ 0.283 for use of corticosteroids
+ 0.982 for respiratory failure
+ 0.018 × urea concentration (mmol/L) at time of ICU admission

The scoring system's intercept is expressed as –3.907; the other numbers represent the regression coefficients (weight) of each predictor

Table 5.3 Prediction rule of the *prediction model for delirium after cardiac surgery*

Risk of delirium = 1/(1+exp – (-3.563))
+ 0.06 × age (years)
+ 0.166 MMSE (points)
+ 0.362 for Charlson's comorbidity index (points)
+ 0.016 × time of bypass (minute)

The scoring system's intercept is expressed as –3.3563; the other numbers represent the regression coefficients (weight) of each predictor

a predicted delirium risk ≤30%, the PRE-DELIRIC model should be used 24 h later to reconfirm the ICU delirium occurrence risk. In this study the E-PRE-DELIRIC model was also validated for use in ICUs where delirium is screened with either the CAM-ICU or the ICDSC [15] .

A Prediction Model for Delirium After Cardiac Surgery

This model was developed at one center using a homogeneous group of 215 cardiac surgery patients aged ≥50 years who required postsurgical ICU care [18]. Although data for many potential delirium risk factors was collected, the specific risk factors included in the prediction model and the rationale for inclusion are unclear. This model, derived using logistic regression with a backward selection procedure, includes four different predictors: age, the mini-mental state examination score at ICU admission, the Charlson's comorbidity index, and duration of cardiac bypass. The prediction rule for this model is provided in Table 5.3.

Although model validation appears to have been completed, the specific group of patients in which validation was performed is not reported. The AUROC of the validated model [0.79 (95% CI 0.73–0.85)] was significantly different from the development model. The optimal risk score cutoff value for patients at high risk for delirium occurrence was 28.9%, resulting in a sensitivity of 71.2%, specificity of 76.3%, a $LR^+ = 3.00$, and a $LR^- = 0.38$. Information surrounding model calibration is not reported. Given the limitations of this model, the exclusion of patients <50 years old, the inclusion of patients from only one center, a sample size that was too small, and the model's static nature, additional model validation studies across cardiac ICUs from multiple centers are required.

ABD-Daily Prediction Model

The Acute Brain Dysfunction-Daily Prediction Model (ABD-pm) evaluated how daily transitions in neurologic status (neither delirium nor coma, awake with delirium, and coma) influence ICU delirium occurrence over the course of the ICU admission [17]. In a group of 810 mixed ICU patients, each patient's daily outcome was categorized to one of five different states: neither delirium nor coma, awake with delirium, coma, ICU discharge, or death. This resulted in a patient having 15 different possible daily transitions. The potential predictors included in this model, based on clear, predefined criteria, were categorized as either ICU admission factors ($n = 5$, i.e., age, ICU type, current use of a medication to treat Alzheimer's disease, APACHE-II score, and use of mechanical ventilation) or daily ICU factors ($n = 10$, [i.e., neurologic status (i.e., presence of neither delirium or coma, presence of delirium, or presence of coma); use of mechanical ventilation; presence of sepsis; modified SOFA score; administration of benzodiazepines, opiates, propofol, antipsychotics, or a statin; and the ICU length of stay].

Using multinomial logistic regression analysis, 14 predictors and 2 interaction terms were included in the final model. With the exception of daily statin use, all of the potential delirium predictors were included in this final model. The daily transition from delirium to ICU death, and from coma to ICU discharge, was under-predicted (i.e., under-estimated) by the model, and the transitions from a normal neurologic status (i.e., neither delirium nor coma) to coma, from a normal neurologic status to ICU death, and from delirium to a normal neurologic status were over-predicted (i.e., over-estimated). For all other transitions, including transitions to delirium, models for each of these daily transitions were found to be well calibrated. In particular, the model yielded very high negative predicted values (NPVs) for "next day" delirium (NPV: 0.82), coma (NPV: 0.89), normal cognitive state (NPV: 0.88), ICU discharge (NPV: 0.91), and mortality (NPV: 0.98). The model demonstrated outstanding calibration when predicting the total number of patients expected to be in any given state across predicted risk and at this time may be useful for predicting the proportion of patients for each outcome state across entire ICU populations to guide quality, safety, and care delivery activities rather than an individual patient's risk. An AUROC was not provided for any of the daily transition models.

The sensitivity of the *transition to delirium (in the ICU) model* was 0.597, specificity 0.792, positive predictive value 0.548, negative predictive value 0.823, LR^+ 2.87, and LR^- 0.51. The likelihood of the transition from a normal to awake with delirium state the next day, using the ABD-pm, is 10%. Delirium prediction rules were not provided, and thus the value, or regression coefficients, for each predictor in each transition model remains unclear.

This ABD-daily prediction model represents the first dynamic model in the ICU delirium field; it should be less affected by residual confounding than the static delirium prediction models previously described in this chapter. The daily ABD-pm can be used regardless of whether patients are admitted to the ICU with delirium.

After validation in a multicenter or preferably multinational study is completed, the ABD prediction model holds great promise for use in routine clinical practice, yet until then it serves better as a surveillance tool for acute brain dysfunction outcomes across ICU populations.

Use of Delirium Prediction Models in Clinical and Research Settings

Clinical Practice

Since 2012, when the first ICU delirium prediction model, PRE-DELIRIC, was described [8], several studies have validated the newer delirium predictions models described in this chapter [14]. Additional studies have evaluated the utility and benefit of using these delirium prediction models in routine clinical practice [4, 16]. While the evidence surrounding ICU delirium risk reduction and prevention continues to increase, the recent SCCM 2018 PADIS guidelines highlight important gaps in our knowledge about how delirium should best be prevented in the ICU [3]. So in some respects, our ability to accurately predict delirium occurrence in the ICU has gotten ahead of our knowledge on how it can best be reduced and prevented.

The optimal cutoff value (for the prediction models reviewed in this chapter) to be able to differentiate patients who are at high risk (vs. moderate risk) for developing delirium during their ICU stay remains unclear. When a delirium prediction tool is being used in daily ICU practice, the prudent clinician should use a cutoff value (for predicted ICU delirium occurrence) of ≥30% to classify a patient at high risk for delirium, given that about 30% of their patients, on average, will develop delirium during their ICU stay. This moderate- vs. high-risk categorization likely influences the degree to which the ICU team implements delirium prevention strategies (both pharmacologic and non-pharmacologic) known to be effective.

Among available ICU delirium prediction models, the E-PRE-DELIRIC and PRE-DELIRIC models have been most extensively studied and validated and are also the models that are ready for use across different ICU settings. As noted above, the E-PRE-DELIRIC model should be used first, and the PRE-DELIRIC model should be considered as confirmation (after 24 h in the ICU) if the E-PRE-DELIRIC model generates a predicted delirium risk ≤30% [15]. Although the ABD-pm model [17] is promising, it is too early to recommend its routine use until it is validated in more ICU settings.

To ease ICU clinician workload and enable ICU delirium prediction models to be implemented in daily practice, the delirium prediction model(s) should be built into existing clinical information systems. This will help automate routine delirium risk prediction efforts, facilitate the real-time implementation of delirium prevention efforts, and allow clinicians to more quickly and accurately inform and educate patients and their families about the risk for delirium in the future.

Research Setting

Building on the recent availability of ICU delirium prediction models, it is critical that cutoff values for delirium risk are established for each model. Delirium risk should be prospectively evaluated during all ICU delirium prevention studies. This data may also help guide decisions about the effectiveness of studied delirium prevention interventions given that the removal of patients with a low calculated risk for delirium from post hoc efficacy analyses will help control for the dilution effects of inclusion of these patients in any investigation. A few studies have been performed [4, 23] or are underway [24] that incorporate ICU delirium prediction model results from these important secondary analyses.

Future Directions

Since the identification of safe and effective treatments for critically ill adults is a never-ending process, and practice changes will continue to be made on an ongoing basis, it is important that ICU delirium prediction models are continuously updated to reflect these changing practice paradigms. For example, mechanically ventilated adults are increasingly maintained at a light level of sedation, benzodiazepines are rarely used, and newer opioids like fentanyl are used (rather than older opioids like morphine) [3]. Therefore, ICU delirium prediction models need to be updated and/or recalibrated regularly.

While most ICUs have a mixed population of patients for which both (E-)PRE-DELIRIC models and the ABD-pm model can be used, there are also specialty ICUs that care for distinct patient populations (e.g., after burn injuries, neurological injuries, or patients having severe decompensated heart failure). Risk factors for delirium in these specialty ICU populations differ from those in medical, surgical, and cardiac surgical ICUs, and thus delirium prediction models need to be developed and validated for this specialty ICUs. This will increase the accuracy of delirium prediction scores in all critically ill subpopulations and facilitate their use in these specialty ICUs.

Conclusions

Four ICU delirium prediction models are available; only the static E-PRE-DELIRIC or the PRE-DELIRIC models should be used in clinical practice at this time for determining an individual patient's risk of delirium. A two-step prediction approach should be used when the E-PRE-DELIRIC generates a delirium prediction score <30%. A currently available prediction model for cardiac surgery patients and the dynamic ABD-pm model, while promising, still need to be validated in multiple different ICU patient cohorts before they should be implemented into routine practice. Delirium prediction can help guide clinicians about which patients should receive the full gamut of delirium prediction strategies early in their ICU stay and help inform their discussions with patients and their families about delirium risk. Delirium prediction models should be incorporated in all ICU delirium prevention studies given their importance in helping to inform secondary analyses focused on efficacy and cost.

References

1. Rood P, Huisman-de Waal G, Vermeulen H, Schoonhoven L, Pickkers P, van den Boogaard M. Effect of organisational factors on the variation in incidence of delirium in intensive care unit patients: a systematic review and meta-regression analysis. Aust Crit Care. 2018;31:180.
2. Ely EW, Gautam S, Margolin R, Francis J, May L, Speroff T, et al. The impact of delirium in the intensive care unit on hospital length of stay. Intensive Care Med. 2001;27(12):1892–900.
3. Devlin JW, Skrobik Y, Gélinas DMN, Slooter AJ, Pandharipande PP, et al. Clinical practice guidelines for the prevention and management of pain, agitation/sedation, delirium, immobility, and sleep disruption in adult patients in the intensive care unit. Crit Care Med. 2018;46:e825–e73.
4. van den Boogaard M, Schoonhoven L, van Achterberg T, van der Hoeven JG, Pickkers P. Haloperidol prophylaxis in critically ill patients with a high risk for delirium. Crit Care. 2013;17(1):R9.
5. Mistraletti G, Pelosi P, Mantovani ES, Berardino M, Gregoretti C. Delirium: clinical approach and prevention. Best Pract Res Clin Anaesthesiol. 2012;26(3):311–26.
6. Steyerberg EW. In: Gail M, Krickeberg K, Samet J, Tsiatis A, Wong W, editors. Clinical prediction models; a practical appraoch to development, validation, ad updating. Rotterdam: Springer Science+Business Media, LCC; 2009.
7. Altman DG, Royston P. What do we mean by validating a prognostic model? Stat Med. 2000;19(4):453–73.
8. van den Boogaard M, Pickkers P, Slooter AJ, Kuiper MA, Spronk PE, van der Voort PH, et al. Development and validation of PRE-DELIRIC (PREdiction of DELIRium in ICu patients) delirium prediction model for intensive care patients: observational multicentre study. BMJ. 2012;344:e420.
9. Van Rompaey B, Elseviers MM, Schuurmans MJ, Shortridge-Baggett LM, Truijen S, Bossaert L. Risk factors for delirium in intensive care patients: a prospective cohort study. Crit Care. 2009;13(3):R77.
10. Zaal IJ, Devlin JW, Peelen LM, Slooter AJ. A systematic review of risk factors for delirium in the ICU. Crit Care Med. 2015;43(1):40–7.
11. Harrell FE Jr, Lee KL, Mark DB. Multivariable prognostic models: issues in developing models, evaluating assumptions and adequacy, and measuring and reducing errors. Stat Med. 1996;15(4):361–87.
12. Ely EW, Girard TD, Shintani AK, Jackson JC, Gordon SM, Thomason JW, et al. Apolipoprotein E4 polymorphism as a genetic predisposition to delirium in critically ill patients. Crit Care Med. 2007;35(1):112–7.
13. Inouye SK, Charpentier PA. Precipitating factors for delirium in hospitalized elderly persons. Predictive model and interrelationship with baseline vulnerability. JAMA. 1996;275(11):852–7.
14. van den Boogaard M, Schoonhoven L, Maseda E, Plowright C, Jones C, Luetz A, et al. Recalibration of the delirium prediction model for ICU patients (PRE-DELIRIC): a multinational observational study. Intensive Care Med. 2014;40(3):361–9.
15. Wassenaar A, Schoonhoven L, Devlin JW, van Haren FMP, Slooter AJC, Jorens PG, et al. External validation of two models to predict delirium in critically ill adults using either the confusion assessment method-ICU or the intensive care delirium screening checklist for delirium assessment. Crit Care Med. 2019. https://doi.org/10.1097/CCM.0000000000003911.
16. Wassenaar A, van den Boogaard M, van Achterberg T, Slooter AJ, Kuiper MA, Hoogendoorn ME, et al. Multinational development and validation of an early prediction model for delirium in ICU patients. Intensive Care Med. 2015;41(6):1048–56.
17. Marra A, Pandharipande PP, Shotwell MS, Chandrasekhar R, Girard TD, Shintani AK, et al. Acute brain dysfunction: development and validation of a daily prediction model. Chest. 2018.

18. Guenther U, Theuerkauf N, Frommann I, Brimmers K, Malik R, Stori S, et al. Predisposing and precipitating factors of delirium after cardiac surgery: a prospective observational cohort study. Ann Surg. 2013;257(6):1160–7.
19. Van Rompaey B, Schuurmans MJ, Shortridge-Baggett LM, Truijen S, Bossaert L. Risk factors for intensive care delirium: a systematic review. Intensive Crit Care Nurs: Off J British Assoc Crit Care Nurs. 2008;24(2):98–107.
20. Azuma K, Mishima S, Shimoyama K, Ishii Y, Ueda Y, Sakurai M, et al. Validation of the prediction of delirium for intensive care model to predict subsyndromal delirium. Acute Med Surg. 2019;6(1):54–9.
21. Spronk PE, Riekerk B, Hofhuis J, Rommes JH. Occurrence of delirium is severely underestimated in the ICU during daily care. Intensive Care Med. 2009;35(7):1276–80.
22. van den Boogaard M, Schoonhoven L, van der Hoeven JG, van Achterberg T, Pickkers P. Incidence and short-term consequences of delirium in critically ill patients: a prospective observational cohort study. Int J Nurs Stud. 2012;49(7):775–83.
23. van den Boogaard M, Slooter AJC, Bruggemann RJM, Schoonhoven L, Beishuizen A, Vermeijden JW, et al. Effect of haloperidol on survival among critically ill adults with a high risk of delirium: the REDUCE randomized clinical trial. JAMA. 2018;319(7):680–90.
24. Wassenaar A, Rood P, Schoonhoven L, Teerenstra S, Zegers M, Pickkers P, et al. The impact of nUrsiNg DEliRium Preventive INnterventions in the Intensive Care Unit (UNDERPIN-ICU): a study protocol for a multi-centre, stepped wedge randomized controlled trial. Int J Nurs Stud. 2017;68:1–8.

Chapter 6
Pediatric Delirium Assessment, Prevention, and Management

Heidi A. B. Smith and Stacey R. Williams

Overview: Pediatric Delirium

Pediatric patients are at risk for delirium, a form of acute brain dysfunction, along with more readily recognized multi-organ failure during critical illness. Delirium is characterized by a primary disturbance in attention (reduced ability to focus, sustain, or shift attention) and awareness (reduced awareness of environment), with secondary perturbations in cognition, which develop acutely (hours to days) and may have a fluctuating course of severity, as described in the *Diagnostic and Statistical Manual of Mental Disorders* (DSM) [1]. Delirium is a direct consequence of a medical and/or surgical condition, and therefore the associated acute disturbances are not part of an established neurocognitive disorder. Delirium has yet to be fully recognized as a distinct entity, historically, considered an unavoidable consequence of critical illness. Many clinicians continue to refer to delirium by nonspecific terms such as ICU psychosis, encephalopathy of critical illness, or ICU syndrome [2–4]. Particularly in children, the advancement of delirium epidemiology research was hindered by the vast differences in cognition, language, and neurobehavioral development in the pediatric population [5–8]. However, over the past decade, the creation and validation of bedside delirium screening tools for pediatric patients have greatly expanded the breadth of knowledge regarding pediatric delirium and associated risk factors and outcomes. Due to these significant advances, there is a growing movement to incorporate routine delirium monitoring to decrease delirium prevalence in the ICU and impact patient care outcomes.

H. A. B. Smith (✉)
Department of Anesthesiology and Pediatrics, Vanderbilt University Medical Center, Nashville, TN, USA
e-mail: heidi.smith@vumc.org

S. R. Williams
Department of Pediatrics, Nurse Practitioner, Division of Pediatric Critical Care, Vanderbilt University Medical Center, Nashville, TN, USA

C. G. Hughes et al. (eds.), *Delirium*, https://doi.org/10.1007/978-3-030-25751-4_6

The implementation of delirium monitoring protocols using valid bedside screening tools and the conduct of numerous large prospective studies in the adult ICU setting have led to a much deeper understanding of delirium epidemiology. Both the high prevalence of delirium and the association with poorer outcomes (e.g., prolonged mechanical ventilation and hospital stay, increased medical cost, long-term cognitive impairment, and greater mortality) in adults [2, 9–17] inspired further need to delineate the impact of delirium on critically ill infants and children. The study of pediatric delirium continues to evolve with an increasingly high number of publications pertaining to the validation and implementation of pediatric-specific delirium screening tools and delirium prevention and management, with the purpose of advancing understanding of this acute organ dysfunction. Yet, there continues to be reluctance among pediatric caregivers to fully embrace the validity and benefit of routine delirium monitoring due, in large part, to inexperience and dearth of knowledge concerning delirium pathophysiology, clinical symptomatology, and treatment options [18, 19]. This chapter is dedicated to advance clinician understanding and confidence in the assessment, prevention, and management of acute brain dysfunction in children.

Etiology of Delirium and Clinical Presentation

Normal brain activity relies on a delicate balance of both excitatory and inhibitory neurotransmission [20]. When critical illness leads to a disruption in this balance (e.g., hypoperfusion, hypoxia, electrolyte disturbance), acute brain dysfunction such as delirium may develop [21]. The causal pathways of neural dysfunction during critical illness and ischemia may lead to (1) an imbalance in neural membrane ionic gradients [22]; (2) altered neurotransmitter synthesis, release, and metabolism [23–25]; and (3) inadequate elimination of neurotoxic by-products [23–25]. Inflammation may also trigger a cascade of activity leading to endothelial dysfunction and microvascular compromise [26]. All patients with delirium exhibit the core DSM criteria (acute change in mental status, inattention, and altered level of consciousness or cognition) due to general acute neuronal dysfunction [1]. Additionally, however, the degree and type of neuronal dysfunction can differ between patients with delirium such that the imbalance in neurotransmission may be either largely excitatory or inhibitory. Dopamine is the chief stimulatory neurotransmitter, whereas acetylcholine and gamma amino butyric acid are key inhibitory neurotransmitters [20]. The disruption of dopaminergic, cholinergic, serotonergic, or glutamatergic receptor activity modulates behavior that can vary patient-to-patient and day-to-day [27–30]. These behavioral manifestations provide for categorization of delirium as hyperactive (often excess dopaminergic activity), hypoactive (often excess cholinergic or glutamatergic activity), or a mixed subtype where a patient may express both hyperactive and hypoactive manifestations [30–34]. Hyperactive or “agitated” delirium is associated with more extreme manifestations including lability in mood, restlessness, agitation, and combativeness that creates a sense of urgency to address. However, hypoactive or "quiet" delirium consists of patients who may be inappropriately sedate or withdrawn and often described by parents as "just not acting like my child." Hypoactive delirium is the most common form (>60%) of ICU delirium in children, whereas hyperactive delirium is the least common (<10%); these parallel motoric subtypes of delirium observed in adults [5, 32]. Patients with hypoactive delirium can often go unrecognized as having brain dysfunction by the medical team. They are commonly paired with other patients, as they require less nursing oversight and are referred to as being "good patients," yet the erroneous patient assessment can be associated with poorer outcomes [35–38]. The clinical diagnosis of delirium can be challenging without the use of a valid tool. Despite core DSM symptoms being present in all patients, the fluctuating course of severity and behavioral manifestations highlights the benefit of routine monitoring [8, 18, 21, 39–41].

Tool Development

The child psychiatrist is considered the reference standard (expert) for delirium diagnosis using DSM criteria. However, the reliance on psychiatry consultation services for routine delirium monitoring is not feasible in the ICU setting due to lack of psychiatry faculty availability and the need for frequent and timely evaluations to optimize diagnosis and management [8, 41–45]. The advancement of pediatric delirium epidemiology research and ICU patient care hinged on the development of efficient and accurate screening tools for use at the bedside.

Evolving cognitive and language skills among infants and younger children initially challenged the medical community to apply delirium criteria, largely pertaining to adult patients, to pediatric patients who expectantly have evolving or atypical neurocognitive skills (infants, toddlers, and those with developmental delay) [20]. The publication of numerous case series involving pediatric delirium has facilitated the development of a symptom profile that consists of both unique aspects of delirium commonly observed in pediatric patients and more uniform signs demonstrated among most patients suffering from delirium regardless of age [34, 45–49]. Distinct neuropsychiatric symptoms such as purposeless actions, inconsolability, and signs of autonomic dysregulation occur more commonly among pediatric patients with delirium [6, 44, 45]. These variations in delirium phenomenology and the techniques to assess for the core DSM criteria for delirium in children highlight the necessity of a pediatric-centered approach to delirium screening [7, 18, 35, 50, 51]. The process of screening tool development in pediatrics required collaboration with child psychiatrists to assure clear translation of the deficit underlying each criterion for delirium and how that is expressed and evaluated in infants and younger children [52]. Indeed, the identification of more subtle symptoms or behaviors consistent with delirium in younger children may require the use of interactive play or consideration of the context of a child's development during delirium evaluation [52, 53]. Though acute brain dysfunction during critical illness may occur in any patient and emerging literature suggests that delirium may occur among premature infants, ongoing scrutiny of currently available diagnostic tools and further validation studies in complicated patient groups, such as infants of prematurity, are necessary to support ongoing research in the epidemiology of pediatric delirium [42, 53–56].

Pediatric Anesthesia Emergence Delirium (PAED) Scale

Emergence delirium (ED) is a dissociative state of consciousness during which patients may exhibit severe irritability and inconsolability or be uncooperative after receiving a general anesthetic [57]. Emergence delirium was first reported in the 1960s following the use of inhalational anesthetics, most commonly in children aged 1–5 years. The Pediatric Anesthesia Emergence Delirium (PAED) scale is an observational tool that identifies "agitated" behavior considered "emergence delirium" in children [58]. Severity scores are provided by the caregiver for five observational domains including (1) degree of eye contact, (2) presence of purposeful actions, (3) awareness of surroundings, (4) restlessness, and (5) inconsolability, using a Likert scale (1–4 points). A positive screen for ED is a final score of 10 or greater based on the original validation study by Sikich and colleagues, in a prospective cohort of 50 patients aged 18 months to 6 years. The consistency of PAED scores of 10 or greater to identify patients clinically perceived to have emergence delirium and treated with dimenhydrinate by the anesthesiologist were analyzed. The PAED performed with a reported sensitivity of 64% in identifying patients treated for emergence delirium based on ROC curve analysis and an interobserver reliability of 0.84 (95% CI 0.76–0.90) [58]. In a subsequent study, the PAED was calculated retrospectively and compared to prospective psychiatry evaluation of pediatric ICU patients using DSM criterion, with reported sensitivity and specificity ranging from 91–100% to 96–98%, respectively [59, 60]. The high sensitivity and specificity in this study were likely due to the patient cohort being largely comprised of patients undergoing consultation by the neuropsychiatric team for "agitated behavior," and therefore the majority of patients diagnosed with delirium by psychiatry had hyperactive delirium, to which the PAED score was compared. With the improved understanding of motoric subtypes of delirium in children, a more recent study screening for all delirium subtypes reported a much lower PAED sensitivity (50%) [61]. Therefore, the validity and generalizability of the PAED for the diagnosis of all delirium subtypes in the pediatric ICU (PICU) setting are uncertain.

The Cornell Assessment for Pediatric Delirium (CAPD)

The Cornell Assessment for Pediatric Delirium (CAPD) is an observational delirium screening tool that is an adaptation of the PAED incorporating three additional assessment domains that detect hypoactive symptoms [62] (Fig. 6.1). The CAPD is

Questions answered based on interactions with the patient over the course of a nursing shift.

1. Does the child make eye contact with the caregiver?
2. Are the child's actions purposeful?
3. Is the child aware of his/her surroundings?
4. Does it take the child a long time to respond to interactions?

→ **Scored 4 (Never), 3 (Rarely), 2 (Sometimes), 1 (Often), 0 (Always)**

5. Is the child restless?
6. Is the child inconsolable?
7. Is the child underactive: very little movement and interaction?
8. Are the child's responses sparse and/or delayed?

→ **Scored 0 (Never), 1 (Rarely), 2 (Sometimes), 3 (Often), 4 (Always)**

Delirium present when total score ≥ 9

Fig. 6.1 Cornell Assessment of Pediatric Delirium . (Adapted schematic of the Cornell assessment for pediatric delirium. Adaptation based from Silver et al. [25])

designed as a purely observational tool for the assessor (the bedside nurse) to score the degree to which they "observe" the presence or absence of delirium symptoms over the course of a nursing shift. The eight assessment domains include (1) eye contact, (2) purposeful actions, (3) awareness of surroundings, (4) communication of needs, (5) restlessness, (6) inconsolability, (7) underactivity while awake, and (8) prolonged response to interactions. These 8 domains are scored using a Likert scale 0–4 (never, rarely, sometimes, often, always), with a total score ≥9 being a positive screen for delirium. The CAPD was validated in a cohort of 111 patients from a mixed surgical/medical PICU, performed with a sensitivity of 94% (95% CI 83–98) and specificity of 79% (95% 73–84) compared to psychiatry assessment using DSM criteria [62]. Consistency of scoring between nurse assessors was high (kappa 0.94, 95% CI 0.68–0.78). In subgroup analysis, the CAPD had a sensitivity of 50% (95% CI 1.3–99%) and specificity of 98% (95% CI 94–100) in children aged greater than 13 years of age, whereas in patients <2 years of age, the CAPD performed with a sensitivity of 100% and a specificity of 68% (95% CI 46–90). The CAPD may detect subtle behaviors over time that may otherwise be missed and does not require active patient participation [63, 64]. Using the CAPD "mid-shift" or at more frequent intervals decreases the length of patient observation and therefore may lead to erroneous screening assessment [62]. The CAPD has been implemented in multiple PICU settings representing ease of use [62, 64, 65].

The Preschool and Pediatric Confusion Assessment Methods for the ICU

The Preschool and Pediatric Confusion Assessment Method for the ICU (ps/pCAM-ICU) is a largely interactive and "point-in-time" delirium assessment that is adapted from the highly valid adult Confusion Assessment Method for the ICU (CAM-ICU) [2, 42, 66] (Fig. 6.2). The adult and pediatric CAM-ICU series is

DELIRIUM = Features 1 AND 2 plus *either* Feature 3 or 4			
Feature 1 Acute Change / Fluctuating Course of Mental Status	Preschool CAM-ICU Pediatric CAM-ICU	(Question 1) Is there an acute change from baseline mental status? (Questions 2) Has the patient's mental status fluctuated during the past 24 hours?	**PRESENT** if **'YES'** to *either* **Question 1 or 2**
If Feature 1 is PRESENT, move onto Feature 2. If NOT present then STOP, DELIRIUM ABSENT			
Feature 2 Inattention	Preschool CAM-ICU	Attention exam showing 10 pictures/mirrors/toys (~ 10 seconds) and assessing for eye contact	**PRESENT** if **3 or more errors** (No eye contact or incorrect response)
	Pediatric CAM-ICU	Vigilance A test (ABADBADAAY) or Attention Screening Exam	
If Feature 2 is PRESENT, move onto Feature 3. If NOT present then STOP, DELIRIUM ABSENT			
Feature 3 Acute Altered Level of Consciousness	Preschool CAM-ICU Pediatric CAM -ICU	(Question) Is the patient currently alert and calm (RASS or SBS = 0)?	**PRESENT** if **'NO'** Not alert and calm
If Feature 3 is PRESENT then STOP, DELIRIUM is PRESENT (Features 1, 2, 3). If NOT present, move onto Feature 4			
Feature 4 Disorganized Thinking or Systems	Preschool CAM-ICU	Symptoms of sleep wake cycle (SWC) disturbance assessed	Present when SWC disturbance present
	Pediatric CAM-ICU	Child asked four simple Yes/No questions and given a 2-step command (5 possible points)	Present if 2 or more errors
If Feature 4 is PRESENT, DELIRIUM is PRESENT (Features 1, 2, 4). If NOT present, DELIRIUM ABSENT			

Fig. 6.2 Preschool and Pediatric Confusion Assessment Method for the ICU. Schematic of the Preschool and Pediatric Confusion Assessment Method for the ICU. (Adaptation based from Smith et al. [5, 52])

founded on DSM criteria for delirium and assesses for the following: feature 1, acute change or fluctuating course of mental status; feature 2, inattention; feature 3, acute altered level of consciousness; and feature 4, presence of disorganized thinking or dysregulated systems [2, 5, 66, 67]. The hierarchal structure of the ps/pCAM-ICU algorithm is efficient and focused on those symptoms, which are most consistent with delirium (i.e., inattention). Delirium is present when features 1 and 2 are present (key DSM criteria) and either feature 3 or 4. The ps/pCAM-ICU allows for a rapid assessment of delirium, taking less than 2 min to complete. Patient care can be personalized by using the ps/pCAM-ICU to monitor brain function at more frequent intervals (every 3 h) when dealing with the highest severity of illness (i.e., delirium screen used as an adjunct or an acute vital sign of decompensation) or decreasing frequency with resolving disease (every 6 h). The emphasis on neurocognition (i.e., patient reaction) as part of delirium screening using the ps/pCAM-ICU diminishes the subjective effect of the examiner's interpretations and thus improves accuracy [68].

The Pediatric Confusion Assessment Method for the Intensive Care Unit (pCAM-ICU) assesses for delirium in children at least 5 years of age, either on or off mechanical ventilation, and with developmental delay. The pCAM-ICU was validated in a prospective cohort of 68 patients admitted to the medical/surgical ICU and performed with a sensitivity of 83% (95% CI 66–93) and specificity of 99% (95% CI 95–100) compared to the reference standard psychiatry assessment using

DSM criteria [67]. The pCAM-ICU is also highly reliable (kappa 0.96, 95%CI 0.74–1.0) regardless of assessor (i.e., nurse or physician). The pCAM-ICU performed well in patients aged ≤12 years (sensitivity 100%, specificity 100%), aged >12 years (sensitivity 80%, specificity 99%), and those on mechanical ventilation (sensitivity 75%, specificity 92%). A second center validation of the pCAM-ICU also reported a sensitivity and specificity of 77% (95% CI 46–95) and 98% (95% CI 90–100) [68]. Additionally, a severity scale for the pCAM-ICU (sspCAM-ICU) is also available, where the severity of inattention and altered mental status is scored ranging from 0 (no delirium) to 19 (delirium with maximum severity). The sspCAM-ICU performed with a sensitivity and specificity of 85% (95% CI 54–98) and 98% (95% CI 90–100), respectively, compared to reference standard assessment a cohort of critically ill children over 5 years of age [68].

The preschool CAM-ICU (psCAM-ICU) diagnoses delirium in critically ill infants and children less than 5 years of age and is a further adaptation of the pCAM-ICU to address the language and cognitive variations expected among infants and younger children [5]. Specific revision included the development of a reliable 10-s assessment for inattention in preverbal infants using pictures, mirrors, or toys (Fig. 6.3) and the use of surrogates for disorganized thinking including (1) sleep-wake cycle disturbance, (2) inconsolability, and (3) unawareness of surroundings [7, 35, 50, 51]. The psCAM-ICU was validated in a cohort of 300 patients admitted to a medical/surgical PICU, aged less than 5 years, with or without developmental delay, and either on or off mechanical ventilation and performed with a sensitivity of 75% (95% CI 72–78) and specificity of 91% (95% CI 90–93) compared to reference standard psychiatry assessment [5]. Reliability was high (kappa 0.79, 95% CI 0.76–0.83). Subgroup analysis revealed that the psCAM-ICU performed well in patients aged <2 years (sensitivity 93%, specificity 78%) and those on mechanical ventilation (sensitivity 96%, specificity 81%).

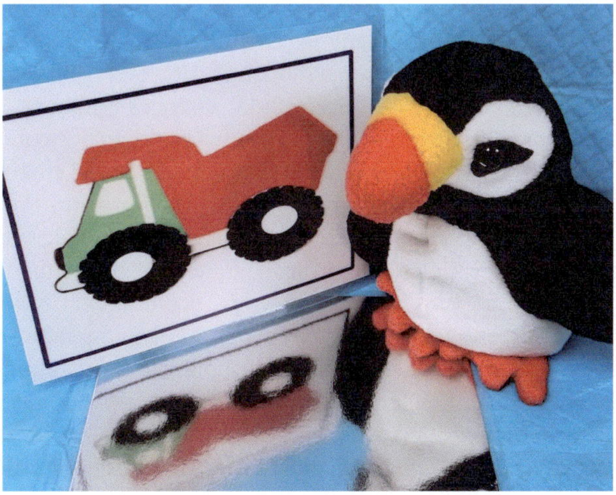

Fig. 6.3 Inattention assessment in infants and children using the psCAM-ICU. Example of picture, mirror, and toy that can be utilized while assessing for inattention in feature 2 of the psCAM-ICU for infants and children. The chosen item is moved back and forth slowly approximately 12 inches from the patient's eyes 10 times, while the assessor observes whether the patient makes eye contact with the item a minimum of 8 times

Pediatric Delirium Prevalence

The prevalence of ICU delirium among infants and children (13–66%) has been well characterized following the implementation of valid pediatric-specific delirium screening tools, supporting the assessment of all motoric subtypes, and conduct of multiple larger prospective pediatric studies [5, 45, 61, 62, 64, 65, 67–72]. A higher delirium prevalence of ~50–70% has been reported in critically ill children less than 5 years of age [5], those receiving mechanical ventilation [5, 71], postoperative cardiac patients [70, 73], and following general anesthesia and elective surgery in the immediate postoperative period [72]. The epidemiology of delirium is described in greater detail in Chap. 7 of this book.

Implementation

The implementation of routine delirium screening may lead to early recognition of acute brain dysfunction and other disease states such as sepsis or low cardiac output. The development of ICU delirium is significantly associated with increases in length of mechanical ventilation, ICU length of stay, hospital costs, and mortality in pediatric patients [42, 65, 69, 74–77]. Therefore, the benefit of early recognition is the opportunity to decrease delirium duration and positively impact the aforementioned short-term outcomes. Additionally, the presence of delirium can be a warning sign of impending decompensation when paired with mean arterial blood pressure, saturations, and/or other end points of oxygen delivery (e.g., lactate or mixed venous saturation). Likewise, the resolution of delirium can be an indicator of improvement following interventions personalized to patient care. Routine delirium monitoring empowers the bedside nurse and provides a sensitive indicator of changing clinical status and a means to discuss necessary reassessment and interventions with the medical team. The long-term implications of ICU delirium on the cognitive and psychological recovery of pediatric survivors of critical illness remain unclear. However, preliminary reports of post-traumatic stress symptoms [77], longer school absences [78], and decreases in spatial and verbal memory and attention in PICU survivors direct attention to the possible long-term impact of critical illness and delirium in infants and children [79].

Successful implementation strategies for delirium monitoring rely heavily on early education for the interdisciplinary team concerning the clinical presentations, etiologies, risk factors, and management of delirium [18]. Furthermore, the beneficial roles for psychiatry, neurology, occupational health, physical therapy, speech therapy, respiratory therapy, rehabilitation, and pharmacy should be appreciated and an opportunity to integrate their input on daily rounds supported by the medical team. Finally, the pertinent role of both the bedside nurse and patient family should be highlighted. The addition of any new patient care initiative may strain available resources including staff and faculty time. The bedside nurses are responsible for the medical care of the patient, accurate and timely documentation, ongoing patient monitoring, and the emotional support of the family [18]. The success of delirium monitoring implementation hinges on the conclusion of the medical team that delirium is important, it is prevalent, and though there may be times it is unavoidable in the setting of severe disease, we can avoid worsening brain dysfunction by averting iatrogenic harm and meeting the challenge of culture change in the PICU. Numerous well-designed prospective cohort studies have demonstrated the successful implementation of pediatric delirium monitoring using the abovementioned delirium tools [5, 45, 61, 62, 64, 65, 67–72]. Patient care becomes more robust as the medical team learns to distinguish anxiety from pain and pain and anxiety from inattention and accurate assessment of level of consciousness. These pieces are paramount to the consideration and management plan for patients both with and without delirium who require relief from painful procedures or ongoing mechanical ventilation. Hence, delirium monitoring, per se, even in the absence of high delirium prevalence, propels the medical team to a higher level of patient assessment and ongoing care.

Obstacles to implementation of delirium monitoring can be experienced upon the initial roll out, upon reassessment of a successful roll out, or months later. Any change in clinical care pathways will require rededication of effort and education at intervals based on the hospital team needs and resources. There are some general suggestions for dealing with common obstacles to practice change regarding delirium that may be useful [8, 41]. First, many clinicians continue to believe that patients can be assessed for delirium without using a valid tool [19, 80, 81]. However, clinicians miss three out of four patients with delirium when not using a valid delirium tool [82]. Delirium monitoring is enhanced when put into the hands of bedside nurses, as their key understanding of the daily schedule of medications, therapies, and care challenges promotes the appropriate timing for neurologic and delirium assessment. Implementation of routine delirium monitoring can complement daily nursing assessments. Integrating a 10-s attention assessment using psCAM-ICU pictures, mirrors, or even a familiar toy into a scheduled neurologic assessment avoids rendering delirium monitoring a daunting added task. Inattention screening is paramount for delirium screening, as inattention is the cardinal feature of delirium. When inattention is present, delirium presence is highly suggestive and empowers the bedside nurse to complete a delirium assessment and communicate the change to the medical team. Knowledge is power for the beside nurse and will ultimately lead to improved patient care. The huge benefit of delirium monitoring is further reinforced when nurses can observe other team members (i.e., nurse practitioner, attending physician) completing an assessment and the importance conveyed through actions and not simply patient care orders. Second, the key for long-term behavioral change in our patient care practices is the intentional modification of response when delirium is present. Nurses are immersed in numerous competing responsibilities that include fulfilling the new demands for delirium monitoring. If the medical team has no response to the presence of delirium, this may lead to future inaction regarding delirium assessment. When delirium is present, the medical team may not be able to reverse the syndrome acutely but will always be able to incorporate plans for reassessment, further evaluate possible causes (e.g., new-onset sepsis or failed mechanical ventilation wean), initiate preventative strategies, or prescribe rescue therapies for severe behavioral manifestations if present. The goal is to not ignore the condition of the patient nor the effort of the team. As part of the response to the presence of delirium, the decrease of, or transition to, new sedatives may be appropriate. Medical team members may be misinformed that a patient with delirium will be awakened and no longer to receive sedation despite being intubated or anxious. The goal here is to support team member concerns but be clear with the intent of decreasing iatrogenic harm while maintaining patient comfort and care which may include ventilator-patient synchrony. As the medical community continues to understand more regarding pediatric delirium, diminishing risks for development of, or increasing duration of, delirium should be considered, such as minimizing benzodiazepine exposure and deep sedation or instituting targeted sedation [8, 18, 41, 74]. It is important to recognize that while delirium can develop or worsen in the setting of sedation exposure, it does not require sedation in order to be present. Just as the expectation is that patients will suffer some degree of renal insufficiency in the setting of severe sepsis or shock, the focus becomes on minimizing iatrogenic harm, as an acute treatment to restore renal function is not available. The neurologic response to critical illness and the response of the medical team to a patient having delirium in many ways parallel this approach. Finally, the care team may be concerned that patients with delirium will be considered psychotic or be placed on antipsychotic therapy for a prolonged period. Education is highlighted here once again as delirium is by nature an acute syndrome of brain dysfunction. Therefore, though a patient may benefit from pharmacologic management of severe behavioral manifestations that sometimes may occur, there is no assumption of prolonged pharmacologic management of delirium [8, 18, 41, 74]. Rather, the focus should always remain on treating the source of delirium, not simply masking symptoms.

Management

One of the key concepts for delirium management lies in the understanding that acute brain dysfunction often occurs due to the same disease-related sequelae (e.g., hypoxia, hypoperfusion, electrolyte imbalances, sedation exposure, sleep-wake cycle disturbance) that lead to multi-organ dysfunction during critical illness. Figure 6.4 demonstrates an easy to use mnemonic – BRAIN MAPS – to remind clinicians of areas to focus on when dealing with a patient with, or at high risk for, delirium. Through the management of critical illness, while judiciously considering other disease or environmental factors that may worsen acute brain dysfunction, the disruption of normal neurologic function will be remedied over time. However, the recognition of delirium and prompt response to decompensation related to delirium has not historically been part of the normal ICU patient care algorithm. As such, practices that lead to worsening of delirium (iatrogenic harm) have ensued [74, 83, 84]. Delirium management can be challenging as the ICU team attempts to meet the often-competing necessary therapies for multi-organ dysfunction. Furthermore, the management process for delirium can be grueling and disappointing to the family and medical team

BRAIN MAPS:
Bring oxygen: hypoxemia, decreased cardiac output, anemia
Remove or Reduce deliriogenic drugs such as benzodiazepine or diphenhydramine
Atmosphere: consider lighting, noise level, schedules, restraints, family, staff
Infection, Immobilization, Inflammation
New organ dysfunction: acute onset of fever, respiratory distress
Metabolic disturbances: electrolyte imbalances, acidosis, alkalosis
Awake: sleep-wake cycle disturbance
Pain: assure assessment, titration or management, and possible withdrawal
Sedation: assure assessment, establish targets, consider titration, and possible withdrawal

Case Scenario: Critically ill child requiring mechanical ventilation (MV) and receiving continuous sedation.

Day 1: Patient admitted for respiratory failure, now intubated on MV, requiring 90% FiO2, PEEP 12.
Target RASS: (-) 3
Actual RASS: **(+) 1** to **(-) 1**, fluctuating mental status, patient struggling against the ventilator
pCAM-ICU: Delirium present
Problem: Patient is under-sedated in the setting of ARDS, ongoing hypoxia, and inadequate end-organ perfusion. Patient-ventilator asynchrony is exacerbating the disease state.
Plan Best approach would be to **increase** sedation. Fentanyl infusion is initiated for pain and to provide mild sedation. Anxiety is treated with intermittent low-dose bolus midazolam on an as needed basis.

Day 4: Patient has demonstrated slow and steady improvement with improving oxygenation indices. He remains on MV, requiring 40% FiO2, PEEP of 6, and the medical goal is to wean ventilation as tolerated. Patient receiving dexmedetomidine and high-dose fentanyl continuous analgesia and sedation.
NEW Target RASS: (-) 1
Actual RASS: **(-) 3**
pCAM-ICU: Delirium present
Problem: Patient is now over-sedated in the setting of a resolving disease state and plan to wean MV.
Plan: Titrate sedation and analgesia towards the target RASS. Wean ventilation as tolerated with aggressive goal of extubation. Consider early mobility, sleep wake cycle considerations, and family involvement.

Day 5: Patient is successfully extubated overnight. The dexmedetomdine and fentanyl infusions were discontinued and replaced with as needed dosing of hydromorphone. Patient has not rested well. Patient is without respiratory distress.
Target RASS: 0
Actual RASS: **(+) 1**
pCAM-ICU: Delirium present
Problem: Patient continues to have delirium despite resolution of HYPOXIA and removal of DRUGS which may cloud the sensorium and exacerbate brain dysfunction. The patient's sleep wake cycle is disturbed.
Plan Consider child life consultation and aggressive move towards initiating a new day/night routine. Consider sleep aide. Reassess pain and anxiety, and consider iatrogenic withdrawal syndrome and treat when appropriate. Consider other causes of delirium (BRAIN MAPS).

Fig. 6.4 Differential diagnosis of delirium. BRAIN MAPS is one of numerous acronyms to recall possible etiologies of delirium. (Adaptation based from Smith et al. [18])

particularly in patients who require continuous sedation while receiving mechanical ventilation. Hence the creation and implementation of consistent and regimented care may impact our patients in a positive manner. The most important aspect of delirium management is routine assessment and "group think" to determine the etiology, ongoing risk factors, and possible modes of prevention and management. Care plans cannot be accurately created or implemented without consistency in patient assessment for level of consciousness, delirium, and pain. One suggested process of rounding follows the "Pediatric Road Map" which is a series of questions that help guide consistent discussions regarding delirium and brain health. Using this paradigm, the ICU team addresses the patient's current condition, how they got to that point, where the team would like to focus care goals, and how they can expedite the patient's clinical status to obtain those goals [8, 18, 41] (*Case scenario in* Fig. 6.4).

The ABCDEF bundle combines protocolized patient care processes with informative daily rounding routines that promote sharing of ideas using an interdisciplinary team with patient/family involvement [85–87]. The ABCDEF bundle includes the following individual bundle elements of (1) assessment, prevention, and management of *pain*; (2) breathing assessment using spontaneous awakening and breathing trials; (3) choice of analgesia and sedation; (4) delirium assessment, prevention, and management; (5) early mobility and consideration of the ICU environment; and (6) family engagement and empowerment. Pun and colleagues were able to demonstrate that as the proportion of ABCDEF bundle elements that are implemented and performed regularly increases, the likelihood of delirium, coma, and death decreases, while the likelihood of ICU and hospital discharge increases [88]. The main goal of this initiative is to liberate the patient from mechanical ventilation and the ICU environment, thereby decreasing exposure to numerous factors that increase the risk for delirium and poorer outcomes. Even in pediatric patients, Simone and colleagues demonstrated that by implementing bundle elements including protocolized sedation and early mobility delirium rates decreased by ~40% in a prospective study of 1875 children [64].

Though studies have not ascertained the full benefit of preventative strategies for delirium in critically ill children, the low risk of many of these environmental modifications, such as supporting sleep hygiene (i.e., minimizing noise, lights off at night), deserves consideration for all patients admitted to the ICU [53, 89–91]. Family involvement in the pediatric ICU has provided abundant opportunities for collaboration between the medical and patient care teams. From creating a calm, familiar, and loving environment utilizing family pictures and cherished toys or blankets to emerging as part of the pain and anxiety comfort care plan, parents are key members of the interdisciplinary team [6, 92]. The connection between physical and cognitive health continues to develop, with numerous studies in adults demonstrating decrease in prevalence and duration of delirium in adult cohorts who are mobilized early, even those that are critically ill [93, 94]. Recent studies have demonstrated both the feasibility and preliminary impact of early mobilization on critically ill pediatric patients including decreasing delirium prevalence [64, 95]. Clearly the historical actions of expecting a sick child to be silent and motion free during their ICU stay directly clash with the now realized pathway for brain health.

Adjuncts to patient care that may ultimately prove to decrease delirium prevalence and improve neurobehavioral outcomes are those that support brain health and sleep hygiene. Critical illness or PICU environmental factors lead to inadequate REM and slow-wave sleep that are necessary for neuronal development in children [91]. Unfortunately, many clinicians assume opioids and sedatives improve sleep; however, these agents often decrease restorative sleep leading to sleep disturbances [91, 95]. Sleep-wake cycle disturbances may initiate or further exacerbate acute brain dysfunction or delirium. A cycle of dysfunction develops where delirium manifestations, such as agitation or restlessness, lead to increased sedation administration to provide "rest" that further aggravates brain function. Numerous nonpharmacologic approaches are available to promote sleep hygiene such as earplugs, eye masks, scheduled sleep/nap times, private rooms, and appropriate light levels depending on the time of day [96]. Pharmacologic strategies to enhance sleep may be beneficial. Melatonin is a hormone that promotes sleep via action on the suprachiasmatic nucleus in the hypothalamus, supporting the day-night cycle [97, 98].

Sedation with dexmedetomidine may also support sleep hygiene at mild to moderate sedative levels as it is associated with EEG patterns that closely mirror natural sleep [99].

In the PICU, continuous sedation is utilized in ~90% of infants and children while receiving mechanical ventilation [100, 101]. ICU sedation can benefit care of the critically ill patient by decreasing anxiety, improving oxygenation, and decreasing oxygen demand [102, 103]. Historically, the gamma-aminobutyric acid (GABA)-ergic benzodiazepines have been the mainstay of sedation in the PICU, frequently resulting in high-dose exposure for multiple days. High-dose benzodiazepine administration is associated with delirium and prolonged ICU length of stay in critically ill infants and children [74]. Furthermore, benzodiazepine exposure and need for mechanical ventilation are independent predictors of delirium as demonstrated in a large pediatric multicenter point prevalence study [65]. Surprisingly, sedation levels in the PICU are commonly assessed as insufficient due to oversedation (30%) rather than under sedation (10%) [104]. Though sedation in the PICU may be unavoidable, routine assessment, targeted sedation, and use of innovative sedatives, such as dexmedetomidine that naturally leads to more moderate sedation, may improve pediatric outcomes. With the significant relationship between sedation choice and delirium prevalence and prolonged ICU and hospital length of stay in adults, the Society of Critical Care Medicine (SCCM) 2018 guidelines recommend maximizing analgesia "first" followed by *non*-benzodiazepine sedation for adult patients receiving mechanical ventilation [93, 94, 105]. Dexmedetomidine, a short-acting alpha-2 agonist, is being used in the PICU setting at an increasing rate for sedation [106–109]. In preliminary studies, dexmedetomidine is associated with decreased opioid and benzodiazepine exposure in critically ill children, as well as increased likelihood of ICU/hospital discharge [110]. Similar to benzodiazepine and opioid use, long-term dexmedetomidine administration can result in physiologic tolerance and withdrawal [111]. Without a transition in PICU culture to include consideration of targeted sedation that encourages patients to be more alert and interactive, there is risk of trading the complication of delirium with others including iatrogenic withdrawal syndrome and adverse effects of other organ systems. Protocolization, targeted, and/or choice of sedation may be some of the most compelling and modifiable iatrogenic risk factors for delirium and short-term outcomes in critically ill children [74, 112]. Patients who are likely to require prolonged continuous sedation may benefit from intermittent administration of sedatives or non-benzodiazepine regimens to minimize risk for delirium. Targeted sedation may impact delirium prevalence by maintaining a higher level of consciousness when able and thereby decreasing drug exposure and allowing for interaction with family and caregivers.

Severe psychomotor behaviors or manifestations of delirium may require more acute treatment for patient safety. The use of typical antipsychotics and atypical antipsychotics has shown little benefit in preventing or treating delirium in adults, though they may diminish the severity of delirium manifestations in some patients [6, 18, 53, 55, 56, 90, 113–120]. Haloperidol blocks primarily dopamine receptors in the brain, preventing excess stimulation of cortical pathways, providing anxiolysis, and restoring attention [6, 31]. Patients with severe behavioral manifestations of agitation or combativeness due to hyperactive delirium may benefit from short-term haloperidol therapy. Atypical antipsychotics, such as quetiapine, risperidone, olanzapine, and ziprasidone, have some dopamine activity in addition to more extensive actions on acetylcholine, serotonin, and norepinephrine receptors [32, 53, 119, 121]. Patients with both hyperactive and hypoactive delirium may benefit from atypical antipsychotics and the multimodal effects. Though there may remain a role for intermittent antipsychotic therapy in patients with severe manifestations of delirium, preventative management has not been shown as effective to decrease delirium prevalence in critically ill adults. Haloperidol and ziprasidone therapy did not reduce delirium, length of mechanical ventilation, ICU or hospital length of stay, or mortality in a large randomized control trial in critically ill adults [122]. The importance of identifying and treating the underlying cause of delirium is even more paramount with the possible diminished role of antipsychotics and atypical antipsychotics for acute brain dysfunction. Furthermore, the decision to use antipsychotics requires careful consideration of the risks and benefits, noting that there is no FDA approval for use in the setting of delirium for any age.

Summary

The implementation of pediatric delirium monitoring and management offers an opportunity to greatly influence the care of critically ill children. Available valid bedside tools, inclusive rounding processes such as the "Pediatric Road Map" or the "ABCDEF" bundle, and preventative strategies for delirium may ultimately impact pediatric outcomes following critical illness. The goal of delirium monitoring and management is fully realized when a child is comfortable, able to interact with their environment and caregivers, while responding to treatment for both delirium and the disease state. This allows for a child who may "experience" critical illness but without the discomfort and apprehension that we all perceive.

References

1. American Psychiatric Association. Diagnostic and statistical manual of mental disorders. 5th ed. Washington, DC: American Psychiatric Publishing; 2013.
2. Ely EW, Margolin R, Francis J, et al. Evaluation of delirium in critically ill patients: validation of the confusion assessment method for the intensive care unit (CAM-ICU). Crit Care Med. 2001;29(7):1370–9.
3. Justic M. Does "ICU psychosis" really exist? Crit Care Nurse. 2000;20(3):28–37; quiz 38–29.
4. McGuire BE, Basten CJ, Ryan CJ, Gallagher J. Intensive care unit syndrome: a dangerous misnomer. Arch Intern Med. 2000;160(7):906–9.
5. Smith HA, Gangopadhyay M, Goben CM, et al. The preschool confusion assessment method for the ICU: valid and reliable delirium monitoring for critically ill infants and children. Crit Care Med. 2016;44(3):592–600.

6. Schieveld JN, Leroy PL, van Os J, Nicolai J, Vos GD, Leentjens AF. Pediatric delirium in critical illness: phenomenology, clinical correlates and treatment response in 40 cases in the pediatric intensive care unit. Intensive Care Med. 2007;33(6):1033–40.
7. LA Schieveld JN. Delirium in severely ill young children in the pediatric intensive care unit (PICU). J Am Acad Child Adolesc Psychiatry. 2005;44(4):392–4.
8. Smith HA, Fuchs DC, Pandharipande PP, Barr FE, Ely EW. Delirium: an emerging frontier in the management of critically ill children. Crit Care Clin. 2009;25(3):593–614.. x
9. Marcantonio ER, Flacker JM, Wright RJ, Resnick NM. Reducing delirium after hip fracture: a randomized trial. J Am Geriatr Soc. 2001;49(5):516–22.
10. Ely EW, Siegel MD, Inouye SK. Delirium in the intensive care unit: an under-recognized syndrome of organ dysfunction. Semin Respir Crit Care Med. 2001;22(2):115–26.
11. Francis MJ, Hastings GZ, Brown AL, et al. Immunological properties of hepatitis B core antigen fusion proteins. Proc Natl Acad Sci U S A. 1990;87(7):2545–9.
12. McNicoll L, Pisani MA, Zhang Y, Ely EW, Siegel MD, Inouye SK. Delirium in the intensive care unit: occurrence and clinical course in older patients. J Am Geriatr Soc. 2003;51(5):591–8.
13. Ely EW, Shintani A, Truman B, et al. Delirium as a predictor of mortality in mechanically ventilated patients in the intensive care unit. JAMA. 2004;291(14):1753–62.
14. Jackson JC, Gordon SM, Hart RP, Hopkins RO, Ely EW. The association between delirium and cognitive decline: a review of the empirical literature. Neuropsychol Rev. 2004;14(2):87–98.
15. Thomason JW, Ely EW. Delirium in the intensive care unit is bad: what is the confusion? Crit Care Med. 2004;32(11):2352–4.
16. Thomason JW, Shintani A, Peterson JF, Pun BT, Jackson JC, Ely EW. Intensive care unit delirium is an independent predictor of longer hospital stay: a prospective analysis of 261 non-ventilated patients. Crit Care. 2005;9(4):R375–81.
17. Pandharipande P, Jackson J, Ely EW. Delirium: acute cognitive dysfunction in the critically ill. Curr Opin Crit Care. 2005;11(4):360–8.
18. Smith HA, Brink E, Fuchs DC, Ely EW, Pandharipande PP. Pediatric delirium: monitoring and management in the pediatric intensive care unit. Pediatr Clin N Am. 2013;60(3):741–60.
19. Staveski SL, Pickler RH, Lin L, et al. Management of pediatric delirium in pediatric cardiac intensive care patients: an international survey of current practices. Pediatr Crit Care Med. 2018;19(6):538–43.
20. Nevid JS. Essentials of psychology: concepts and applications. 5th ed. Cengage Learning: Australia; 2018.
21. Trzepacz P. Update on the neuropathogenesis of delirium. Dement Geriatr Cogn Disord. 1999;10:330–4.
22. Basarsky TA, Feighan D, MacVicar BA. Glutamate release through volume-activated channels during spreading depression. J Neurosci. 1999;19(15):6439–45.
23. Busto R, Globus MY, Dietrich WD, Martinez E, Valdes I, Ginsberg MD. Effect of mild hypothermia on ischemia-induced release of neurotransmitters and free fatty acids in rat brain. Stroke. 1989;20(7):904–10.
24. Globus MY, Alonso O, Dietrich WD, Busto R, Ginsberg MD. Glutamate release and free radical production following brain injury: effects of posttraumatic hypothermia. J Neurochem. 1995;65(4):1704–11.
25. Globus MY, Busto R, Dietrich WD, Martinez E, Valdes I, Ginsberg MD. Effect of ischemia on the in vivo release of striatal dopamine, glutamate, and gamma-aminobutyric acid studied by intracerebral microdialysis. J Neurochem. 1988;51(5):1455–64.
26. Wheeler AP, Bernard GR. Treating patients with severe sepsis. N Engl J Med. 1999;340(3):207–14.
27. Pavlov VAWH, Czura CJ, Friedman SG, Tracey KJ. The cholinergic anti-inflammatory pathway: a missing link in neuroimmunomodulation. Mol Med. 2003;9:125–34.
28. Flacker JM, Lipsitz LA. Neural mechanisms of delirium: current hypotheses and evolving concepts. J Gerontol A Biol Sci Med Sci. 1999;54(6):B239–46.
29. Bloom FEKD, Bunney BS. Amines. Psychopharmacology: the fourth generation of progress. New York: Raven Press, Ltd.; 1995. p. 1287–359.

30. Gunther ML, Morandi A, Ely EW. Pathophysiology of delirium in the intensive care unit. Crit Care Clin. 2008;24(1):45–65.. viii
31. Meagher DJ, Trzepacz PT. Motoric subtypes of delirium. Semin Clin Neuropsychiatry. 2000;5(2):75–85.
32. Peterson JF, Pun BT, Dittus RS, et al. Delirium and its motoric subtypes: a study of 614 critically ill patients. J Am Geriatr Soc. 2006;54(3):479–84.
33. Pandharipande P, Cotton BA, Shintani A, et al. Motoric subtypes of delirium in mechanically ventilated surgical and trauma intensive care unit patients. Intensive Care Med. 2007;33(10):1726–31.
34. Turkel SB, Trzepacz PT, Tavare CJ. Comparing symptoms of delirium in adults and children. Psychosomatics. 2006;47(4):320–4.
35. Turkel SBTP, Tavare CJ. Comparing symptoms of delirium in adults and children. Psychosomatics. 2006;47(4):320–4.
36. Francis JMD, Kapoor WN. A prospective study of delirium in hospitalized elderly. JAMA. 1990;263(8):1097–101.
37. O'Keefe STCA. Postoperative delirium in the elderly. Br J Anaesth. 1994;73:673–87.
38. Inouye SKSM, Lydon TJ. Delirium: a symptom of how hospital care is failing older persons and a window to improve quality of hospital care. Am J Med. 1999;106(5):565–73.
39. Pandharipande PJJ, Ely EW. Delirium: acute cognitive dysfunction in the critically ill. Curr Opin Crit Care. 2005;11:360–8.
40. Trzepacz PT. Delirium. Advances in diagnosis, pathophysiology, and treatment. Psychiatr Clin North Am. 1996;19(3):429–48.
41. Smith HA, Fuchs DC, Pandharipande PP, Barr FE, Ely EW. Delirium: an emerging frontier in the management of critically ill children. Anesthesiol Clin. 2011;29(4):729–50.
42. Paterson RS, Kenardy JA, De Young AC, Dow BL, Long DA. Delirium in the critically ill child: assessment and sequelae. Dev Neuropsychol. 2017;42(6):387–403.
43. Grover S, Agarwal M, Sharma A, et al. Symptoms and aetiology of delirium: a comparison of elderly and adult patients. East Asian Arch Psychiatry. 2013;23(2):56–64.
44. Grover S, Ghosh A, Kate N, et al. Do motor subtypes of delirium in child and adolescent have a different clinical and phenomenological profile? Gen Hosp Psychiatry. 2014;36(2):187–91.
45. Grover S, Kate N, Malhotra S, Chakrabarti S, Mattoo SK, Avasthi A. Symptom profile of delirium in children and adolescent--does it differ from adults and elderly? Gen Hosp Psychiatry. 2012;34(6):626–32.
46. Turkel SB, Braslow K, Tavare CJ, Trzepacz PT. The delirium rating scale in children and adolescents. Psychosomatics. 2003;44(2):126–9.
47. Hatherill S, Flisher AJ. Delirium in children and adolescents: a systematic review of the literature. J Psychosom Res. 2010;68(4):337–44.
48. Mattoo SK, Grover S, Chakravarty K, Trzepacz PT, Meagher DJ, Gupta N. Symptom profile and etiology of delirium in a referral population in northern India: factor analysis of the DRS-R98. J Neuropsychiatry Clin Neurosci. 2012;24(1):95–101.
49. Leentjens AF, Schieveld JN, Leonard M, Lousberg R, Verhey FR, Meagher DJ. A comparison of the phenomenology of pediatric, adult, and geriatric delirium. J Psychosom Res. 2008;64(2):219–23.
50. Martini DR. Commentary: the diagnosis of delirium in pediatric patients. J Am Acad Child Adolesc Psychiatry. 2005;44(4):395–8.
51. Smith HABJ, Fuchs DC. Diagnosing delirium in critically ill children: validity and reliability of the pediatric confusion assessment method for the intensive care unit. Crit Care Med. 2011;39(1):150–7.
52. Gangopadhyay M, Smith H, Pao M, et al. Development of the Vanderbilt assessment for delirium in infants and children to standardize pediatric delirium assessment by psychiatrists. Psychosomatics. 2017;58(4):355–63.
53. Silver GH, Kearney JA, Kutko MC, Bartell AS. Infant delirium in pediatric critical care settings. Am J Psychiatry. 2010;167(10):1172–7.

54. Turkel SB, Tavare CJ. Delirium in children and adolescents. J Neuropsychiatry Clin Neurosci. 2003;15(4):431–5.
55. Edwards LE, Hutchison LB, Hornik CD, Smith PB, Cotten CM, Bidegain M. A case of infant delirium in the neonatal intensive care unit. J Neonatal Perinatal Med. 2017;10(1):119–23.
56. Madden K, Turkel S, Jacobson J, Epstein D, Moromisato DY. Recurrent delirium after surgery for congenital heart disease in an infant. Pediatr Crit Care Med. 2011;12(6):e413–5.
57. Coté CJ, Lerman J, Anderson BJ. A practice of anesthesia for infants and children. 6th ed. Philadelphia: Elsevier; 2019.
58. Sikich N, Lerman J. Development and psychometric evaluation of the pediatric anesthesia emergence delirium scale. Anesthesiology. 2004;100(5):1138–45.
59. Blankespoor RJ, Janssen NJ, Wolters AM, Van Os J, Schieveld JN. Post-hoc revision of the pediatric anesthesia emergence delirium rating scale: clinical improvement of a bedside-tool? Minerva Anestesiol. 2012;78(8):896–900.
60. Janssen NJ, Tan EY, Staal M, et al. On the utility of diagnostic instruments for pediatric delirium in critical illness: an evaluation of the pediatric anesthesia emergence delirium scale, the delirium rating scale 88, and the delirium rating scale-revised R-98. Intensive Care Med. 2011;37(8):1331–7.
61. Silver G, Traube C, Kearney J, et al. Detecting pediatric delirium: development of a rapid observational assessment tool. Intensive Care Med. 2012;38(6):1025–31.
62. Traube C, Silver G, Kearney J, et al. Cornell assessment of pediatric delirium: a valid, rapid, observational tool for screening delirium in the PICU*. Crit Care Med. 2014;42(3):656–63.
63. Bettencourt A, Mullen JE. Delirium in children: identification, prevention, and management. Crit Care Nurse. 2017;37(3):e9–e18.
64. Simone S, Edwards S, Lardieri A, et al. Implementation of an ICU bundle: an Interprofessional quality improvement project to enhance delirium management and monitor delirium prevalence in a single PICU. Pediatr Crit Care Med. 2017;18(6):531–40.
65. Traube C, Silver G, Reeder RW, et al. Delirium in critically ill children: an international point prevalence study. Crit Care Med. 2017;45(4):584–90.
66. Ely EW, Inouye SK, Bernard GR, et al. Delirium in mechanically ventilated patients: validity and reliability of the confusion assessment method for the intensive care unit (CAM-ICU). JAMA. 2001;286(21):2703–10.
67. Smith HA, Boyd J, Fuchs DC, et al. Diagnosing delirium in critically ill children: validity and reliability of the pediatric confusion assessment method for the intensive care unit. Crit Care Med. 2011;39(1):150–7.
68. Luetz A, Gensel D, Muller J, et al. Validity of different delirium assessment tools for critically ill children: covariates matter. Crit Care Med. 2016;44(11):2060–9.
69. Traube C, Silver G, Gerber LM, et al. Delirium and mortality in critically ill children: epidemiology and outcomes of pediatric delirium. Crit Care Med. 2017;45(5):891–8.
70. Alvarez RV, Palmer C, Czaja AS, et al. Delirium is a common and early finding in patients in the pediatric cardiac intensive care unit. J Pediatr. 2018;195:206–12.
71. Londoño EMC, Gil ICM, Hernández KU, Ramírez CR, Gómez MLA, Peña RAC, Vélez CAA, Penagos SZ, Parra ME, Vásquez JGF. Delirium during the first evaluation of children aged five to 14 years admitted to a paediatric critical care unit. Intensive Crit Care Nurs. 2018;45:37.
72. Meyburg J, Dill ML, Traube C, Silver G, von Haken R. Patterns of postoperative delirium in children. Pediatr Crit Care Med. 2017;18(2):128–33.
73. Patel AK, Biagas KV, Clarke EC, et al. Delirium in children after cardiac bypass surgery. Pediatr Crit Care Med. 2017;18(2):165–71.
74. Smith HAB, Gangopadhyay M, Goben CM, et al. Delirium and benzodiazepines associated with prolonged ICU stay in critically ill infants and young children. Crit Care Med. 2017;45(9):1427–35.
75. Traube C, Mauer EA, Gerber LM, et al. Cost associated with pediatric delirium in the ICU. Crit Care Med. 2016;44(12):e1175–9.

76. Smeets IA, Tan EY, Vossen HG, et al. Prolonged stay at the paediatric intensive care unit associated with paediatric delirium. Eur Child Adolesc Psychiatry. 2010;19(4):389–93.
77. Colville G, Kerry S, Pierce C. Children's factual and delusional memories of intensive care. Am J Respir Crit Care Med. 2008;177(9):976–82.
78. Rees G, Gledhill J, Garralda ME, Nadel S. Psychiatric outcome following paediatric intensive care unit (PICU) admission: a cohort study. Intensive Care Med. 2004;30(8):1607–14.
79. Al-Timari UA, Fisera L, Goljer I, Ertl P. Regio- and stereo-selective synthesis of carbohydrate isoxazolidines by 1,3-dipolar cycloaddition of nitrones to 5,6-dideoxy-1,2-O-isopropylidene-alpha-D-xylo-hex-5-enofuranose. Carbohydr Res. 1992;226(1):49–56.
80. Patel RP, Gambrell M, Speroff T, et al. Delirium and sedation in the intensive care unit: survey of behaviors and attitudes of 1384 healthcare professionals. Crit Care Med. 2009;37(3):825–32.
81. Ely EW, Stephens RK, Jackson JC, et al. Current opinions regarding the importance, diagnosis, and management of delirium in the intensive care unit: a survey of 912 healthcare professionals. Crit Care Med. 2004;32(1):106–12.
82. Spronk PE, Riekerk B, Hofhuis J, Rommes JH. Occurrence of delirium is severely underestimated in the ICU during daily care. Intensive Care Med. 2009;35(7):1276–80.
83. Pandharipande PP, Girard TD, Jackson JC, et al. Long-term cognitive impairment after critical illness. N Engl J Med. 2013;369(14):1306–16.
84. Pandharipande PP, Pun BT, Herr DL, et al. Effect of sedation with dexmedetomidine vs lorazepam on acute brain dysfunction in mechanically ventilated patients: the MENDS randomized controlled trial. JAMA. 2007;298(22):2644–53.
85. Ely EW. The ABCDEF bundle: science and philosophy of how ICU liberation serves patients and families. Crit Care Med. 2017;45(2):321–30.
86. Barnes-Daly MA, Pun BT, Harmon LA, et al. Improving health care for critically ill patients using an evidence-based collaborative approach to ABCDEF bundle dissemination and implementation. Worldviews Evid-Based Nurs. 2018;15(3):206–16.
87. Barnes-Daly MA, Phillips G, Ely EW. Improving hospital survival and reducing brain dysfunction at seven California community hospitals: implementing PAD guidelines via the ABCDEF bundle in 6,064 patients. Crit Care Med. 2017;45(2):171–8.
88. Pun BT, Balas MC, Barnes-Daly MA, et al. Caring for critically ill patients with the ABCDEF bundle: results of the ICU liberation collaborative in over 15,000 adults. Crit Care Med. 2018;47:3.
89. Practice guideline for the treatment of patients with delirium. American Psychiatric Association. Am J Psychiatry 1999;156(5 Suppl):1–20.
90. Van Tuijl SG, Van Cauteren YJ, Pikhard T, Engel M, Schieveld JN. Management of pediatric delirium in critical illness: a practical update. Minerva Anestesiol. 2015;81(3):333–41.
91. Kudchadkar SR, Aljohani OA, Punjabi NM. Sleep of critically ill children in the pediatric intensive care unit: a systematic review. Sleep Med Rev. 2014;18(2):103–10.
92. Inouye SK, Bogardus ST Jr, Charpentier PA, et al. A multicomponent intervention to prevent delirium in hospitalized older patients. N Engl J Med. 1999;340(9):669–76.
93. Barr J, Fraser GL, Puntillo K, et al. Clinical practice guidelines for the management of pain, agitation, and delirium in adult patients in the intensive care unit. Crit Care Med. 2013;41(1):263–306.
94. Devlin JW, Skrobik Y, Gelinas C, et al. Clinical practice guidelines for the prevention and management of pain, agitation/sedation, delirium, immobility, and sleep disruption in adult patients in the ICU. Crit Care Med. 2018;46(9):e825–73.
95. Kudchadkar SR, Yaster M, Punjabi NM. Sedation, sleep promotion, and delirium screening practices in the care of mechanically ventilated children: a wake-up call for the pediatric critical care community*. Crit Care Med. 2014;42(7):1592–600.
96. Hu RF, Jiang XY, Hegadoren KM, Zhang YH. Effects of earplugs and eye masks combined with relaxing music on sleep, melatonin and cortisol levels in ICU patients: a randomized controlled trial. Crit Care. 2015;19:115.

97. Bagci S, Horoz OO, Yildizdas D, Reinsberg J, Bartmann P, Muller A. Melatonin status in pediatric intensive care patients with sepsis. Pediatr Crit Care Med. 2012;13(2):e120–3.
98. Bruni O, Alonso-Alconada D, Besag F, et al. Current role of melatonin in pediatric neurology: clinical recommendations. Eur J Paediatr Neurol. 2015;19(2):122–33.
99. Mason KP, O'Mahony E, Zurakowski D, Libenson MH. Effects of dexmedetomidine sedation on the EEG in children. Paediatr Anaesth. 2009;19(12):1175–83.
100. Best KM, Wypij D, Asaro LA, Curley MA. Randomized evaluation of sedation titration for respiratory failure study I. patient, process, and system predictors of iatrogenic withdrawal syndrome in critically ill children. Crit Care Med. 2017;45(1):e7–e15.
101. Best KM, Boullata JI, Curley MA. Risk factors associated with iatrogenic opioid and benzodiazepine withdrawal in critically ill pediatric patients: a systematic review and conceptual model. Pediatr Crit Care Med. 2015;16(2):175–83.
102. Playfor S, Jenkins I, Boyles C, et al. Consensus guidelines on sedation and analgesia in critically ill children. Intensive Care Med. 2006;32(8):1125–36.
103. Twite MD, Rashid A, Zuk J, Friesen RH. Sedation, analgesia, and neuromuscular blockade in the pediatric intensive care unit: survey of fellowship training programs. Pediatr Crit Care Med. 2004;5(6):521–32.
104. Vet NJ, Ista E, de Wildt SN, van Dijk M, Tibboel D, de Hoog M. Optimal sedation in pediatric intensive care patients: a systematic review. Intensive Care Med. 2013;39(9):1524–34.
105. Jacobi J, Fraser GL, Coursin DB, et al. Clinical practice guidelines for the sustained use of sedatives and analgesics in the critically ill adult. Crit Care Med. 2002;30(1):119–41.
106. Whalen LD, Di Gennaro JL, Irby GA, Yanay O, Zimmerman JJ. Long-term dexmedetomidine use and safety profile among critically ill children and neonates. Pediatr Crit Care Med. 2014;15(8):706–14.
107. Ahmed SS, Unland T, Slaven JE, Nitu ME. High dose dexmedetomidine: effective as a sole agent sedation for children undergoing MRI. Int J Pediatr. 2015;2015:397372.
108. Andreolio C, Piva JP, Baldasso E, Ferlini R, Piccoli R. Prolonged infusion of dexmedetomidine in critically-ill children. Indian Pediatr. 2016;53(11):987–9.
109. Burbano NH, Otero AV, Berry DE, Orr RA, Munoz RA. Discontinuation of prolonged infusions of dexmedetomidine in critically ill children with heart disease. Intensive Care Med. 2012;38(2):300–7.
110. Gupta P, Whiteside W, Sabati A, et al. Safety and efficacy of prolonged dexmedetomidine use in critically ill children with heart disease*. Pediatr Crit Care Med. 2012;13(6):660–6.
111. Tobias JD. Dexmedetomidine: are tolerance and withdrawal going to be an issue with long-term infusions? Pediatr Crit Care Med. 2010;11(1):158–60.
112. Mody K, Kaur S, Mauer EA, et al. Benzodiazepines and development of delirium in critically ill children: estimating the causal effect. Crit Care Med. 2018;46(9):1486–91.
113. Turkel SB, Jacobson JR, Tavare CJ. The diagnosis and management of delirium in infancy. J Child Adolesc Psychopharmacol. 2013;23(5):352–6.
114. Turkel SB, Jacobson J, Munzig E, Tavare CJ. Atypical antipsychotic medications to control symptoms of delirium in children and adolescents. J Child Adolesc Psychopharmacol. 2012;22(2):126–30.
115. Turkel SB, Hanft A. The pharmacologic management of delirium in children and adolescents. Paediatr Drugs. 2014;16(4):267–74.
116. Turkel SB. Pediatric delirium: recognition, management, and outcome. Curr Psychiatry Rep. 2017;19(12):101.
117. Page VJ, Ely EW, Gates S, et al. Effect of intravenous haloperidol on the duration of delirium and coma in critically ill patients (Hope-ICU): a randomised, double-blind, placebo-controlled trial. Lancet Respir Med. 2013;1(7):515–23.
118. Neufeld KJ, Yue J, Robinson TN, Inouye SK, Needham DM. Antipsychotic medication for prevention and treatment of delirium in hospitalized adults: a systematic review and meta-analysis. J Am Geriatr Soc. 2016;64(4):705–14.

119. Joyce C, Witcher R, Herrup E, et al. Evaluation of the safety of quetiapine in treating delirium in critically ill children: a retrospective review. J Child Adolesc Psychopharmacol. 2015;25(9):666–70.
120. van den Boogaard M, Schoonhoven L, van Achterberg T, van der Hoeven JG, Pickkers P. Haloperidol prophylaxis in critically ill patients with a high risk for delirium. Crit Care. 2013;17(1):R9.
121. Karnik NS, Joshi SV, Paterno C, Shaw R. Subtypes of pediatric delirium: a treatment algorithm. Psychosomatics. 2007;48(3):253–7.
122. Girard TD, Exline MC, Carson SS, et al. Haloperidol and ziprasidone for treatment of delirium in critical illness. N Engl J Med. 2018;379:2506.
123. Smith HA, Berutti T, Brink E, et al. Pediatric critical care perceptions on analgesia, sedation, and delirium. Semin Respir Crit Care Med. 2013;34(2):244–61.

Chapter 7
Epidemiology of Delirium in Children: Prevalence, Risk Factors, and Outcomes

Sean S. Barnes, Christopher Gabor, and Sapna R. Kudchadkar

Introduction

Although the *Diagnostic and Statistical Manual of Mental Disorders* (DSM) established diagnostic criteria for delirium in 1980, delirium research in the pediatric population has lagged significantly behind the mounting evidence in adults. A 2009 systematic review of the literature on delirium in children and adolescents identified only case series and a few case reports totaling 217 children or adolescents [1]. However, the last decade has seen an explosion in pediatric delirium research resulting from the introduction of validated pediatric-specific delirium screening tools [2]. Several research groups have shown that the prevalence of delirium in critically ill children approaches estimates in adults, and a growing body of literature has begun to identify the risk factors and outcomes associated with delirium development in children. While many of these risk factors and outcomes are parallel to those adults, there are specific predictors unique to the pediatric population.

In the latest edition of the DSM (DSM-5), the definition of delirium was modified to emphasize the cardinal features of diagnosis: (1) disturbances in attention or awareness, (2) changes in cognition, and (3) fluctuation in symptoms [3]. However, even this definition can be challenging to apply in the pediatric setting given

S. S. Barnes (✉)
Department of Anesthesiology and Critical Care Medicine, Johns Hopkins Charlotte R. Bloomberg Children's Center, Baltimore, MD, USA
e-mail: sbarne21@jhmi.edu

C. Gabor
Department of Emergency & Community Medicine, Hamilton Health Sciences, Hamilton, ON, Canada

S. R. Kudchadkar
Department of Anesthesiology and Critical Care Medicine, Pediatrics and Physical Medicine and Rehabilitation, Johns Hopkins Charlotte R. Bloomberg Children's Center, Baltimore, MD, USA

C. G. Hughes et al. (eds.), *Delirium*, https://doi.org/10.1007/978-3-030-25751-4_7

substantial variability in the premorbid neurocognitive state and language abilities of children. Neither the DSM-5 nor International Classification of Diseases (10th edition) definitions include pediatric-specific delirium definitions [4], highlighting the importance of having validated pediatric-specific delirium screening tools, as was discussed in Chap. 6.

In order to understand the clinical burden and implications of delirium in children, it is imperative to review the epidemiology of delirium including prevalence, risk factors, and outcomes in a vulnerable group of patients undergoing active neurocognitive development.

Description of Studies

While there are a small number of studies that have examined delirium in the pediatric emergency department [5], neonatal intensive care unit [6] (NICU), and children with oncological disease [7], delirium in children is most frequently studied in the pediatric intensive care unit (PICU). A recent systematic review on pediatric delirium from Holly et al. identified 21 studies investigating how delirium is recognized in hospitalized children [8]. The overwhelming majority (90%) of these studies included PICU patients. Furthermore, only a small number of studies were prospective, with many case reports and case series included, providing a window into the current status of pediatric delirium research and future opportunities.

Prevalence

Prevalence is defined as the number of existing cases at a single point in time, while incidence is defined as the number of new cases population at risk in a given time period. Historically, the prevalence of delirium in children was largely extrapolated from referrals to child psychiatry services [9]. Children and adolescents accounted for 10% of consultation-liaison psychiatry services and between 17% and 66% of psychiatry referrals from PICUs. Furthermore, early case reports seemed to underestimate the burden of delirium in critically ill children with an incidence of 4–5%, likely due to under diagnosis [1]. The introduction of validated pediatric-specific delirium screening tools has propelled the field of pediatric delirium research into the modern day. The majority of literature describes the prevalence of delirium in critically ill children often admitted to the PICU.

In 2011, Smith et al. introduced one of the first validated pediatric-specific delirium screening tools [10]. In this study, a total of 68 pediatric critically ill patients, at least 5 years of age, were included in a prospective study to validate the Pediatric Confusion Assessment Method for Intensive Care Unit (pCAM-ICU). As detailed in Chap. 6, the pCAM-ICU was adapted from the well-established Confusion Assessment Method-ICU (CAM-ICU). The pCAM-ICU validation study identified a prevalence of 13.2% among a mixed population of pediatric intensive care patients including medical, surgical, and cardiac diagnoses. Recognizing the pCAM-ICU was excluding a large population of critically ill children, Smith et al. went on to create and validate the Preschool Confusion Assessment Method for the ICU (psCAM-ICU) in 2016 [11]. This study included 281 critically ill children aged 6 months to 5 years admitted to the PICU. In this younger population, the overall delirium prevalence was 44%. Interestingly, rates of delirium were 53% in patients <2 years of age versus 33% in patients 2–5 years of age.

The other major validated pediatric-specific delirium screening tool is the Cornell Assessment for Pediatric Delirium (CAPD). In the initial validation study by Silver et al. in 2014 [12], 111 patients of ages ranging from 0 to 21 years admitted to a tertiary PICU were found to have a delirium prevalence of 20.6%. Other notable findings from this study include higher prevalence for delirium in critically ill children with developmental delay and higher severity of illness. The authors noted that children with developmental delay were diagnosed with delirium almost three times as often as children without delay (38.8% vs 13.9%). Additionally, those with a higher severity of illness, as determined by the Pediatric Index of Mortality II score, were also noted to have a higher likelihood of being diagnosed with delirium (29.7% vs 12.3%).

The largest study to establish the prevalence of delirium in the pediatric population was published by Traube et al. in 2017 [13], with an overall objective to determine the prevalence of delirium in critically ill children and explore associated risk factors. The study was a multi-institutional point prevalence study including 25 pediatric critical care units in the United States, the Netherlands, New Zealand, Australia, and Saudi Arabia. The majority of units were affiliated with universities; however, three were part of community hospitals. At the conclusion of the study, 994 subjects were enrolled, and an overall point prevalence was 25%. These findings were consistent with those of prior single-center studies that reported pediatric delirium rates ranging from 10% to 30% [14–16]. Of note, the delirium prevalence increased significantly (up to 38%) for those children admitted to the PICU for 6 or more days.

Risk Factors

Current literature has identified many risk factors for the development of delirium in critically ill children (Fig. 7.1). Despite the physiological and developmental differences between children (i.e., infants, toddlers, school age children, and adolescence), there is significant overlap in the risk factors for developing delirium across these groups.

The point prevalence study described above is one of the largest studies examining pediatric delirium to date, identifying many risk factors included in Fig. 7.1. These include age (less than 2 years), mechanical ventilation, exposure to vasopressor medications (potentially a marker for severity of illness), and antiepileptics.

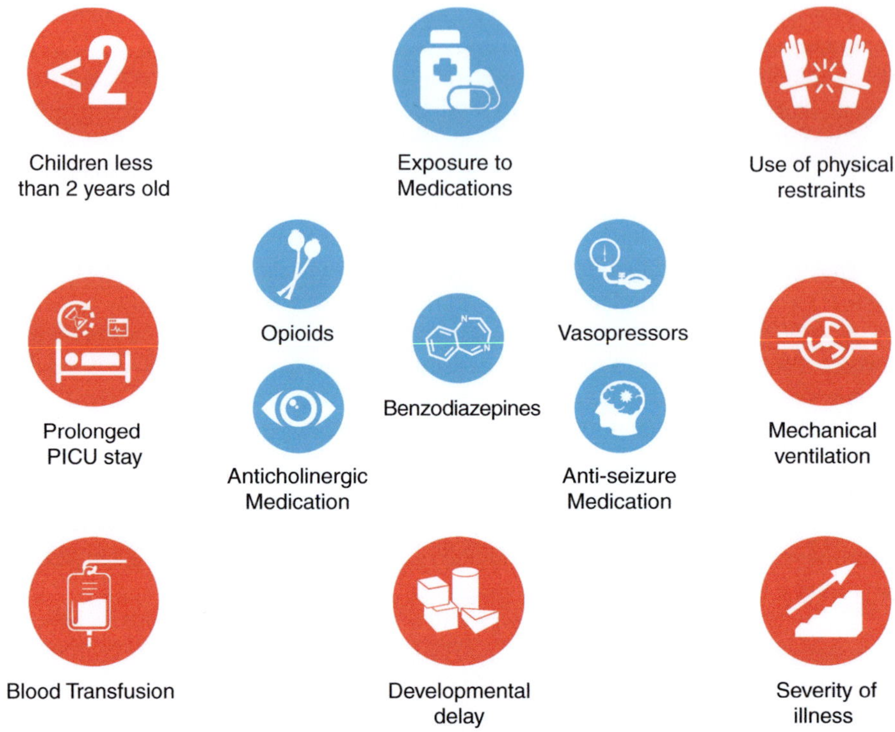

Fig. 7.1 Risk factors associated with delirium in critically ill children

Additionally, exposure to benzodiazepines, opioids, and use of physical restraints was strongly associated with delirium. Furthermore, the point prevalence study noted that the risk for developing delirium increased with the length of PICU admission [17]. Children admitted to the PICU with an infectious or inflammatory disorder had the highest rate of developing delirium (42%). These risk factors highlight how the most vulnerable patients are susceptible to developing delirium. In adults, the elderly are often most at risk for developing delirium; however, in children, it is the youngest who are most at risk. Similar to adults, those receiving mechanical ventilation are at significant risk for developing delirium. While adult studies are conflicting, early pediatric studies have shown that blood transfusions in the critically ill child are independently associated with the development of delirium.

A recent study by Nellis et al. identified that children who were transfused red blood cells (RBCs) were more than twice as likely to develop delirium during their admission compared with children who were never transfused. The authors observed a temporal relationship among transfused children, and for each additional 10 mL/kg of RBCs transfused, recipients were 90% more likely to develop delirium [18].

Medication exposure can also be a risk factor for the development of delirium in critically ill children. Fortunately, medication exposure is also one of the most common potentially modifiable risk factors.

Approaches in minimal but effective sedation in pediatric critical care have lagged behind adults. Many PICUs around the world still implement a combination of opioid and benzodiazepine as the primary sedatives for critically ill children [19]. Both opioids and benzodiazepines are known independent risk factors for the development of delirium in children. Traube et al. demonstrated that benzodiazepines were strongly associated with transition from normal cognitive status to delirium. In a retrospective observational study, they found that benzodiazepine use more than quadrupled delirium rates with an odds ratio of 4.4 [20]. In a secondary analysis of the psCAM-ICU validation study, Smith et al. demonstrated that greater benzodiazepine exposure was significantly associated with a lower likelihood of ICU discharge, longer delirium duration, and increased risk for delirium the following day [21]. Additionally, exposure to anticholinergic drugs may potentiate the effects of benzodiazepines and increase the risk of developing delirium [22]. While sedatives are often needed for mechanical ventilation in postoperative pediatric patients, the postoperative period in and of itself is a known risk factor for the development of delirium.

In fact, the postoperative period is a particularly vulnerable time for children to develop delirium. Meyberg et al. have published two articles on the same cohort of children investigating delirium in the postoperative period [23, 24] and identified specific risk factors for developing delirium in the postoperative period. Younger children develop delirium more frequently and with more pronounced symptoms. Interestingly, the number of preceding operations did not influence the risk of delirium. Of note, the authors identified that patients receiving total intravenous anesthesia had a lower risk of developing delirium than those who had received inhalational anesthesia. Lastly, invasive catheters, respiratory devices, and the development of an infection all increased the risk of developing delirium. A secondary analysis of this cohort described two different patterns of delirium in postoperative children admitted to the PICU. One pattern was an early short-lasting delirium (24 h), and the other was a longer more severe course. Overall the incidence of delirium was 66%, and the group was evenly split in each pattern.

There are special pediatric populations that are more likely to develop delirium. Two notable populations are children requiring extracorporeal membrane oxygenation (ECMO) and cardiac surgery. In a prospective observational longitudinal cohort study, Patel et al. describe delirium in children requiring ECMO [25]. In this study, eight patients accounted for 72 days of ECMO, and all patients developed delirium. The authors found that only 13% of ECMO days were categorized as delirium-free and coma-free, and the majority of patient days on ECMO were spent in coma (65%). Children undergoing cardiac surgery, and specifically surgery with cardiopulmonary bypass, are particularly susceptible to development of postoperative delirium [26]. In a prospective observational single-center study, Patel et al. report delirium prevalence of 49% in children after cardiac surgery with cardiopulmonary bypass [27]. The authors note that delirium often lasted 1–2 days and developed within the first 1–3 days after surgery. Similar to other postoperative pediatric delirium studies, age less than 2 years was a risk factor for developing delirium. Other unique risk factors included developmental delay, higher Risk Adjustment for Congenital Heart Surgery-1 (RACHS-1) score, cyanotic disease, and albumin less than 3 g/dL.

Outcomes

There is a paucity of studies examining outcomes in pediatric delirium. However, emerging literature would suggest that children share many of the same unfavorable outcomes associated with delirium as adults (Fig. 7.2). In a prospective longitudinal cohort study of 1547 consecutive patients, Traube et al. characterized the epidemiology and outcomes of pediatric delirium [28]. In this study, delirium was diagnosed in 17% of all subjects and lasted a median of 2 days. Similar to adults, most cases of delirium were of the hypoactive and mixed subtypes, 46% and 45%, respectively. Core outcome measures such as length of stay were increased in children with

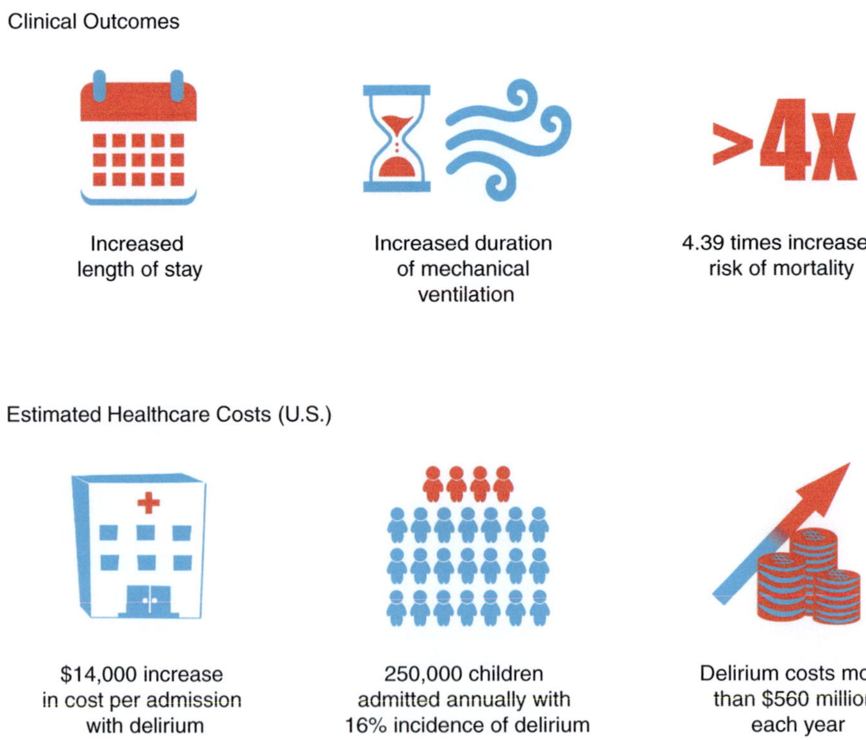

Fig. 7.2 Outcomes associated with delirium in children in the ICU

delirium, as was duration of mechanical ventilation. Finally, the authors identified that delirium was a strong and independent predictor of mortality with an adjusted odds ratio of 4.39. While other studies had identified that prolonged stay in the PICU was associated with delirium, this is one of the first studies to highlight the impact of delirium on mortality.

Another emerging outcome of interest in the study of delirium is the cognitive and behavioral consequences of delirium. Recent evidence supports the concern that adults who develop delirium are at an increased risk for a decline in cognitive and adaptive functioning. To begin to explore this topic in critically ill children, Meyburg et al. conducted a single-center point prevalence study to investigate the long-term neurocognitive impact of delirium on children [29]. Contrary to the findings in adults, the authors found no clear association between pediatric delirium and long-term neurocognitive outcomes. Larger multicenter studies are now required to further evaluate this relationship.

An often overlooked outcome in delirium is healthcare costs. Delirium in adults has been associated with an increase in healthcare costs, with some estimates at over 4 billion dollars annually [30]. While on a smaller scale, pediatric delirium likely contributes to an overall increase in healthcare costs in the United States. In a single-center study, Traube et al. found that a diagnosis of delirium is associated with an 85% increase in PICU costs, and at their institution, this increase in cost was approximately $14,000 per admission [31]. With an incidence of delirium of 16% (in their cohort) and roughly 250,000 children admitted to critical care units in the United States annually, this would translate into an increase in hospital charges of more than $560 million each year.

Conclusion

Much has been learned about the epidemiology of pediatric delirium over the last decade. Due to advances in delirium screening methods in children, we now know that one in four children admitted to the PICU are likely to suffer from delirium. Delirium itself significantly impacts length of stay in the hospital and dramatically increases overall hospital cost. The prevalence is even higher in special pediatric populations, such as those who require ECMO or cardiac surgery. However, much less is known about delirium in children outside the PICU. With emerging literature on the benefits of the ABCDEF bundle and extrapolated data from our adult colleagues, Fig. 7.3 highlights potential practices for prevention and management of delirium in children. Significant contributions have been made to the study of pediatric delirium, but much work is still to be done.

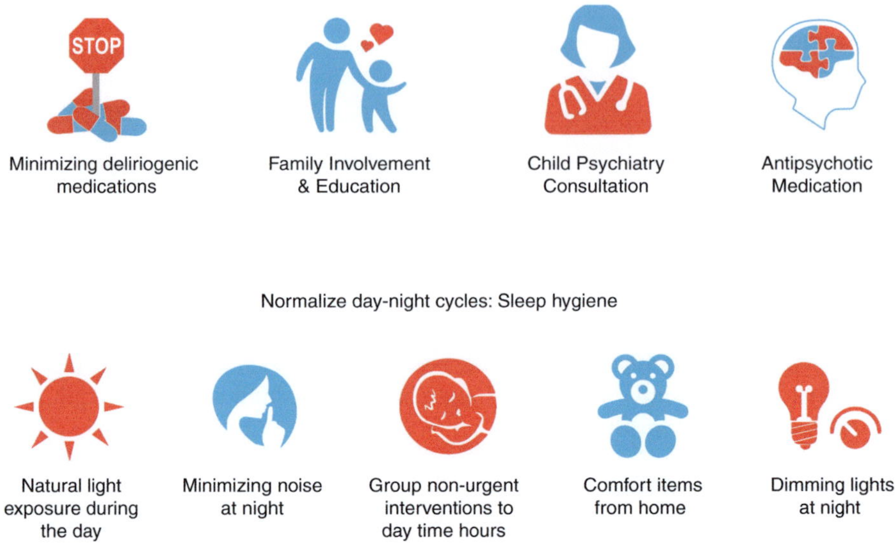
STOP
Minimizing deliriogenic medications
Family Involvement & Education
Child Psychiatry Consultation
Antipsychotic Medication
Normalize day-night cycles: Sleep hygiene
Natural light exposure during the day
Minimizing noise at night
Group non-urgent interventions to day time hours
Comfort items from home
Dimming lights at night

Fig. 7.3 Potential practices for prevention and management of delirium in children

References

1. Hatherill S, Flisher AJ. Delirium in children and adolescents: a systematic review of the literature. J Psychosom Res. 2010;68:337–44.
2. Walker T, Kudchadkar SR. Pain and sedation management: 2018 update for the Rogers' textbook of pediatric intensive care. Pediatr Crit Care Med. 2019;20(1):54–61.
3. American Psychiatric Association. Diagnostic and statistical manual of mental disorders. 5th ed. Arlington: American Psychiatric Association; 2013.
4. Thom R. Pediatric Delirium. Am J Psychiatry Residents' J. 2017;12:6–8.
5. Augenstein JA, Klein EJ, Traube C. Delirium upon presentation to the pediatric emergency department: a case series. Pediatr Emerg Care. 2018;34:e147–e9.
6. Groves A, Traube C, Silver G. Detection and management of delirium in the neonatal unit: a case series. Pediatrics. 2016;137:e20153369.
7. Traube C, Ariagno S, Thau F, et al. Delirium in hospitalized children with cancer: incidence and associated risk factors. J Pediatr. 2017;191:212–7.
8. Holly C, Porter S, Echevarria M, Dreker M, Ruzehaji S. CE: original research: recognizing delirium in hospitalized children: a systematic review of the evidence on risk factors and characteristics. Am J Nurs. 2018;118:24–36.
9. Barnes SS, Grados MA, Kudchadkar SR. Child psychiatry engagement in the management of delirium in critically ill children. Crit Care Res Pract. 2018;2018:9135618.
10. Smith HA, Boyd J, Fuchs DC, et al. Diagnosing delirium in critically ill children: validity and reliability of the pediatric confusion assessment method for the intensive care unit. Crit Care Med. 2011;39:150–7.
11. Smith HA, Gangopadhyay M, Goben CM, et al. The preschool confusion assessment method for the ICU: valid and reliable delirium monitoring for critically ill infants and children. Crit Care Med. 2016;44:592–600.
12. Traube C, Silver G, Kearney J, et al. Cornell assessment of pediatric delirium: a valid, rapid, observational tool for screening delirium in the PICU∗. Crit Care Med. 2014;42:656–63.

13. Traube C, Silver G, Reeder RW, et al. Delirium in critically ill children: an international point prevalence study. Crit Care Med. 2017;45:584–90.
14. Creten C, Van Der Zwaan S, Blankespoor RJ, Leroy PL, Schieveld JN. Pediatric delirium in the pediatric intensive care unit: a systematic review and an update on key issues and research questions. Minerva Anestesiol. 2011;77:1099–107.
15. Silver G, Traube C, Gerber LM, et al. Pediatric delirium and associated risk factors: a single-center prospective observational study. Pediatr Crit Care Med. 2015;16:303–9.
16. Smith HA, Brink E, Fuchs DC, Ely EW, Pandharipande PP. Pediatric delirium: monitoring and management in the pediatric intensive care unit. Pediatr Clin N Am. 2013;60:741–60.
17. Smeets IA, Tan EY, Vossen HG, et al. Prolonged stay at the paediatric intensive care unit associated with paediatric delirium. Eur Child Adolesc Psychiatry. 2010;19:389–93.
18. Nellis ME, Goel R, Feinstein S, Shahbaz S, Kaur S, Traube C. Association between transfusion of RBCs and subsequent development of delirium in critically ill children. Pediatr Crit Care Med. 2018;19:925–9.
19. Kudchadkar SR, Yaster M, Punjabi NM. Sedation, sleep promotion, and delirium screening practices in the care of mechanically ventilated children: a wake-up call for the pediatric critical care community∗. Crit Care Med. 2014;42:1592–600.
20. Mody K, Kaur S, Mauer EA, et al. Benzodiazepines and development of delirium in critically ill children: estimating the causal effect. Crit Care Med. 2018;46:1486–91.
21. Smith HAB, Gangopadhyay M, Goben CM, et al. Delirium and benzodiazepines associated with prolonged ICU stay in critically ill infants and young children. Crit Care Med. 2017;45:1427–35.
22. Madden K, Hussain K, Tasker RC. Anticholinergic medication burden in pediatric prolonged critical illness: a potentially modifiable risk factor for delirium. Pediatr Crit Care Med. 2018;19:917–24.
23. Meyburg J, Dill ML, Traube C, Silver G, von Haken R. Patterns of postoperative delirium in children. Pediatr Crit Care Med. 2017;18:128–33.
24. Meyburg J, Dill ML, von Haken R, et al. Risk factors for the development of postoperative delirium in pediatric intensive care patients. Pediatr Crit Care Med. 2018;19:e514–e21.
25. Patel AK, Biagas KV, Clark EC, Traube C. Delirium in the pediatric cardiac extracorporeal membrane oxygenation patient population: a case series. Pediatr Crit Care Med. 2017;18:e621–e4.
26. Leroy PL, Schieveld JN. Mind the heart: delirium in children following cardiac surgery for congenital heart disease. Pediatr Crit Care Med. 2017;18:196–8.
27. Patel AK, Biagas KV, Clarke EC, et al. Delirium in children after cardiac bypass surgery. Pediatr Crit Care Med. 2017;18:165–71.
28. Traube C, Silver G, Gerber LM, et al. Delirium and mortality in critically ill children: epidemiology and outcomes of pediatric delirium. Crit Care Med. 2017;45:891–8.
29. Meyburg J, Ries M, Zielonka M, et al. Cognitive and behavioral consequences of pediatric delirium: a pilot study. Pediatr Crit Care Med. 2018;19:e531–e7.
30. Barr J, Fraser GL, Puntillo K, et al. Clinical practice guidelines for the management of pain, agitation, and delirium in adult patients in the intensive care unit. Crit Care Med. 2013;41:263–306.
31. Traube C, Mauer EA, Gerber LM, et al. Cost associated with pediatric delirium in the ICU. Crit Care Med. 2016;44:e1175–e9.

Chapter 8
Delirium After Primary Neurological Injury

Mina F. Nordness, Diane N. Haddad, Shayan Rakhit, and Mayur B. Patel

M. F. Nordness
Critical Illness, Brain Dysfunction, and Survivorship Center, Vanderbilt University Medical Center, Nashville, TN, USA

Division of Trauma, Surgical Critical Care, and Emergency General Surgery, Section of Surgical Sciences, Department of Surgery, Vanderbilt University Medical Center, Nashville, TN, USA
e-mail: mina.f.mirhoseini@vumc.org

D. N. Haddad
Critical Illness, Brain Dysfunction, and Survivorship Center, Vanderbilt University Medical Center, Nashville, TN, USA

Division of Trauma, Surgical Critical Care, and Emergency General Surgery, Section of Surgical Sciences, Department of Surgery, Nashville, TN, USA
e-mail: diane.n.haddad@vumc.org

S. Rakhit
Critical Illness, Brain Dysfunction, and Survivorship Center, Vanderbilt University Medical Center, Nashville, TN, USA

Division of Trauma, Surgical Critical Care, and Emergency General Surgery, Section of Surgical Sciences, Department of Surgery, Nashville, TN, USA

Vanderbilt University School of Medicine, Nashville, TN, USA
e-mail: shayan.rakhit.1@vumc.org

M. B. Patel (✉)
Critical Illness, Brain Dysfunction, and Survivorship Center, Vanderbilt University Medical Center, Nashville, TN, USA

Division of Trauma, Surgical Critical Care, and Emergency General Surgery, Section of Surgical Sciences, Department of Surgery, Nashville, TN, USA

Vanderbilt University Medical Center, Nashville, TN, USA

Geriatric Research Education and Clinical Center, Tennessee Valley Veterans Affairs Healthcare System, Nashville, TN, USA

Departments of Neurosurgery, and Hearing & Speech Sciences, Vanderbilt Brain Institute, Nashville, TN, USA

Surgical Service, Department of Veterans Affairs Medical Center, Tennessee Valley Healthcare System, Nashville, TN, USA
e-mail: mayur.b.patel@vumc.org

C. G. Hughes et al. (eds.), *Delirium*, https://doi.org/10.1007/978-3-030-25751-4_8

Introduction

Over the last two decades, delirium has been identified as a major morbidity of critical illness leading to increased hospital length of stay, ICU days, mortality, and long-term cognitive impairment with loss of independence and quality of life [1–4]. Much of delirium research has been repeatedly validated in medical, surgical, and cardiovascular critical care patients. Delirium metrics, however, are not as widely applied in patients with acute primary brain dysfunction, also known as primary neurologic injury (PNI) related to stroke (ischemic and hemorrhagic) or traumatic brain injury (TBI) [2, 5–7].

Until recent years, the limited investigations and application of delirium in PNI are likely rooted in the assumption that delirium cannot be assessed in these patients. PNI can result in permanent structural injury to the brain leading to lifelong changes in cognition, language, perception, motor ability, and sensorium. These acute changes can make delineating secondary cerebral dysfunction, such as delirium, from the primary injury very difficult. However, a growing number of studies have shown delirium assessment in neurologically injured patients is possible and that delirium after PNI has similar poor outcomes compared to non-PNI cohorts.

In this chapter, we hope to better clarify the existing data on prevalence and outcomes of delirium in PNI patients. Further, we hope to provide a platform for future studies and delineate what is still not understood from the available literature.

Delirium Assessment in Primary Brain Injury

Even after PNI, delirium assessment is still based on four main criteria (i.e., acute onset with fluctuating course, inattention, disorganized thinking, altered level of consciousness) derived from the Diagnostic and Statistical Manual of Mental Disorders version IIIR (DSM-IIIR), DSM-IV, and more recently DSM-V. In patients with PNI, Inouye's Confusion Assessment Method (CAM) [8] has been studied, as has Ely's Confusion Assessment Method for ICU (CAM-ICU) [9]. The CAM-ICU utilizes the Richmond Agitation-Sedation Scale (RASS) as part of its assessment for consciousness. Patients with coma (RASS scores of −4 and −5) are unable to be assessed for delirium with the CAM-ICU. This challenge exists for many patients with severe PNI, as they often start and/or progress to a comatose state.

Other assessment methods have been used in patients with PNI, including the Intensive Care Delirium Screening Checklist (ICDSC) [10, 11] and the 4-A Test (4AT) rapid clinical test for delirium [12, 13]. We note that there are currently no delirium assessment tools that are specifically tailored toward patients with PNI.

Assessment of delirium in patients with PNI has been performed less universally than in other critically ill patient cohorts. Elements contributing to this difference

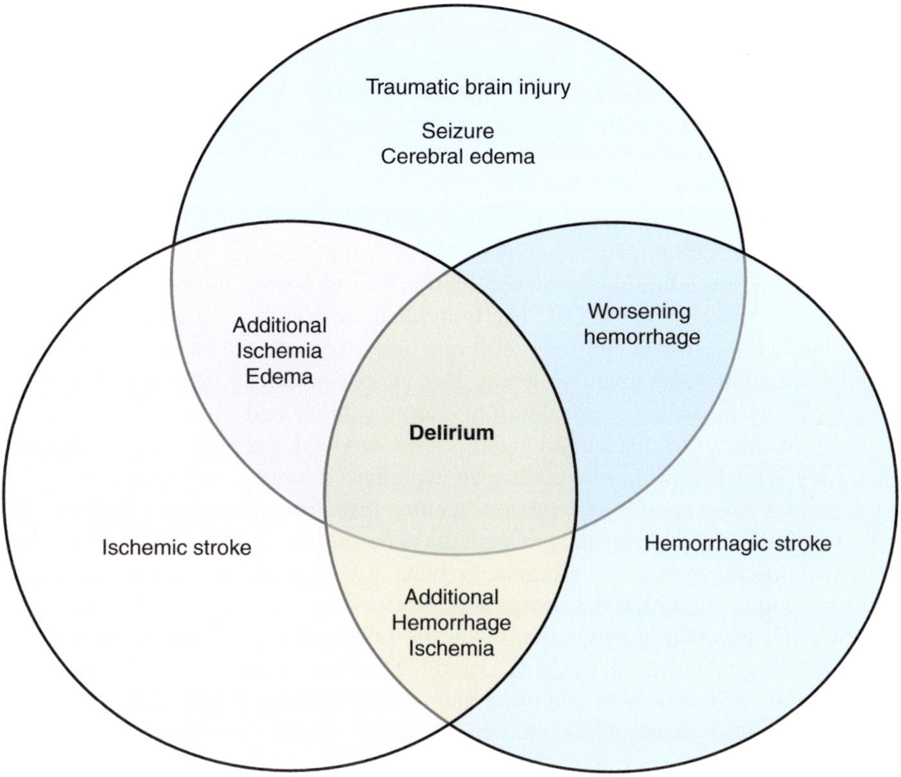

Fig. 8.1 Differential diagnoses for mental status change in the neurologically injured

include comatose state, unclear neurologic baselines after PNI, and communication difficulties such as aphasia limiting ability for interactive assessment. Most importantly, acute mental status changes in patients with PNI must first be assessed for acute processes such as further ischemia, cerebral edema, hemorrhage, seizures, or encephalitis (Fig. 8.1). Once these have been ruled out, additional sources of changes of mental status from new baseline are relevant to delirium measurement.

Review of the Primary Literature

Building on a recent systematic review on delirium in neurologically injured patients [14], we hope to further detail the primary literature on the evaluation of delirium in patients with PNI. We specifically focus on delirium findings as it relates to three subcategories of neurologic injury: TBI, intracerebral hemorrhage, and ischemic stroke.

Traumatic Brain Injury

TBI, defined as an alteration in brain function caused by an external force, is a major public health concern, with an incidence exceeding two million individuals annually in the USA alone [15]. Only two studies were identified in the most recent literature on the evaluation of delirium in a TBI population. These studies both confirm the ability to assess delirium in individuals with TBI.

The first is a 2008 retrospective review by Scherer et al. of 132 patients admitted to an inpatient brain injury neurorehabilitation unit post-hospital discharge from an acute hospital admission for TBI [16]. Individuals with confusion while in rehabilitation had worse clinical and long-term outcomes. Using their own internally validated Confusion Assessment Protocol, the authors noted a longer acute hospital length of stay in patients with delirium. Employability and productivity status at 1-year post-injury for discharged patients who survived, the primary outcomes for this study, were lower in individuals who experienced longer confusion times.

A second study sought to validate screening tests for delirium in a TBI population. In a 2016 prospective study of patients with mild to moderate TBI admitted to an ICU following multisystem trauma, Frenette et al. assessed patients at three separate time points during the ICU hospitalization for delirium with the CAM-ICU, the ICDSC, and psychiatric evaluation using the DSM-IV-TR [17]. Compared to the DSM-IV-TR gold standard, CAM-ICU and ICDSC had sensitivities of 62 and 64%, specificities of 74 and 79%, and good inter-rater reliability (kappa 0.64 and 0.68), respectively. Both assessments had similar positive predictive values (63 vs 74%) and negative predictive values (70 vs 69%). Of note, the assessment of delirium with CAM-ICU and ICDSC assessments in the second study was done by pharmacists and then compared to the assessment of intensivists and psychiatrists. Although in clinical practice these assessments are traditionally completed by bedside nurses, the high inter-rater reliability again demonstrates the capability of a wide range of providers to administer these tests.

Overall there is a paucity of data describing delirium in the TBI population. The INSIGHT-ICU (Illuminating Neuropsychological dysfunction and Systemic Inflammatory mechanisms Gleaned after Hospitalization in Trauma-ICU Study, clinicaltrials.gov NCT03098459) [18] is an accruing prospective cohort of critically ill trauma patients, which will better define the impact of delirium in trauma ICU patients with and without TBI.

Hemorrhagic Stroke

Nontraumatic intracerebral hemorrhage, (ICH) or hemorrhagic stroke, affects approximately 100,000 new individuals per year in the USA [19]. The following studies show that delirium can be adequately assessed in individuals with nontraumatic ICH and that delirium after this form of PNI is associated with worse long-term outcomes.

In a 2013 study by Naidech et al., patients (*n* = 114) with nontraumatic hemorrhagic stroke in the ICU were assessed twice daily for delirium via the CAM-ICU by bedside nurses [20]. Delirium prevalence was 27%, and symptoms were nearly always hypoactive rather than hyperactive. The presence of delirium led to a statistically significant increase in both ICU and hospital length of stay even after controlling for patient age, benzodiazepine use, and admission National Institute of Health Stroke Scale (NIHSS). Delirium was also associated with worse quality of life, poor executive function, and decreased cognition at 1-year assessments even after adjusting for other factors. Of note, this population had lower reported baseline levels of dementia than other stroke populations.

In 2017, Rosenthal et al. examined another prospective cohort of patients with spontaneous nontraumatic ICH (*n* = 174), with 30% of patients developing delirium, as assessed twice daily by trained nursing staff using the CAM-ICU [21]. Patients with delirium had worse cognitive function and quality of life at 28-days and 1-year post-hospital discharge even after controlling for severity of neurologic injury, age, and time of assessment. There was no documented association between medication or infection and delirium. They also noted a close association of delirium with agitation (as assessed by the RASS) in this hemorrhagic stroke population and worse outcomes in those with documented delirium and agitation. This study, like others, excluded individuals with severe ICH as they were unable to be assessed due to coma.

Ischemic Stroke

There are approximately 700,000 individuals affected by cerebrovascular accident, or ischemic stroke, annually in the USA. Combined with the aforementioned ICH, stroke is the fifth leading cause of death in the USA [19]. Assessing delirium in this population has been documented in a larger number of studies than other PNI populations. Six studies documented an 11.8–43% prevalence of delirium in the ischemic stroke population (sometimes admixed with hemorrhagic stroke). A number of delirium risk factors were identified, including age, stroke severity, and certain stroke characteristics [22–27]. Delirium was also associated with worse outcomes in this stroke population [22, 24, 26].

In a 2011 study, patients admitted to a Netherlands stroke unit (n = 527) were assessed for delirium via CAM at two separate time points in the hospitalization, reporting an 11.8% overall prevalence [22]. Oldenbeuving et al. attributed the low delirium prevalence to the limited time frame for assessment (two time points vs multiple daily assessments) given that acute onset and fluctuating course is a hallmark delirium feature. Risk factors for delirium included pre-stroke cognitive decline, infection, higher NIHSS, and brain atrophy. Delirium was independently associated with higher length of stay and worse functional outcomes but not with mortality.

In a 2012 study by Kostalova et al., patients (*n* = 119) with either ischemic or hemorrhagic stroke admitted to an ICU were followed up to 1 week [23]. Daily delirium assessments were completed by trained professionals using DSM-IV criteria and CAM-ICU. Delirium prevalence was 43%, with 67% of cases within the first 24 h of poststroke admission. Onset of delirium occurred within the first 5 days of stroke onset, with a median duration of 5 days. Risk factors for delirium included increasing age, suspected or diagnosed pre-stroke dementia, lab markers associated with chronic alcoholism (elevated gamma-glutamyl transferase and thrombocytopenia), and increased severity of illness via metabolic derangements (hyponatremia, creatinine, hyperbilirubinemia). Stroke characteristics associated with increased delirium risk were hemorrhagic stroke, large ischemic volume (>40 cm^3), and large hemispheric infarctions (total anterior circulation infarction).

Also in 2012, Mitasova et al. reported a delirium prevalence of 24% with daily CAM-ICU assessment in patients with either ischemic or hemorrhagic stroke evaluated in the ICU for 1 week post-event ($n = 129$) [24]. As compared to the study era's DSM-IV gold standard, the CAM-ICU assessment in this population demonstrated high sensitivity and specificity (76% and 98%), accuracy (94%), and inter-rater reliability (kappa 0.94). Delirium in this poststroke population was independently associated with longer hospital length of stay, even after adjusting for other clinical factors (e.g., age, gender, prestrike dementia, NIHSS on admission, severity of illness score, aphasia). Patients with stroke and delirium had worse functional status than non-delirious stroke patients, but delirium was not an independent risk factor for mortality after adjusting for clinical characteristics.

In 2013, Lees et al. assessed patients ($n = 111$) with acute stroke for delirium at one time point between day 1 and 4 post admission to a dedicated stroke unit with a variety of screening tests [25]. This sample population, which excluded individuals with severe stroke, included a high prevalence of individuals with pre-stroke dementia (41%) as assessed by the Informant Questionnaire on Cognitive Decline in the Elderly (IQCODE) and high levels of cognitive impairment as assessed by Montreal Cognitive Assessment (MoCA), up to 85% using the most sensitive cutoff (MoCA <26). Using the CAM assessment as the reference standard, the 4AT test demonstrated high sensitivity (1.0, 95% CI [0.74–1.0]) and specificity (0.82, 95% CI [0.72–0.89]) for delirium detection. Abbreviated mental tests (AMT-10 and AMT-4) had lower sensitivity (0.75, 0.83) and specificity (0.61, 0.61) for delirium detection.

In a 2018 prospective cohort study, patients ($n = 261$) admitted with initial or recurrent ischemic stroke were assessed for delirium using CAM assessments at two different times during their first hospital week, with a reported 14.6% delirium prevalence [26]. Of note, Qu et al. excluded preexisting cognitive disorders such as dementia. Risk factors for delirium were increased age, higher NIHSS at admission, and prior stroke. Stroke-specific characteristics that were predictors of delirium included left cortical infarcts, larger infarct volume, and more severe medial temporal lobe atrophy – all of which are also associated with advanced age. A smaller number of patients with and without poststroke delirium were assessed at 3 and 6 months. Poststroke delirious patients ($n = 38$) showed trends toward worse functional outcomes, but this was not statistically significant likely due to small sample size.

A 2018 study by Pasinska et al. assessed patients ($n = 750$) admitted with ischemic or hemorrhagic stroke with the abbreviated CAM (bCAM) or CAM-ICU [27]. Prevalence of delirium was 27% with hypoactive and mixed subtype being the most common (41.9% and 39.9%, respectively), while a small number developed hyperactive delirium (15.3%). Independent risk factors for delirium that were identified included pre-stroke mental status, cumulative illness rating score, and admission cognitive dysfunction (MoCA score). Elevated white blood cell count and urinary tract infection during admission were risk factors for developing delirium. Of note, right-sided lesions were more suggestive of future delirium with a trend toward significance.

Discussion

A review of the literature emphasizes that delirium after PNI is a clinically relevant phenomenon and deserves further scientific inquiry. From the available studies, delirium after PNI likely has an impact on functional outcomes but with an unclear impact on mortality. The lack of association of delirium after PNI with survival may be related to the use of improved biostatistical techniques and covariate adjustment. Common risk factors that may potentiate delirium included pre-stroke dementia or functional impairment, age, medical comorbidities, degree of neurologic impairment after stroke (NIHSS scores), and certain anatomic areas of injury.

Individuals with PNI have a unique risk for delirium, as there are actual structural disturbances within the brain, compared to other critically ill populations without PNI. Several of these studies remarked on structural components as possible risk factors for delirium [21–23, 26, 27]. The larger prospective studies evaluating a post-stroke population, such as those by Qu et al. [26], Pasinska et al. [27], and Oldenbeuving et al. [22], were the most robust investigations on the structural components of poststroke delirium. Separately identified in these different studies, regions of the brain that have potentially increased delirium risk when injured include parahippocampal regions [21], anterior circulation strokes [22, 23], and both right [21, 22, 27] and left [26] hemisphere strokes. One explanation for these variable findings is that any larger insult may facilitate either profound language and cognitive deficits or visuospatial abnormalities, such as hemineglect that may either promote delirium and/or make it more difficult to diagnose in light of our current delirium assessment methods being dependent on language production, comprehension, and visuospatial reasoning. Kostalova et al. alluded to these suggestions and showed that the volume of brain injured correlated with risk of delirium development [23].

The primary structural insult in these patients, differing them from other critically ill cohorts, creates a perpetual confounder, as it can be unclear whether the clinical constellation we evaluate is a result of this underlying structural abnormality, as opposed to true secondary brain dysfunction of delirium caused by infectious, metabolic, and/or hypoxic reasons. As always, delirium must be a diagnosis of exclusion after other life-threatening PNI-related causes of altered mental status are considered (Fig. 8.1).

An important item to note in the assessment of delirium in PNI is the establishment of a "new baseline." This was explicitly mentioned in two works from the same group [23, 24] on the evaluation of patients with stroke. These patients were evaluated on admission for a "new baseline." This baseline was adjusted upward if their mental status improved to its pre-hospital state, but otherwise delirium was identified with fluctuations in mental status from this new post-PNI baseline, not from what is considered "normal" or pre-PNI.

Another important factor affecting the bedside assessment of delirium is the impact of aphasia or communication deficits after PNI. Mitasova et al. noted false-positive assessments of delirium with the CAM-ICU, as compared to DSM-IV, due to underlying global or receptive (i.e., Wernicke's) aphasia [24]. Assessment of delirium with bedside tests in this subset of patients must take into account the patient's ability to understand verbal or written instructions and respond to visual, auditory, or tactile stimuli. Further work is needed in this realm for better rapid delirium assessments in the aphasic or sensory-deprived PNI patient population.

Conclusion

The current literature on delirium after PNI is not as robust as that for other critically ill patients, but the emerging literature suggests similar findings to non-neurologically injured delirium cohorts hailing from medical and/or surgical ICUs. Delirium is measurable after PNI with reasonable test characteristics for a number of delirium assessment tools. After PNI, there is a significant impact of delirium on hospital and ICU length of stay, as well as cognitive and functional outcomes, but delirium's impact on mortality in PNI has yet to be properly established [14]. The best data are in poststroke delirium, with a significant paucity of large prospective studies in patients with TBI. The INSIGHT-ICU Study is an accruing prospective cohort that will better define the impact of delirium in a critically ill trauma cohort with and without TBI [18]. Further work needs to be done both on confirming the outcomes of delirium and potentially different subsets of risk factors in patients with PNI, as well as the development of delirium assessment methods tailored to patients with altered language processing and visuospatial deficits from their underlying brain injury.

Acknowledgment Federal sources include the National Institutes of Health R01 GM120484 and R01 AG058639 (Bethesda, MD).

References

1. Salluh JIF, Wang H, Schneider EB, Nagaraja N, Yenokyan G, Damluji A, et al. Outcome of delirium in critically ill patients: systematic review and meta-analysis. BMJ. 2015;350:h2538.
2. Pandharipande PP, Girard TD, Jackson JC, Morandi A, Thompson JL, Pun BT, et al. Long-term cognitive impairment after critical illness. N Engl J Med. 2013;369(14):1306–16.

3. Girard TD, Jackson JC, Pandharipande PP, Pun BT, Thompson JL, Shintani AK, et al. Delirium as a predictor of long-term cognitive impairment in survivors of critical illness. Crit Care Med. 2010;38(7):1513–20.
4. Mehta S, Cook D, Devlin JW, Skrobik Y, Meade M, Fergusson D, et al. Prevalence, risk factors, and outcomes of delirium in mechanically ventilated adults. Crit Care Med. 2015;43(3):557–66.
5. Zaal IJ, Devlin JW, Peelen LM, Slooter AJ. A systematic review of risk factors for delirium in the ICU. Crit Care Med. 2015;43(1):40–7.
6. Veliz-Reissmuller G, Aguero Torres H, van der Linden J, Lindblom D, Eriksdotter Jonhagen M. Pre-operative mild cognitive dysfunction predicts risk for postoperative delirium after elective cardiac surgery. Aging Clin Exp Res. 2007;19(3):172–7.
7. Vaurio LE, Sands LP, Wang Y, Mullen EA, Leung JM. Postoperative delirium: the importance of pain and pain management. Anesth Analg. 2006;102(4):1267–73.
8. Inouye SK, van Dyck CH, Alessi CA, Balkin S, Siegal AP, Horwitz RI. Clarifying confusion: the confusion assessment method. A new method for detection of delirium. Ann Intern Med. 1990;113(12):941–8.
9. Ely EW, Margolin R, Francis J, et al. Evaluation of delirium in critically ill patients: validation of the Confusion Assessment Method for the Intensive Care Unit (CAM-ICU). Crit Care Med. 2001;29(7):1370–9.
10. Bergeron N, Dubois MJ, Dumont M, et al. Intensive care delirium screening checklist: evaluation of a new screening tool. Intensive Care Med. 2001;27(5):859–64.
11. Tomasi CD, Grandi C, Salluh J, Soares M, Giombelli VR, Cascaes S, et al. Comparison of cam-Icu and Icdsc for the detection of delirium in critically ill patients focusing on relevant clinical outcomes. J Crit Care. 2012;27(2):212–7.
12. Bellelli G, Morandi A, Davis DH, Mazzola P, Turco R, Gentile S, et al. Validation of the 4at, a new instrument for rapid delirium screening: a study in 234 hospitalised older people. Age Ageing. 2014;43(4):496–502.
13. Shenkin SD, Fox C, Godfrey M, Siddiqi N, Goodacre S, Young J, et al. Protocol for validation of the 4AT, a rapid screening tool for delirium: a multicentre prospective diagnostic test accuracy study. BMJ Open. 2018;8(2):e015572.
14. Patel MB, Bednarik J, Lee P, Shehabi Y, Salluh JI, Slooter AJ, et al. Delirium monitoring in neurocritically ill patients: a systematic review. Crit Care Med. 2018;46(11):1832–41.
15. Roozenbeek B, Maas AIR, Menon DK. Changing patterns in the epidemiology of traumatic brain injury. Nat Rev Neurol. 2013;9(4):231–6.
16. Sherer M, Yablon SA, Nakase-Richardson R, Nick TG. Effect of severity of post-traumatic confusion and its constituent symptoms on outcome after traumatic brain injury. Arch Phys Med Rehabil. 2008;89(1):42–7.
17. Frenette AJ, Bebawi ER, Deslauriers LC, Tessier AA, Perreault MM, Delisle MS, et al. Validation and comparison of CAM-ICU and ICDSC in mild and moderate traumatic brain injury patients. Intensive Care Med. 2016;42(1):122–3.
18. Patel MB. Illuminating Neuropsychological Dysfunction and Systemic Inflammatory Mechanisms Gleaned after Hospitalization in Trauma-ICU Study (INSIGHT-ICU): ClinicalTrials.gov; Last Accessed 11/5/2018. Available from: https://clinicaltrials.gov/ct2/show/NCT03098459.
19. Benjamin EJ, Blaha MJ, Chiuve SE, Cushman M, Das SR, Deo R, et al. Heart disease and stroke statistics-2017 update: a report from the American Heart Association. Circulation. 2017;135(10):e146–603.
20. Naidech AM, Beaumont JL, Rosenberg NF, et al. Intracerebral hemorrhage and delirium symptoms: length of stay, function and quality of life in a 114-patient cohort. Am J Respir Crit Care Med. 2013;188(11):1331–7.
21. Rosenthal LJ, Francis BA, Beaumont JL, Cella D, Berman MD, Maas MB, et al. Agitation, delirium, and cognitive outcomes in intracerebral hemorrhage. Psychosomatics. 2017;58(1):19–27.
22. Oldenbeuving AW, de Kort PL, Jansen BP, Algra A, Kappelle LJ, Roks G. Delirium in the acute phase after stroke: incidence, risk factors, and outcome. Neurology. 2011;76(11):993–9.

23. Kostalova M, Bednarik J, Mitasova A, Dusek L, Michalcakova R, Kerkovsky M, et al. Towards a predictive model for poststroke delirium. Brain Inj. 2012;26(7–8):962–71.
24. Mitasova A, Kostalova M, Bednarik J, Michalcakova R, Kasparek T, Balabanova P, et al. Poststroke delirium incidence and outcomes: validation of the Confusion Assessment Method for the Intensive Care Unit (Cam-Icu). Crit Care Med. 2012;40(2):484–90.
25. Lees R, Corbet S, Johnston C, Moffitt E, Shaw G, Quinn TJ. Test accuracy of short screening tests for diagnosis of delirium or cognitive impairment in an acute stroke unit setting. Stroke. 2013;44(11):3078–83.
26. Qu J, Chen Y, Luo G, Zhong H, Xiao W, Yin H. Delirium in the acute phase of ischemic stroke: incidence, risk factors, and effects on functional outcome. J Stroke Cerebrovasc Dis. 2018;27(10):2641–7.
27. Pasinska P, Kowalska K, Klimiec E, Szyper-Maciejowska A, Wilk A, Klimkowicz-Mrowiec A. Frequency and predictors of poststroke delirium in Prospective Observational Polish Study (PROPOLIS). J Neurol. 2018;265(4):863–70.

Chapter 9
Neuroimaging Findings of Delirium

Robert Sanders and Paul Rowley

Introduction

The clinical significance of delirium may be contrasted with our limited understanding of its pathogenesis [1]. In particular, how the symptoms of delirium may arise so suddenly and severely, and yet then often dissipate days later, is perplexing. The lack of robust animal models that mimic the behavioral and cognitive changes in delirium further hampers our insights. This has led many groups to turn to neuroimaging as a tool to gain a greater understanding of the pathogenesis of delirium. Up front, it is important to acknowledge the limited gains that may be expected from this approach. Firstly, delirious patients are unlikely to cooperate with imaging (though hypoactive delirious patients may) [2]. Secondly, it is expensive, logistically complex, and occasionally unpleasant for the patient to undergo imaging, making this research hard to perform, often leading to limited sample sizes in imaging studies. Thirdly, delirium is a heterogeneous condition, and thus it is likely that it may be provoked by diverse pathological mechanisms, making imaging research more difficult again [3].

That said, providing insight into vulnerable brain regions in delirium or altered neuronal dynamics may illuminate the "black box" that is our understanding of delirium pathogenesis. Given the constraints above, research must proceed (at least initially) in a focused, hypothesis-driven manner. Recently the Cognitive Disintegration model [4] has been proposed wherein delirium is proposed to result from a breakdown in connectivity in higher order "cognitive" brain regions, such as

R. Sanders (✉) · P. Rowley
Department of Anesthesiology, University of Wisconsin School of Medicine and Public Health, Madison, WI, USA
e-mail: robert.sanders@wisc.edu; prowley@wisc.edu

C. G. Hughes et al. (eds.), *Delirium*, https://doi.org/10.1007/978-3-030-25751-4_9

frontoparietal networks like the default mode network [4]. As such prior to delirium, weakened connectivity in these networks could bring someone closer to a "delirium threshold" in connectivity making them more vulnerable to any subsequent precipitant for delirium. Some predisposing factors for delirium, for example, have been associated with impaired functional and structural connectivity, and delirium has been associated with impaired functional connectivity on electroencephalogram (EEG) monitoring. While the literature to date is perhaps inconclusive, neuroimaging research in delirium certainly warrants further study, especially when combined with clear hypotheses about the nature of the pathogenesis of delirium.

Materials and Methods

Search Strategy

A PubMed search using the terms "delirium, imaging" was performed on 28 November 2018 (Fig. 9.1). This query returned 548 results which were initially screened based on their titles and abstracts. Five hundred twenty-two publications were excluded from further evaluation if they were editorials, commentaries, reviews, case reports, or irrelevant. Studies deemed irrelevant included those investigating disorders other than delirium defined as an acute confusional state. The full texts of 50 publications were read and included if quantitative analytic or reliable

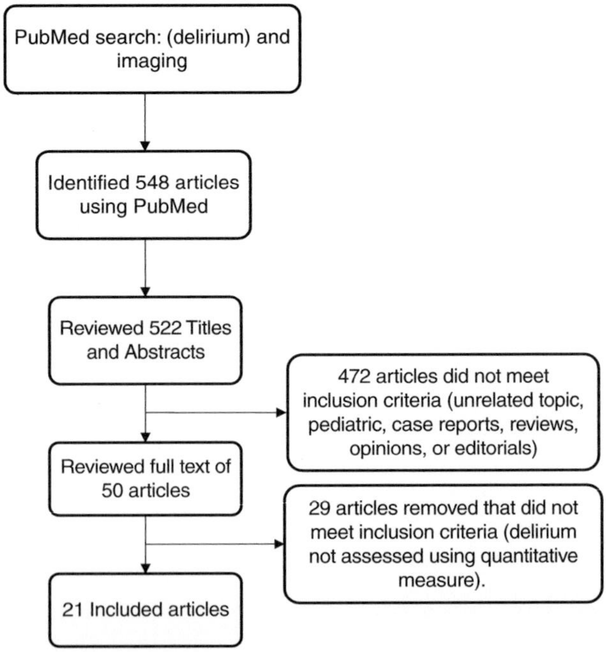

Fig. 9.1 Systematic review flow diagram

qualitative neuroimaging disease classification scales were reported. Twenty-one publications met all these criteria (Table 9.1).

Inclusion Criteria

Studies were considered for inclusion if (1) imaging modalities such as computerized tomography (CT), functional magnetic resonance imaging (fMRI), diffusion tensor imaging (DTI), or positron emission tomography (PET) were used, and (2) the study reported quantitative measures such as cerebral blood flow (CBF), diffusion metrics (e.g., fractional anisotropy [FA]), volumetric analyses (e.g., gray matter volume), glucose metabolism (e.g., standardized uptake value ratios [SUVR]), or measured brain pathology using reliable disease classification scales (e.g., Fazekas scale for characterizing white matter lesions [29]).

Outcome Measures

Studies included described delirium incidence and severity using at least one of the following delirium assessment methods: Confusion Assessment Method (CAM), Confusion Assessment Method Short Form (CAM-S), Confusion Assessment Method for the ICU (CAM-ICU), Delirium Rating Scale-Revised-98 (DRS-98), and/or Diagnostic and Statistical Manual for Mental Disorders (DSM-IV) criteria. Studies were included if delirium diagnosis was based on prospective diagnosis and/or validated methods for retrospective diagnosis of delirium by chart review [30, 31].

Associations Between Delirium and Cerebrovascular Pathology

We identified 12 studies that investigated associations between cerebrovascular pathology (e.g., white matter hyperintensity burden [WMHB], brain atrophy) and delirium.

A prospective study of delirium in 47 intensive care unit (ICU) patients (median age = 58 years) involved baseline cognitive assessments (IQCOD-SF), 1-year follow-up cognitive testing, and volumetric MRIs at discharge and 3 months after discharge [8]. This study found greater brain atrophy (as measured by a larger ventricle-to-brain ratio [VBR]) associated with delirium duration at discharge ($p = 0.03$). Longer duration of delirium was also correlated with smaller superior frontal lobe ($p = 0.03$) and hippocampal volumes ($p < 0.001$). Furthermore, worse cognitive performance on the RBANS battery at 1 year after discharge was

Table 9.1 Associated neuroimaging findings of delirium

Reference	Sample size (D+/n)	Methods (scan time point)	Outcome measures	Quantitative metric/ analytic method	Study conclusions
Yokoto et al. [5]	10/10 (100%)	Xe-CT in ICU patients during and after delirium	Delirium incidence (delirium assessment test not listed)	Regional CBF	Regional (cortical and subcortical) and global CBF significantly lower during delirium compared to after delirium resolved
Shioiri et al. [6]	19/116 (16%)	Presurgical DTI, pre-, peri-, and postoperative factors collected	Delirium severity (DRS-98)	FA/voxel-based analysis	Incidence of POD correlated with significantly lower FA in bilaterally widespread deep white matter and bilateral thalamus on preoperative scan
Choi et al. [7]	22*/44 (50%)	Resting-state fMRI during and after delirium *14/22 completed follow-up scans after delirium resolved	Incidence and severity of delirium (MDAS, DRS-98)	Cortical functional connectivity assessed using seed region of PCC and a priori subcortical regions related to Ach and DA	DLPFC activity and PCC activity were inversely related in control subjects but strongly correlated in delirious patients. Precuneus activity positively correlated with PCC in both groups, but more so in delirium, and the increment was associated with less severity and shorter duration of delirium
Gunther et al. [8]	33/47 (70%)	Baseline cognitive assessment (IQCODE-SF), volumetric brain MRI at discharge and 3-month follow-up	Delirium incidence (CAM-ICU), sedation level (RASS), cognitive performance (RBANS)	VBR, TBV, regional volumetric analysis based on a priori regional assignments	Increased duration of delirium associated with smaller brain volumes up to 3 months after discharge and smaller brain volumes associated with LTCI up to 12 months

Morandi et al. [9]	32/47 (68%)	DTI at discharge and 3 months follow-up	Delirium incidence and duration (CAM-ICU), pre-hospitalization cognitive assessment (IQCODE-SF), sedation level (RASS), cognitive performance (RBANS)	FA	Increased duration of delirium associated with decreased FA in the genu and splenium of corpus callosum and anterior limb of internal capsule at discharge
Root et al. [10]	23/47 (49%)	Retrospective analysis of preoperative structural MRI from 23 delirious patients to 24 age- and gender-matched control patients	Delirium assessments performed within 4 days postoperatively (delirium assessment test not listed)	Global WMHB, global CA	Delirium group exhibit greater WMHB, with advancing age being significantly associated with greater WMHB. (No significant difference in CA between groups)
Hatano et al. [11]	18/130 (14%)	Retrospective chart review of preoperative brain MRIs of patients undergoing cardiac surgery	Delirium incidence inferred by two psychiatrists reviewing medical charts using DSM-IV diagnostic criteria for delirium	WMH (Fazekas criteria)	WMH significantly higher in patients with delirium. Three independent predictors of delirium identified abnormal creatinine, severe WMH, and duration of surgery
Brown et al. [12]	28/79 (35%)	Postoperative brain MRI	Delirium assessed using a validated chart review method, preoperative neuropsychological testing	Validated method for grading WMH, ventricular size, and cerebral sulcal size; binary assessment of new ischemic lesions	In an unadjusted analysis, patients who developed POD had significantly higher ventricular size compared to patients without delirium
Omiya et al. [13]	55/80 (66%); 48/80 (60%) DRS between 1 and 7, 7/80 (9%) score DRS = 8	Preoperative (within 3 days) and postoperative (within 2 weeks) MRI and MR angiography (MRA)	Delirium incidence and severity (DRS-R98)	WMH (Fazekas criteria)	The presence of new deep subcortical white matter hyperintensities (DSWMH) following surgery was significantly associated with POD

(continued)

Table 9.1 (continued)

Reference	Sample size (D+/n)	Methods (scan time point)	Outcome measures	Quantitative metric/ analytic method	Study conclusions
Cavallari et al. [14]	32/146 (22%)	Preoperative brain MRI (1 month before surgery), baseline cognitive assessment (SF-12, 3MS, CAM, GDS, and multipart cognitive battery) 2 weeks before surgery	POD incidence (CAM and chart review) and delirium severity (CAM-S) during hospital stay	WMH volume (WM pathology), BPV (brain atrophy), hippocampal volume (regional atrophy)	No statistically significant differences in WMH, whole brain, or hippocampal volume between delirious and non-delirious groups. No statistically significant association between any MRI measure and delirium incidence or severity
Naidech et al. [15]	25/89 (28%)	CT	Delirium incidence (CAM-ICU)	Hematoma volume and location (voxel-wise analysis)	Patients with hematoma in the right parahippocampal gyrus, right anterior SLF, and right posterior SLF were significantly associated with the delirium group
Cavallari et al. [16]	29/136 (21%)	Presurgical DTI (median = 7 days before surgery)	POD incidence (CAM and chart review) and delirium severity (CAM-S long form) during hospital stay	DTI metrics (AD, FA, MD, RD)	Presurgical diffusion tensor imaging abnormalities of the cerebellum, cingulum, corpus callosum, internal capsule, thalamus, basal forebrain, occipital, parietal, and temporal lobes, including the hippocampus, were associated with delirium incidence and severity, after adjusting for covariates. After further controlling for general cognitive performance, diffusion tensor imaging abnormalities of the cerebellum, hippocampus, thalamus, and basal forebrain remained associated with delirium incidence and severity

Hshieh et al. [17]	32/146 (22%)	Preoperative brain MRI (1 month before surgery), baseline cognitive assessment (SF-12, 3MS, CAM, GDS, and multipart cognitive battery) 2 weeks before surgery	POD incidence (CAM and chart review) and delirium severity (CAM-S) during hospital stay	Whole-brain and globally normalized voxel-wise analysis of CBF	No significant association between CBF measures with delirium incidence or severity in both unadjusted and adjusted analyses. CBF globally and regionally (notably precuneus and posterior cingulate) was correlated with performance on several neuropsychological tests
Shioiri et al. [18]	19/116 (16%)	Presurgical MRI, pre-, peri-, and postoperative factors collected	Delirium severity (DRS-98)	Gray matter volume, evaluated as a fraction (%) of the total ICV	Delirium patients displayed a significant reduction in gray matter volume in the define gyri of the temporal and limbic lobes. A receiver operating characteristic curve revealed the gyri of the temporal lobe to display moderate value (>0.8) in predicting POD
Haggstrom et al. [19]	13/13 (100%)	FDG-PET during delirium (13/13) and post-delirium (6/13)	CAM	Cerebral glucose metabolism	Glucose metabolism was significantly higher post-delirium in the whole brain and bilateral PCC compared to during delirium
Cavallari et al. [20]	25/113 (22%)	Presurgical DTI (median = 7 days) and 1-year postoperative DTI (median = 378 days)	POD incidence (CAM and chart review) and delirium severity (CAM-S)	DTI metrics (FA, MD)	Positive association between GCP changes over 1 year and FA changes, and a negative association with MD changes, predominantly in the posterior temporal, parietal, and occipital white matter

(continued)

Table 9.1 (continued)

Reference	Sample size (D+/n)	Methods (scan time point)	Outcome measures	Quantitative metric/ analytic method	Study conclusions
Rolandi et al. [21]	5/11 (45%)	Postoperative PET (^{18}F-Flutematamol), DTI and rs-fMRI	POD assessed daily for 3 days after surgery using CAM and chart review	GM atrophy, WMH volumes, DTI metrics (AD, FA, MD, RD), DMN functional connectivity	5/5 (100%) POD+ were amyloid negative, while 6/11 (54%) POD- were amyloid positive. POD+ compared to POD- displayed significantly lower gray matter volumes in amygdala, middle temporal gyrus, and ACC, increased diffusivity in the genu of corpus callosum and anterior corona radiata, and higher functional connectivity within the Default Mode Network (DMN) (i.e., R and L superior parietal cortex)
Detweiler et al. [22]	100/200 (50%)	CT	Delirium diagnosis (retrospective chart review for ICD-IX code for delirium during hospitalization, later verified using DSM-IV criteria)	White matter lesions (WML), atrophy, intracranial extravascular calcifications	Patients with delirium were found to have significantly more WMLs in the periventricular temporal lobe, subcortical temporal lobe, globus pallidus, putamen, and internal capsule. Atrophy in the parietal lobes and cerebellum was significantly associated with the delirium group
Kyeong et al. [23]	34/72 (47%)	rs-fMRI	Severity of delirium assessed using Korean version of the Delirium Rating Scale-Revised-98 (KDRS), KDRS sleep-wake cycle disturbances, and MMSE	Correlation analysis between SCN and regions associations between FC strengths	Resting-state functional connectivity between the suprachiasmatic nucleus (SCN) and right cerebellum was significantly decreased in delirious patients compared to non-delirium group

Matano et al. [24]	29/200 (13%)	MRI on admission to neuro ICU	Intensive care delirium screening checklist	Global WMH (Fazekas criteria)	Patients with severe white matter disease (per Fazekas criteria) were significantly more likely to become delirious than those without severe white matter disease
Racine et al. [25]	32/145 (22%)	Preoperative MRI	Delirium incidence (CAM), delirium severity (CAM-S), cognitive function (GCP)	Regional cortical thickness	Patients who developed delirium displayed significantly thinner superior parietal cortex than patients who did not develop delirium. Among patients who developed delirium, delirium severity was predicted by a significant reduction in cortical thickness of the middle frontal gyrus, superior frontal gyrus, supramarginal gyrus, and superior parietal cortex
van Montfort et al. [26]	*22/44 (50%)	rs-fMRI *Of 22 patients in delirium cohort, only 16 imaging exams were acquired. Of these 16 patients, 9 were imaged while delirious and 7 imaged post-delirium	Diagnosis of delirium based on DSM-IV, delirium severity assessed by DRS-R-98, delirium duration based on days	Global and regional network analysis	Connectivity strength was significantly decreased in the post-delirium group compared to control and delirium group. Longer diameter and lower leaf fraction were found during delirium compared to control. Betweenness centrality of left anterior cingulum and right palladium was lower in the post-delirium group compared to control. Betweenness centrality of the orbital part of the right middle frontal gyrus, right medial orbitofrontal cortex, and left anterior cingulate was lower in the delirium group compared to the post-delirium group

(continued)

Table 9.1 (continued)

Reference	Sample size (D+/n)	Methods (scan time point)	Outcome measures	Quantitative metric/ analytic method	Study conclusions
Qu et al. [27]	38/261 (15%)	Neurologic deficit assessment (National Institutes of Health Stroke Scale (NIHSS)) on admission, MRI	Delirium incidence (CAM) and delirium severity (DRS-98) during 1st week after admission for acute ischemic stroke	Regional infarction (ROI area measurement), WML (Fazekas criteria), medial temporal lobe atrophy (MTLA) (Scheltens' scale)	Univariate analysis revealed patients with poststroke delirium (PSD) displayed significantly greater infarct volume and MTLA than patients without PSD. Multivariate logistic regression of risk factors for PSD found prior stroke and L-cortical infarction to be significantly associated with patients with PSD
Hijazi et al. [28]	1653/32,725 (5%)	CT, MRI –457/1653 (28%) D+ CT only –10/1653 (1%) D+ MRI only –71/1653 (4%) CT and MRI –1115 (75%) no imaging	Retrospective chart review (ICD-10)	Pathological changes on radiology report noting at least one finding from a set of 10 a priori selected diseases considered "positive" as possible delirium etiology	11% of CT brain scans from delirious patients were positive; diagnoses included hemorrhage ($n = 23$), infarct ($n = 18$), suspected neoplasm ($n = 15$), and posterior reversible encephalopathy syndrome ($n = 1$)

Postoperative delirium (POD), Xenon-enhanced computed tomography (Xe-CT), intensive care unit (ICU), cerebral blood flow (CBF), diffusion tensor imaging (DTI), Delirium Rating Scale-Revised-98 (DRS-R98), fractional anisotropy (FA), functional magnetic resonance imaging (fMRI), Memorial Delirium Assessment Scale (MDAS), posterior cingulate cortex (PCC), acetylcholine (ACh), dopamine (DA), dorsolateral prefrontal cortex (DFC), Short Informant Questionnaire on Cognitive Decline in the Elderly (IQCODE-SF), Confusional Assessment Method (CAM), Repeatable Battery for the Assessment of Neuropsychological Status (RBANS), ventricle-to-brain ratio (VBR), total brain volume (TBV), long-term cognitive impairment (LTCI), white matter hyperintensity burden (WMHB), cerebral atrophy (CA), The Fourth Edition of the *Diagnostic and Statistical Manual of Mental Disorders* (DSM-IV), Short Form 12 (SF-12), Modified Mini-Mental State Examination (MMSE), Geriatrics Depression Scale (GDS), Cognitive Assessment Method Severity (CAM-S), general cognitive performance (GCP), brain parenchymal volume (BPV), axial diffusivity (AD), mean diffusivity (MD), radial diffusivity (RD), arterial spin labelling (ASL), intracranial volume (ICV), default mode network (DMN), resting-state functional MRI (rs-fMRI), MR angiography (MRA) associated with greater brain atrophy (i.e., VBR) at 3 months after discharge ($p = 0.04$). Analysis of volumetric brain MRIs acquired 3 months after discharge compared to imaging at 1 year follow-up found smaller frontal lobe, thalamic, and cerebellar volumes at 3 months associated with worse performance on executive function and visual attention assessments at 12 months after discharge. Associations between brain volumes and cognitive outcomes (global RBANS score, memory, executive functioning, attention and concentration, visual spatial construction, and language) were adjusted for age at study enrollment and presence of sepsis at any time during ICU stay; however, analyses were not corrected for multiple comparisons.

A retrospective analysis of preoperative brain MRIs from 130 cardiac surgery patients (mean age = 66.9 years) found white matter hyperintensity burden (WMHB) in the 18 patients (14%) who developed delirium was significantly greater than in those without delirium ($p = 0.03$) [11]. Relative to patients without delirium, patients who developed postoperative delirium (POD) were also found to have a significantly greater proportion of severe periventricular white matter disease (Fazekas score 3) ($p = 0.04$). Multiple logistic regression analysis additionally identified severe deep WMH (Fazekas score 3) (odds ratio (OR) 3.9, $p = 0.02$), abnormal creatinine level (creatinine >1.1 mg/dL) (OR 4.5, $p = 0.01$), and duration of surgery (OR 1.4, $p = 0.02$) as independent predictors of delirium.

A retrospective analysis of preoperative brain MRIs from 47 age- and gender-matched patients (23 delirious, 23 not delirious, mean = 74 years) who had surgical resection of non-small cell cancer found patients who developed POD displayed greater presurgical global WMHB ($p = 0.017$) than patients without delirium [10]. WMHB was calculated as the ratio of WMH to total intracranial volume, whereas cerebral atrophy was calculated by percent cerebrospinal fluid (CSF) as a fraction of intracranial volume (ICV). While this study found greater WMHB associated with advanced aging ($p = 0.002$), it did not find a significant difference in cerebral atrophy between delirious patients and those without delirium. Advanced aging for all patients was significantly associated with cerebral atrophy ($p = 0.007$).

A prospective study involving 116 cardiac surgical patients (mean age = 64.3 years) reported a significant reduction in temporal and limbic gray matter volume in the 16% (19/116) of patients who developed POD relative to 65 age-controlled non-delirium patients [18]. Delirium was diagnosed using DSM-IV criteria. Delirium severity was quantified using the DRS-98 score. Brain volumes were calculated using automatic atlas-based and voxel-based morphometry. Relative to patients without delirium, the delirium cohort demonstrated significant reductions in gray matter volume in the temporal transverse gyrus ($F = 13.615$, $p < 0.0036$), middle temporal gyrus ($F = 14.033$, $p < 0.0036$), fusiform gyrus ($F = 18.424$, $p < 0.0036$), and hippocampus ($F = 9.539$, $p < 0.0036$). There was no significant decrease in global white matter volume among patients with delirium. A receiver operating characteristic (ROC) analysis revealed atrophy of the fusiform gyrus, middle temporal gyrus, and limbic lobe to be moderately predictive of POD ([AUC = 0.824, $p < 0.001$], [AUC = 0.813, $p < 0.001$], [AUC = 0.764. $p < 0.001$], respectively). Linear regression analysis found weak, albeit statistically significant correlations between age of the non-delirium group and associated gray matter volumes for the fusiform gyrus ($r = 0.316$, $p = 0.010$) and middle temporal gyrus ($r = 0.378$, $p = 0.002$). In a similar analysis for the delirium group, linear regression analysis found a statistically significant correlation between age and middle temporal gyrus volume reduction ($r = 0.516$, $p = 0.024$).

A prospective cohort study of 88 patients undergoing elective off-pump coronary artery bypass (OPCAB) reported 66% (55/80) of patients developed POD [13]. Postoperative brain MRI revealed 7.9% (7/88) of patients had new ischemic lesions that were not present on preoperative brain MRI. Multivariate logistic regression analysis found new ischemic lesions (OR 11.07, 95% confidence interval [CI] = 1.53–80.03; $p = 0.017$) and deep subcortical WMH (OR 3.04, 95% CI = 1.14–8.12; $p = 0.027$) were significantly associated with POD.

A retrospective chart review study examining the association of brain MRI characteristics and POD in cardiac surgery patients reported a delirium prevalence of 35.4% (28/79) [12]. An unadjusted analysis found patients who developed POD had significantly higher ventricular size compared to patients who did not develop delirium ($p = 0.002$).

An analysis from a subsample of the Successful Aging after Elective Surgery (SAGES) study found that in 146 elderly patients (≥70 years) without dementia, there was no statistically significant difference in WMHB ($p = 0.710$), brain atrophy ($p = 0.334$), and hippocampal atrophy ($p = 0.862$) between the 22% (32/146) of patients who developed POD and those who did not (114/146) [14]. All patients completed baseline cognitive testing within 2 weeks prior to surgery. Incidence and severity of delirium were measured by either CAM alone (0/32), a validated chart review method (9/32), or both (23/32). Presurgical MRI indices of brain damage, which included WMHB (by proxy of white matter hyperintensity volume), brain atrophy (by proxy of brain parenchymal volume [BPV]), and hippocampal volume, were found to have no significant impact on POD incidence; this lack of effect was robust in both an unadjusted and adjusted regression model which included the following covariates: intracranial cavity volume (ICV), age, gender, global cognitive performance (GCP), and vascular comorbidity. However, there was an effect of presurgical MRI indices (WMH volume, brain atrophy, and hippocampal) on delirium severity (as measured by CAM-S test Long Form); in the fully adjusted model, white matter hyperintensity volume was found to be significantly reduced in the delirium group ($p = 0.045$).

A prospective study of 90 patients with intracerebral hemorrhage used voxel-based lesion-symptom mapping with acute CT to identify hematoma locations associated with delirium symptoms ($N = 89$ patients included in analysis) [15]. Delirium was assessed using CAM-ICU and occurred in 28% (25/89) of patients. Patients with hematoma in the right parahippocampal gyrus, right anterior superior longitudinal fasciculus (SLF), and right posterior SLF were significantly associated with the delirium group. Based on the results of voxel-based lesion-symptom mapping analysis, hematoma locations were treated as regions of interest (ROI) to assess the increased likelihood of delirium symptoms given hematoma location. The investigators found hematoma within the ROI increased relative risk for delirium by 6.8

(95% CI = 2.7–17.0, $Z = 4.1$, $P < 0.0001$; OR 13.0, 95% CI = 3.9–43.3, $Z = 4.2$, $P < 0.0001$). Relative risk for hematoma within separate ROIs was calculated and found statistically significant associations for each region: parahippocampal gyrus relative risk = 7.8, 95% CI = 1.7–36.1, $Z = 2.6$, $P = 0.009$; posterior white matter relative risk = 6.9, 95% CI = 2.0–24.1, $Z = 3.1$, $P = 0.002$; and anterior white matter relative risk = 6.5, 95% CI = 1.5–28.6, $Z = 2.5$, $P = 0.01$.

A case-control retrospective chart review of $n = 200$ military veterans (100 delirious, 100 age-, sex-, race-matched controls) examined the association of white matter lesions (WML), cerebral atrophy, intracranial extravascular calcifications, and ventricular-communicating hydrocephalus discovered on CT with delirium [22]. Patients with delirium were found to have significantly more WMLs in the periventricular temporal lobe, subcortical temporal lobe, globus pallidus, putamen, and internal capsule ($p = 0.001$, $p = 0.038$, $p = 0.036$, $p = 0.005$, $p = 0.019$, respectively). Logistic regression for various sizes of WML in brain areas in military veterans with and without delirium revealed significant associations between temporal periventricular WML of <1 cm, 1–2 cm, and >2 cm and delirium occurrence ([OR 20.1, $p = 0.024$], [OR 30.7, $p = 0.009$], [OR 120.9, $p = 0.018$], respectively). Military veterans with WML less than 1 cm in the globus pallidus, putamen, and internal capsule were also significantly associated with the delirium group ([OR 0.005, $p = 0.039$], [OR 00.3, $p = 0.002$], [OR 00.4, $p = 0.010$]). There was also a significant association between parietal and cerebellar atrophy and delirium occurrence among military veterans ($p = 0.044$, $p = 0.041$, respectively).

A prospective study examining environmental and clinical risk factors for delirium in a neurosurgical center reported a delirium incidence of 13.2% (29/200) [24]. MRI on admission to the neurological intensive care unit and global WMH was assessed using Fazekas criteria; univariate analysis revealed patients with severe white matter disease were significantly more likely to become delirious than those without severe white matter disease (OR 7.826, $p = 0.0001$). Additionally, the univariate analysis showed patients diagnosed with subarachnoid hemorrhage on admission were also significantly more likely to become delirious than patients without subarachnoid hemorrhage (OR 4.933, $p = 0.0293$).

As a sub-analysis of the Successful Aging after Elective Surgery (SAGES) study, an investigation into the association between Alzheimer's-related cortical atrophy and POD reported a delirium incidence of 22% (32/145) in a population of elderly patients without dementia who underwent elective surgery [25]. There was no significant association between preoperative MRI estimates of cortical thickness within a set of nine regions associated with Alzheimer's disease (termed the "AD signature") and delirium incidence. However patients who developed delirium were found to have significantly thinner superior parietal cortex than patients without delirium ($p = 0.018$) at baseline. Among patients who developed delirium, delirium severity was predicted by a significant reduction in cortical thickness of the middle frontal gyrus, superior frontal gyrus, supra marginal gyrus, and superior parietal cortex ($p = 0.028$, $p = 0.011$, $p = 0.012$, $p = 0.004$, respectively).

Delirium occurred in 14.6% (38/261) of patients enrolled in a prospective cohort study assessing the incidence of and risk factors for delirium following acute ischemic stroke [27]. A univariate analysis of MRI data acquired within 7 days of admission revealed patients with poststroke delirium (PSD) displayed significantly greater infarct volume and medial temporal lobe atrophy than patients without PSD ($p < 0.001$, $p < 0.001$, respectively). Furthermore, multivariate logistic regression analysis of risk factors for PSD revealed patients with previous stroke and left cortical infarct were significantly more likely to develop delirium than patients without either risk factor ($p = 0.006$, $p = 0.001$).

Cerebrovascular pathology, such as age-related atrophy, white matter disease, and ischemic lesions, is common among patients with delirium and seem to cluster in regions critical to memory and attention. However, the evidence does not point to a discrete pattern of vascular brain lesions to reliably predict or retrospectively explain delirium.

Association Between Delirium and Cerebral Blood Flow

In a study of ten ICU patients (mean age = 47.5 years) diagnosed with hypoactive delirium [2], regional cerebral blood flow (rCBF) was measured using xenon-enhanced computer tomography (Xe-CT) during delirium and after delirium resolved [5]. Global cerebral blood flow (CBF) was significantly decreased during delirium compared to after delirium resolved ($p = 0.0056$). Cortical CBF was also significantly decreased during delirium across all reported regions. The most significant decreases in cortical CBF occurred in bilateral frontal ($p = 0.0010$) and right frontal regions ($p = 0.007$). Subcortical CBF was also significantly diminished during delirium with the most significant decreases observed in the left lenticular nucleus ($p = 0.0038$), left thalamus ($p = 0.0044$), and bilateral thalami ($p = 0.0045$).

A study demonstrated cerebral blood flow MRI in the nondemented elderly is not predictive of POD but is correlated with cognitive performance [17]. Preoperative brain MRIs from 146 patients (ages ≥70 years) were acquired within 1 month of surgery, and baseline cognitive assessments were performed within 2 weeks prior to surgery. Twenty-two percent (32/146) of patients were prospectively diagnosed with delirium based on confusional assessment method (CAM) alone (0/32), retrospectively based on chart review (9/32), or both (23/32). Delirium severity was prospectively measured during hospital stay using the CAM short form (CAM-S). This study found no significant association between voxel-wise cerebral blood flow measures with delirium incidence or severity. This negative finding was robust in follow-up analyses which included other covariates such as vascular comorbidities and years of education. Positive associations were however found between CBF of the posterior cingulate and precuneus and baseline performance on cognitive tests such as the Hopkins Verbal Learning Test Total Recall (HVLT-R Total Recall), Visual Search and Attention Test (VSAT), and the general cognitive performance measure (GCP). Thus, differences in cerebral blood flow before delirium do not seem to predispose to delirium, but studies suggest that CBF may be reduced during delirium.

Associations Between Delirium and Impaired Functional Connectivity

We identified several studies which investigated impaired functional connectivity (FC) in delirium.

In a case-control functional MRI (fMRI) study, 22 actively delirious patients (mean age = 73.6 years) and 22 age-matched comparison patients received resting-state fMRI scans [7]. Of the 22 delirious patients, 14 completed follow-up scans after delirium resolved. Functional connectivity was assessed by seeding the posterior cingulate cortex (PCC) and measuring FC between the PCC seed and "a priori subcortical regions related to acetylcholine and dopamine." Differences in FC were assessed between 18 of the 20 initial scans (2 excluded due to head movement) and 13 follow-up scans in the delirium group. Follow-up scans were acquired an average of 5.8 days after the initial scan. FC differences between the 18/20 of the delirious and 20 comparison patient scans were also evaluated. The investigators reported that fMRI data from comparison subjects revealed inversely correlated activity between the PCC and the dorsolateral prefrontal cortex bilaterally. Actively delirious patients (also referred to as "during-episode patients") showed a positive correlation between these two regions as well as the left inferior frontal gyrus and precuneus bilaterally. Data acquired from actively delirious patients also showed significantly decreased connectivity between the PCC and left cerebellum compared to the comparison group ($T_{max} = -5.333$). Patients who had previously been delirious showed no correlation with any dorsolateral prefrontal cortex region on fMRI scans acquired after delirium resolved.

Analyses of FC strengths between subcortical regions revealed similar patterns of positively correlated activity between regions in control patients and post-resolution delirium patients. Actively delirious patients, however, lacked significantly correlated FC between several pairs of regions. These pairs of regions include the intralaminar thalamic nuclei and nucleus basalis ($p = 0.888$), the intralaminar thalamic nuclei and ventral tegmental area ($p = 0.103$), the caudate and mesencephalic tegmentum ($p = 0.225$), and the caudate and nucleus basalis ($p = 0.065$). Relative to comparison subjects, during-episode patients had reduced correlation between the intralaminar thalamic nuclei and the mesencephalic tegmentum, nucleus basalis, and ventral tegmental area. Decreased correlation coefficients for connections of the mesencephalic tegmentum with the ventral tegmentum area were also detected ($p = 0.049$) in during-episode patients relative to comparison subjects.

Greater FC between the bilateral precuneus and PCC in during-episode patients was correlated with delirium severity, as measured by Memorial Delirium Assessment Scale (MDAS) (left precuneus $r = -0.47$, $p < 0.05$; right precuneus $r = -0.58$, $p < 0.01$). This FC association with delirium was also detected when delirium severity was measured by the Delirium Rating Scale-Revised-98 (left precuneus = -0.58, $p < 0.01$; right precuneus $r = -0.62$, $p < 0.01$). Delirium duration was negatively correlated with the increased FC between PCC and bilateral precuneus (left precuneus $r = -0.80$, $p < 0.01$; right precuneus $r = -0.66$, $p < 0.05$).

Resting-state functional MRI was collected from 34 delirious patients and 38 non-delirious controls to assess differences in FC of the circadian clock and neural substrates of sleep-wake disturbances in delirium [23]. Seed-based connectivity of the suprachiasmatic nucleus (SCN) was compared between groups. Analysis of the FC data found connectivity between the SCN and right cerebellum was significantly decreased in delirious patients compared to controls without delirium ($p = 0.02$).

In a study investigating network disintegration during delirium, resting-state functional MRI were collected from 22 delirious and 22 age- and sex-matched non-delirious controls [26]. Controls were also matched on degree of white matter hyperintensity burden. Of the 22 patients in the delirium cohort, imaging exams were acquired from 16 patients. Of these 16 imaging exams, 9 were acquired from delirious patients, whereas 7 were collected from patients after delirium resolution. Global network analysis revealed connectivity strength was significantly reduced in the post-delirium group (M 0.16, SD 0.01) compared to the control group (M 0.19, SD 0.02) with a difference of −0.04 (95% CI −0.05, −0.02, corrected $p = 0.001$) and compared to the delirium group (M 0.17, SD 0.03) with a difference of −0.02 (95% CI −0.02–0.00, corrected $p = 0.027$). Diameter, a measure of the efficiency of global network organization, was significantly increased during delirium (M 0.03, SD 0.05) compared to the control group (M 0.28, SD 0.04) with a difference of 0.04 (95% CI −0.01–0.08, corrected $p = 0.024$). Leaf fraction reflects the extent to which the network has central, integrated organization and was found to be significantly decreased during delirium (M 0.32, SD 0.03) compared to control group (M 0.35, SD 0.03), with a difference of −0.02 (95% CI −0.04–0.02, corrected $p = 0.027$). There were significant negative correlations between delirium duration and leaf fraction (rho = −0.73, $p = 0.039$) and between delirium duration and tree hierarchy (rho = −0.92, $p = 0.001$). Analysis of regional measures by degree, an indication of the importance of a node in the network, found the degree of right posterior cingulate cortex was lower in the delirium group compared to the control group (corrected $p = 0.039$). Betweenness centrality is defined as the fraction of shortest paths that pass through a particular node and was found to be lower in the right inferior temporal gyrus in the delirium group compared to the control group (corrected $p = 0.004$). There was decreased betweenness centrality of the orbital part of the right middle frontal gyrus, right medial orbitofrontal cortex, and left anterior cingulate in the delirium group compared to the post-delirium group (corrected $p = 0.030$, corrected $p = 0.016$, corrected $p = 0.031$, respectively).

Disturbances in functional connectivity during and after episodes of delirium are observed in the limited set of functional imaging studies on delirium. In particular, breakdown in short- and long-range connections, especially those involving the posterior cingulate cortex (PCC), appears to be a common feature of delirium.

Associations Between Delirium and White Matter Integrity

Five studies used diffusion tensor imaging (DTI) to examine white matter tract characteristics associated with delirium. A study of 116 surgical patients (mean age 64.3 years) reported 19 of the 116 patients (16.4%) were delirious [6]. Of these 19 patients with delirium, 18 (94.7%) were older than 60 years. Voxel-wise analysis of preoperative DTI brain scans revealed a significantly increased incidence of POD in individuals with lower fractional anisotropy (FA) in widespread deep white matter structures bilaterally, bilateral thalamus, and corpus callosum compared to non-delirious patients ($p < 0.001$ uncorrected). When the analysis was adjusted for age, a significant decrease in FA was only detected in the left frontal lobe white matter and left thalamus when compared to the non-delirium group.

A two-center, prospective cohort study used DTI to examine the relationship between delirium duration, white matter integrity, and cognitive impairment in 47 ICU survivors (median age 58 years) [9]. Patients were scanned at discharge and at 3 months follow-up. Increased duration of delirium (3 vs 0 days) was associated with decreased FA in the genu (−0.02; $p = 0.04$) and splenium (−0.01; $p = 0.02$) of corpus callosum and anterior limb of internal capsule (−0.02; $p = 0.01$) at discharge. Neuroimaging at 3 months after discharge demonstrated persistent reductions for the genu (−0.02; $p = 0.02$) and splenium (−0.01; $p = 0.004$).

In another DTI study, presurgical diffusion MRIs were collected from 136 elderly patients (≥70 years). Twenty-one percent (29/136) of these patients developed POD [16]. POD diagnosis was made prospectively using the confusional assessment method (CAM) (24/29) or retrospectively based on chart review (5/29). After adjusting for variables such as age, gender, and vascular comorbidity, abnormalities in white matter tracts (as indicated by decreased fractional anisotropy (FA), increased axial diffusivity (AD), increased mean diffusivity (MD), and increased radial diffusivity (RD)) were positively associated with delirium incidence and severity across several brain regions. FA in the cingulum and corpus callosum was significantly decreased in the delirious group compared to patients without delirium ($p = 0.002$, $p = 0.002$, respectively). Delirious patients were found to have significantly greater AD in corpus callosum ($p = 0.004$) and right temporal lobe ($p = 0.015$) compared to patients without delirium. MD was significantly increased in delirious patients in the cingulum ($p = 0.008$), left frontal lobe ($p = 0.013$), left cerebellum ($p = 0.002$), and right parietal lobe ($p = 0.001$). Compared to patients without delirium, delirious patients were found to have significantly increased RD in the cingulum ($p = 0.001$), frontal lobe ($p = 0.006$), and left and right cerebellum ($p = 0.001$, $p = 0.001$).

An additional analysis of a subset of the Successful Aging after Elective Surgery (SAGES) study examined longitudinal diffusion changes in a cohort of older adults (≥70 years) without dementia who underwent elective surgery [20]. Postoperative delirium occurred in 22% (25/113) of participants who had DTI before and 1 year after surgery. Multiple linear regression analysis adjusted for age, sex, education, and baseline general cognitive performance (GCP) found a positive association between changes in GCP over 1 year and reductions in FA and increases in MD, predominantly in the posterior temporal, parietal, and occipital white matter ($p = 0.02$).

A retrospective chart review investigating CT and MRI findings among hospitalized patients identified delirium occurrence in 5% (1653/32,725, median age = 80 years, IQR 71–86, 54% male) of the study population [28]. Within the cohort of delirious patients who had cerebral imaging (538/1653, 33%), 11% ($n = 57$) of CT brain scans most commonly showed evidence of hemorrhage ($n = 23$), followed by infarct ($n = 18$), suspected neoplasm ($n = 15$), and posterior reversible encephalopathy ($n = 1$). Brain MRI was completed in 17 delirious patients with evidence of pathologic changes on brain CT (17/57); in two cases of suspected neoplasm based on CT, diagnoses were changed after brain MRI to an abscess and an infarct.

Diffusion tensor imaging studies of delirium have shown patients with delirium often demonstrate decreased white matter integrity within the prefrontal cortex, cingulum, and corpus callosum. Nevertheless, future studies are needed to clarify the relationship between DTI measures and delirium pathogenesis.

Associations Between Delirium and Amyloid Positron Emission Tomography

We identified two studies that center on positron emission tomography (PET) imaging findings associated with delirium.

A multimodal imaging study used ^{18}F-Flutemetamol PET, DTI, and resting state functional MRI to investigate the association of POD with markers of neurodegeneration and brain amyloidosis [21]. The study found 45% (5/11) of patients developed POD. All delirious patients in this study were amyloid negative, and 54% (6/11) patients without delirium displayed brain amyloid positivity. Compared to patients without delirium, patients who developed POD displayed significantly lower gray matter volumes in the amygdala ($p = 0.003$) and in the middle temporal gyrus and in the anterior cingulate cortex ($p < 0.001$) and increased diffusivity in the genu of the corpus callosum and in the anterior corona radiata ($p < 0.05$). Analysis of functional connectivity data revealed high functional connectivity within the default mode network, particularly in the right and left superior parietal cortex, in the patients without delirium compared to those with delirium. Voxel-wise tract-based analysis showed no significant difference between groups in FA; however, POD patients were found to have higher mean, axial, and radial diffusivity in the genu of corpus callosum and anterior corona radiata compared to patients without delirium.

One study investigated disturbances in cerebral glucose metabolism in elderly inpatients (median age = 84 years) during delirium ($N = 13/13$) and after delirium resolution ($N = 6/6$) using 2-^{18}F-fluoro-2-deoxyglucose (FDG) positron emission tomography (PET) [19]. All participants ($N = 13$) showed evidence of cortical hypometabolism during delirium that improved upon delirium resolution ($N = 6/6$). The authors report glucose metabolism was higher post-delirium in the whole brain and bilateral posterior cingulate cortex (PCC) compared to during delirium ($p < 0.05$).

Despite constituting the smallest category of imaging studies on delirium, PET is already proving to be a promising approach for tracing disturbances in brain glucose metabolism to cognitive changes during and after delirium.

Discussion

In general, these studies demonstrate that delirious patients have sicker brains prior to a stimulus than non-delirious subjects, but these associations are slightly fragile as there is little consideration for the precipitating event that actually induces the delirium. Nonetheless, they provide important preliminary insights about what makes a delirious subject's brain vulnerable to delirium. It seems consistent that both gray and white matter degeneration may predispose to delirium. In particular, differences in structural connectivity appear to be associated with subsequent delirium; whether this can be meaningfully used to predict delirium in other cohorts should be tested. These changes are broadly consistent with our Cognitive Disintegration model, but the role of degenerating gray matter was not covered in our model and may be critically important, especially if specific cell types or synaptic loss can be identified to be selectively degenerating. Perhaps most intriguing is the recent paper suggesting that amyloid beta deposition is not associated with delirium, contrasting with strong evidence that dementia predisposes to delirium. While this study was very small and prone to selection bias, it seems to oppose the view that dementia pathology is associated with delirium based on studies of cerebrospinal fluid markers of dementia [32]. A large amyloid PET study is required to resolve this ambiguity.

In contrast, differences in cerebral blood flow before delirium do not seem to predispose to delirium. Studies of the critical dynamic phase of delirium (i.e., during delirium) are rare. Studies suggest that CBF may be reduced during delirium, and functional connectivity may shift from baseline patterns to a new network orientation with greater connectivity in posterior cortex and impaired connectivity of subcortical regions. These latter studies are remarkably difficult due to motion artifact, and this makes reproducing these results of particular importance. Nonetheless the fact there are changes in CBF and connectivity during delirium is an important insight. Of course, decreases in CBF may also make interpretation of changes in fMRI connectivity (a measure that is dependent on blood flow) more complicated, and this confound requires that other imaging modalities are considered when assessing the pathophysiology of delirium. While CBF studies suggest frontal cortical involvement, fMRI studies suggest that the most relevant connectivity changes may occur posteriorly in cortex or at a subcortical level in delirium. This discordance is intriguing and may yield important clues about the pathophysiology of delirium. However, a key issue is to understand the direction of causality (if any) between these findings. Assuming causation from observational imaging studies is clearly dangerous and warrants cautious interpretation. Nonetheless it appears biologically plausible that changes in blood flow (presumably indicating changes in neuronal activity) and functional connectivity (presumably reflecting integration of information across neurons) may be associated with delirium.

Future Directions

Future studies must concentrate on reproducing prior findings and consideration of both imaging and confounding factors including the severity of the precipitating event. Ideally, longitudinal scanning designs will be adopted to improve the likelihood that any factor identified changed contemporaneously with delirium symptoms. In particular, resolving the role of amyloid pathology and delirium seems a key issue for the field.

References

1. Salluh JI, Wang H, Schneider EB, Nagaraja N, Yenokyan G, Damluji A, Serafim RB, Stevens RD. Outcome of delirium in critically ill patients: systematic review and meta-analysis. BMJ. 2015;350:h2538.
2. Hosker C, Ward D. Hypoactive delirium. BMJ. 2017;357:j2047.
3. Sanders RD, Pandharipande PP, Davidson AJ, Ma D, Maze M. Anticipating and managing postoperative delirium and cognitive decline in adults. BMJ. 2011;343:d4331.
4. Sanders RD. Hypothesis for the pathophysiology of delirium: role of baseline brain network connectivity and changes in inhibitory tone. Med Hypotheses. 2011;77(1):140–3.
5. Yokota H, Ogawa S, Kurokawa A, Yamamoto Y. Regional cerebral blood flow in delirium patients. Psychiatry Clin Neurosci. 2003;57(3):337–9.
6. Shioiri A, Kurumaji A, Takeuchi T, Matsuda H, Arai H, Nishikawa T. White matter abnormalities as a risk factor for postoperative delirium revealed by diffusion tensor imaging. Am J Geriatr Psychiatry. 2010;18(8):743–53.
7. Choi SH, Lee H, Chung TS, Park KM, Jung YC, Kim SI, Kim JJ. Neural network functional connectivity during and after an episode of delirium. Am J Psychiatr. 2012;169(5):498–507.
8. Gunther ML, Morandi A, Krauskopf E, Pandharipande P, Girard TD, Jackson JC, Thompson J, Shintani AK, Geevarghese S, Miller RR III, Canonico A. The association between brain volumes, delirium duration and cognitive outcomes in intensive care unit survivors: a prospective exploratory cohort magnetic resonance imaging study. Crit Care Med. 2012;40(7):2022.
9. Morandi A, Rogers BP, Gunther ML, Merkle K, Pandharipande P, Girard TD, Jackson JC, Thompson J, Shintani AK, Geevarghese S, Miller RR III. The relationship between delirium duration, white matter integrity, and cognitive impairment in intensive care unit survivors as determined by diffusion tensor imaging. Crit Care Med. 2012;40(7):2182.
10. Root JC, Pryor KO, Downey R, Alici Y, Davis ML, Holodny A, Korc-Grodzicki B, Ahles T. Association of pre-operative brain pathology with post-operative delirium in a cohort

of non-small cell lung cancer patients undergoing surgical resection. Psycho-Oncology. 2013;22(9):2087–94.

11. Hatano Y, Narumoto J, Shibata K, Matsuoka T, Taniguchi S, Hata Y, Yamada K, Yaku H, Fukui K. White-matter hyperintensities predict delirium after cardiac surgery. Am J Geriatr Psychiatry. 2013;21(10):938–45.
12. Brown CH IV, Faigle R, Klinker L, Bahouth M, Max L, LaFlam A, Neufeld KJ, Mandal K, Gottesman RF, Hogue CW Jr. The association of brain MRI characteristics and postoperative delirium in cardiac surgery patients. Clin Ther. 2015;37(12):2686–99.
13. Omiya H, Yoshitani K, Yamada N, Kubota Y, Takahashi K, Kobayashi J, Ohnishi Y. Preoperative brain magnetic resonance imaging and postoperative delirium after off-pump coronary artery bypass grafting: a prospective cohort study. Can J Anesth/J C d'anesthésie. 2015;62(6):595–602.
14. Cavallari M, Hshieh TT, Guttmann CR, Ngo LH, Meier DS, Schmitt EM, Marcantonio ER, Jones RN, Kosar CM, Fong TG, Press D. Brain atrophy and white-matter hyperintensities are not significantly associated with incidence and severity of postoperative delirium in older persons without dementia. Neurobiol Aging. 2015;36(6):2122–9.
15. Naidech AM, Polnaszek KL, Berman MD, Voss JL. Hematoma locations predicting delirium symptoms after intracerebral hemorrhage. Neurocrit Care. 2016;24(3):397–403.
16. Cavallari M, Dai W, Guttmann CR, Meier DS, Ngo LH, Hshieh TT, Callahan AE, Fong TG, Schmitt E, Dickerson BC, Press DZ. Neural substrates of vulnerability to postsurgical delirium as revealed by presurgical diffusion MRI. Brain. 2016;139(4):1282–94.
17. Hshieh TT, Dai W, Cavallari M, Guttmann CR, Meier DS, Schmitt EM, Dickerson BC, Press DZ, Marcantonio ER, Jones RN, Gou YR. Cerebral blood flow MRI in the nondemented elderly is not predictive of post-operative delirium but is correlated with cognitive performance. J Cereb Blood Flow Metab. 2017;37(4):1386–97.
18. Shioiri A, Kurumaji A, Takeuchi T, Nemoto K, Arai H, Nishikawa T. A decrease in the volume of gray matter as a risk factor for postoperative delirium revealed by an atlas-based method. Am J Geriatr Psychiatry. 2016;24(7):528–36.
19. Haggstrom LR, Nelson JA, Wegner EA, Caplan GA. 2-18F-fluoro-2-deoxyglucose positron emission tomography in delirium. J Cereb Blood Flow Metab. 2017;37(11):3556–67.
20. Cavallari M, Dai W, Guttmann CR, Meier DS, Ngo LH, Hshieh TT, Fong TG, Schmitt E, Press DZ, Travison TG, Marcantonio ER. Longitudinal diffusion changes following postoperative delirium in older people without dementia. Neurology. 2017;89(10):1020–7.
21. Rolandi E, Cavedo E, Pievani M, Galluzzi S, Ribaldi F, Buckley C, Cunningham C, Guerra UP, Musarra M, Morzenti S, Magnaldi S. Association of postoperative delirium with markers of neurodegeneration and brain amyloidosis: a pilot study. Neurobiol Aging. 2018;61:93–101.
22. Detweiler MB, Sherigar RM, Bader G, Sullivan K, Kenneth A, Kalafat N, Reddy P, Lutgens B. Association of white matter lesions, cerebral atrophy, intracranial extravascular calcifications, and ventricular-communicating hydrocephalus with delirium among veterans. South Med J. 2017;110(6):432–9.
23. Kyeong S, Choi SH, Shin JE, Lee WS, Yang KH, Chung TS, Kim JJ. Functional connectivity of the circadian clock and neural substrates of sleep-wake disturbance in delirium. Psychiatry Res Neuroimaging. 2017;264:10–2.
24. Matano F, Mizunari T, Yamada K, Kobayashi S, Murai Y, Morita A. Environmental and clinical risk factors for delirium in a neurosurgical center: a prospective study. World Neurosurg. 2017;103:424–30.
25. Racine AM, Fong TG, Travison TG, Jones RN, Gou Y, Vasunilashorn SM, Marcantonio ER, Alsop DC, Inouye SK, Dickerson BC. Alzheimer's-related cortical atrophy is associated with postoperative delirium severity in persons without dementia. Neurobiol Aging. 2017;59:55–63.
26. van Montfort SJ, van Dellen E, van den Bosch AM, Otte WM, Schutte MJ, Choi SH, Chung TS, Kyeong S, Slooter AJ, Kim JJ. Resting-state fMRI reveals network disintegration during delirium. NeuroImage: Clinical. 2018;20:35–41.

27. Qu J, Chen Y, Luo G, Zhong H, Xiao W, Yin H. Delirium in the acute phase of ischemic stroke: incidence, risk factors, and effects on functional outcome. J Stroke Cerebrovasc Dis. 2018;27(10):2641–7.
28. Hijazi Z, Lange P, Watson R, Maier AB. The use of cerebral imaging for investigating delirium aetiology. Eur J Intern Med. 2018;52:35–9.
29. Helenius J, Henninger N. Leukoaraiosis burden significantly modulates the association between infarct volume and National Institutes of Health Stroke Scale in ischemic stroke. Stroke. 2015;46(7):1857–63.
30. Inouye SK, Leo-Summers L, Zhang Y, Bogardus ST Jr, Leslie DL, Agostini JV. A chart-based method for identification of delirium: validation compared with interviewer ratings using the confusion assessment method. J Am Geriatr Soc. 2005;53(2):312–8.
31. Saczynski JS, Kosar CM, Xu G, Puelle MR, Schmitt E, Jones RN, Marcantonio ER, Wong B, Isaza I, Inouye SK. A tale of two methods: chart and interview methods for identifying delirium. J Am Geriatr Soc. 2014;62(3):518–24.
32. Cunningham EL, McGuinness B, McAuley DF, Toombs J, Mawhinney T, O'Brien S, Beverland D, Schott JM, Lunn MP, Zetterberg H, Passmore AP. CSF beta-amyloid 1–42 concentration predicts delirium following elective arthroplasty surgery in an observational cohort study. Annals of surgery. 2019;269(6):1200–5.

Chapter 10
Inflammatory Biomarkers and Neurotransmitter Perturbations in Delirium

José R. Maldonado

Introduction

Delirium is an acute neuropsychiatric syndrome characterized by acute changes in cognition (e.g., perceptual distortions, impairment in abstract thinking, memory impairment, disorientation), psychomotor alterations (e.g., hyper- or hypoactivity), disturbances in the circadian sleep-wake cycle, emotional disturbance (e.g., irritability, anger, fear, anxiety, perplexity), and altered level of consciousness and attention (e.g., reduced ability to direct, focus, sustain, and shift attention) [1]. Delirium's prevalence surpasses that of all other psychiatric syndromes in every medical unit in which it has been studied [2], from the general medical setting (between 15% and 60%) [3, 4], among the elderly admitted to a general hospital (between 6% and 46%) [5], in the postoperative setting (between 10% and 74%) [6, 7], and in up to 87% of critically ill patients in the intensive care units [8].

Delirium is a neurobehavioral syndrome caused by the transient disruption of normal neuronal activity secondary to systemic disturbances [9–11]. Over the years, multiple theories have been proposed to explain the processes leading to the development of delirium [12, 13]. Most of these theories are complementary, rather than competing, as there is significant interdependence among most of them (see Fig. 10.1). It is likely that none of the previously postulated theories by itself explains the phenomena of delirium but rather that a multitude of them act together to lead to the biochemical derangement we know as delirium. The latest such theory is the *Systems Integration Failure Hypothesis (SIFH)* which proposes that individuals have varying degrees of non-modifiable factors, or substrates, and that this "load" will determine the basic frailty of the system in an inverse relationship with acute "precipitants and modifiable" factors (e.g., infection and inflammation, sleep

J. R. Maldonado (✉)
Division of Psychosomatic Medicine, Emergency Psychiatry Service,
Stanford University School of Medicine, Stanford, CA, USA
e-mail: jrm@stanford.edu

C. G. Hughes et al. (eds.), *Delirium*, https://doi.org/10.1007/978-3-030-25751-4_10

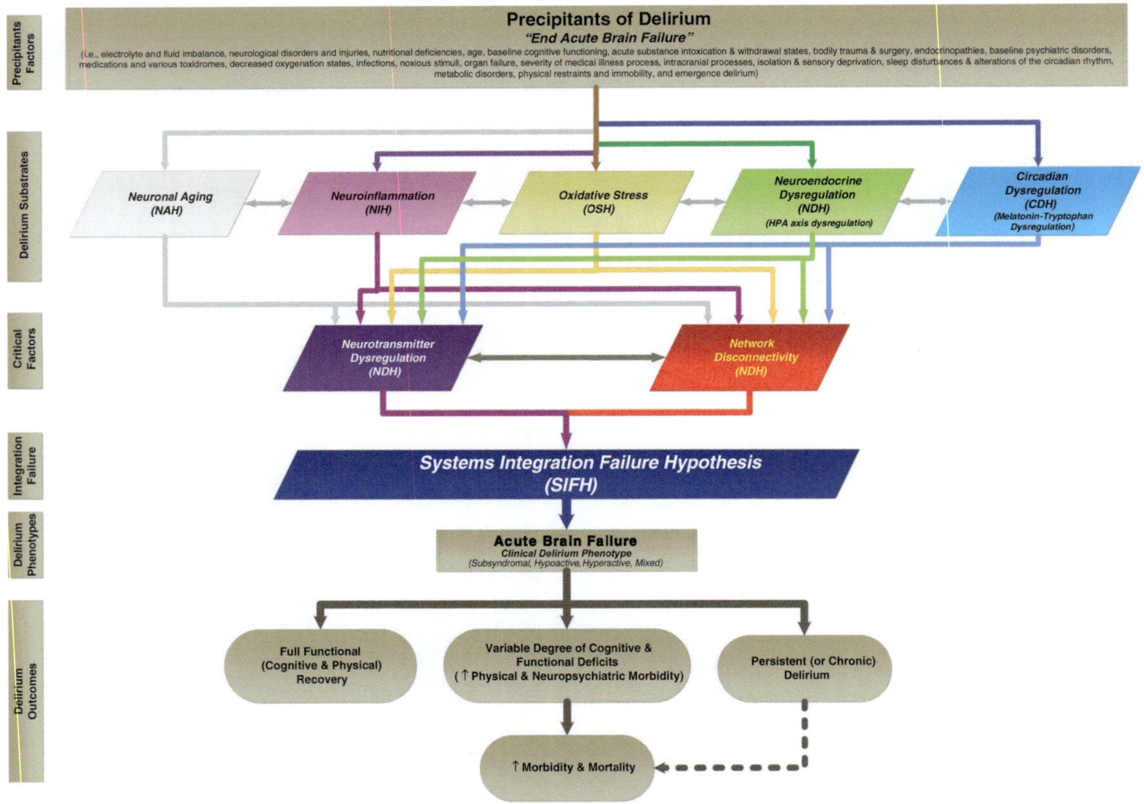

Fig. 10.1 Systems Integration Failure Hypothesis (SIFH). According to the *Systems Integration Failure Hypothesis (SIFH)*, there are multiple important determinants that eventually predict a subject's vulnerability to delirium: (**a**) the presence of physiological vulnerabilities (the substrate); (**b**) an acute insult (precipitant) further taxing an already fragile system with limited functional reserves. The various vulnerabilities make it more likely that a patient may experience a derangement in functional metabolism leading to (**c**) an alteration in neurotransmitter synthesis, function, and/or availability, and (**d**) a dysregulation of neuronal activity and connectivity secondary to systemic disturbances, which mediates the complex phenotypic and neurocognitive changes observed in delirium. (Courtesy of José R. Maldonado. Used with permission. Source: [13])

deprivation, trauma, surgery, hypoxia, medication use, substances of abuse, organ failure, electrolyte imbalance, metabolic derangement) [13]. Ultimately, the SIFH proposes that the specific combination of neurotransmitter dysfunction and the variability in integration and appropriate processing of sensory information and motor responses, as well as the degree of breakdown in cerebral network connectivity, directly contributes to the various cognitive and behavioral changes and clinical motoric phenotype observed in delirium [13]. There are a number of patient-specific physiological characteristics that serve as substrate to the development of delirium (Fig. 10.2). Of these, this article will focus on neuroinflammation as a substrate for delirium and its relationship to the development of specific neurotransmitter perturbations characteristic of the syndrome of delirium.

The Neuroinflammatory Hypothesis of Delirium

The "neuroinflammatory hypothesis" (NIH) of delirium theorized a pathophysiological link between delirium and a broad array of infectious and inflammatory abnormalities, suggesting that the central nervous system (CNS) and the peripheral immune system maintain a dynamic cross talk to tightly coordinate the innate immune response [14]. Accordingly, the NIH proposes that delirium represents the CNS manifestation of a systemic disease state that has crossed the blood-brain barrier (BBB) [12, 15]. Even though there are circumstances associated with a high occurrence of delirium (e.g., infections, postoperative states) which are associated with compromise of BBB integrity, a physical failure of the BBB is not required. In fact, there are many illness processes (e.g., bodily trauma, peripheral infections, surgical procedures, use of extracorporeal circulation, hypoxia) which may introduce triggering factors leading to the activation of the inflammatory cascade (reviewed by Maldonado 2008, 2013) [12, 13].

Systemic inflammation has long been recognized as a trigger for episodes of delirium, particularly in elderly or demented patients, even though their deliriogenic effect seems to be lessened in younger and non-demented patients [16–26]. In fact, the Greeks used the term *phrenitis*, meaning "acute inflammation of mind and body" to describe an acute alteration of brain functioning (mind or thinking) associated to a bodily disease process as opposed to conventional madness, or what we would describe nowadays as mental illness [23, 27, 28].

This does not mean that there needs to be an infectious or inflammatory process in the CNS, as in the case of meningitis, but rather that the brain monitors the presence of peripheral inflammation. Instead, the NIH suggests that acute peripheral inflammatory processes (e.g., infections, surgery, trauma) are able to induce activation of brain parenchymal cells and expression of proinflammatory cytokines and inflammatory mediators in the CNS (e.g., CRP, IL-6, TNF-alpha, IL-1RA, IL-10, and IL-8 [16, 29]), which in turn induces neuronal and synaptic dysfunction that may serve as the substrate for the neurobehavioral and cognitive symptoms characteristic of delirium (Fig. 10.3) [14, 24, 30–35].

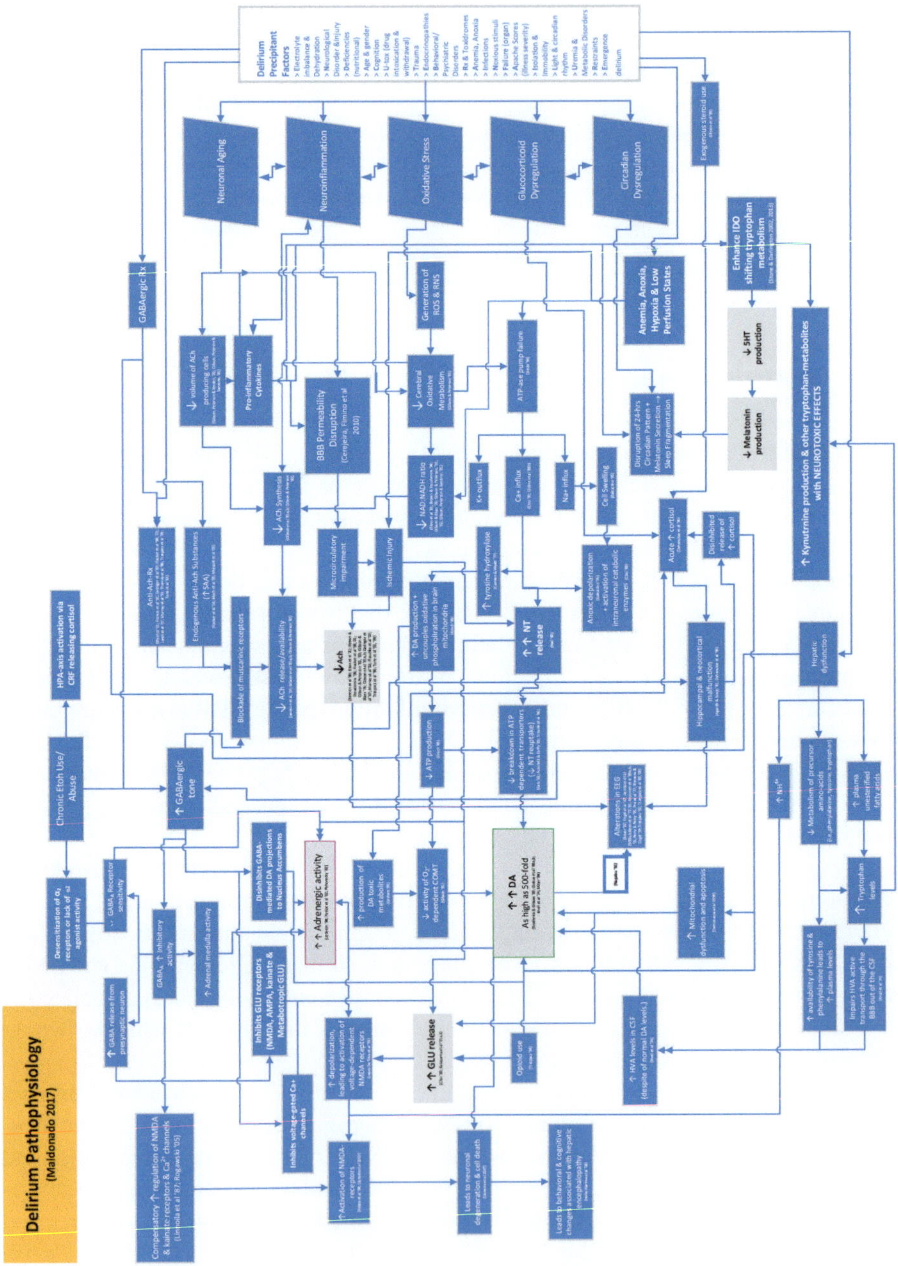
Delirium Pathophysiology
(Maldonado 2017)
Delirium Precipitant Factors
Neuronal Aging
Neuroinflammation
Oxidative Stress
Glucocorticoid Dysregulation
Circadian Dysregulation
GABAergic Rx
Chronic Etoh Use/ Abuse
HPA-axis activation via CRF releasing cortisol
↑ GABAergic tone
BBB Permeability Disruption
Anemia, Anoxia, Hypoxia & Low Perfusion States
Enhance IDO shifting tryptophan metabolism
↑ Kynutrnine production & other tryptophan-metabolites with NEUROTOXIC EFFECTS
↓ Ach
↑↑ NT release
↑↑ DA
As high as 500-fold
↑↑ Adrenergic activity
↑↑ GLU release

Fig. 10.2 Pathophysiology of delirium. The *Systems Integration Failure Hypothesis (SIFH)* suggests that most of the previously available theories of delirium pathophysiology are complementary, rather than mutually exclusive, with many areas of intersection and reciprocal influence, which is more akin the complexities of the human brain. The SIFH suggests that individuals have varying degrees of critical etiological factors and that this "load" will determine the basic fragility of the system in an inverse relationship with acute "precipitants and modifiable" factors (e.g., infection and inflammation, sleep deprivation, trauma, surgery, hypoxia, medication use, substances of abuse, organ failure, electrolyte imbalance, metabolic derangement). Eventually, the interplay between the alterations in neurotransmitter dysfunction and which network emerges as dominant or unchecked gives rise to the various clinical manifestations observed in the various motoric phenotypes (e.g., hyperactive, hypoactive, mixed). Thus, the manifestations of the specific delirium picture (i.e., phenotype) result from a combination of the alteration in neurotransmitter function and availability and the variability in integration and appropriate processing of sensory information and motor responses, mediated by an acute breakdown in brain network connectivity. In other words, the form of delirium that ensues will depend upon how and which networks breaks down, influenced by both the individual's baseline network connectivity and the degree of change in inhibitory tone produced. Thus, the SIFH predicts that failure of one system will undoubtedly affect others. (Courtesy of José R. Maldonado. Used with permission. Source: [13])

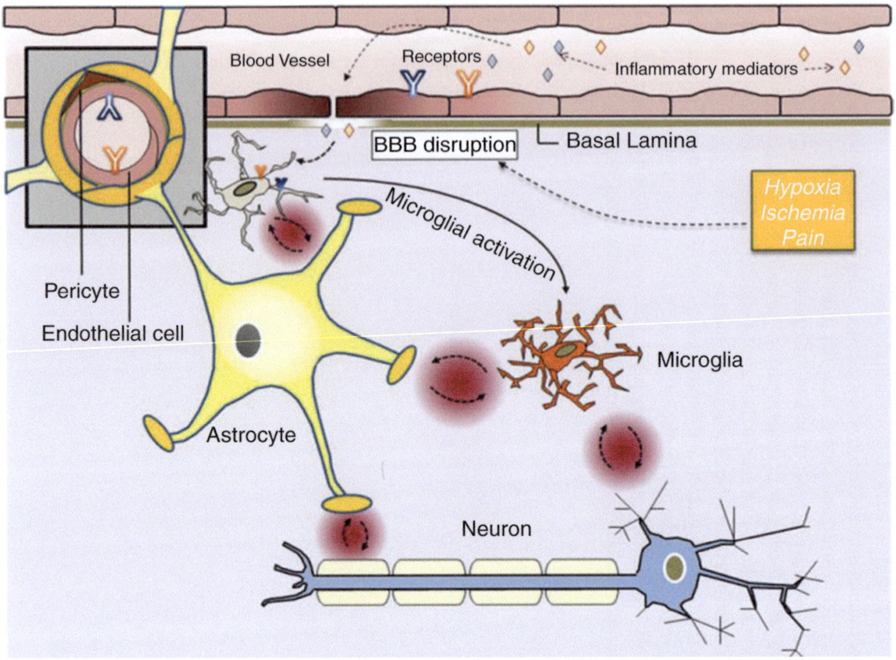

Fig. 10.3 Recognition and propagation of peripheral immune stimuli in the CNS. The interaction of circulating inflammatory mediators (e.g., cytokines and lipopolysaccharide) with the neurovascular unit is associated with increased permeability of the BBB. Recognition of peripheral inflammatory stimuli in the BBB is followed by a cascade of events leading to microglia activation and subsequent modulation of adjacent cells including astrocytes and neurons. (Source: [14])

Systemic Inflammation Leading to Acute Brain Dysfunction and Sickness Behavior

Multiple studies have demonstrated the brain's ability to monitor the presence of systemic inflammatory processes (i.e., outside the BBB) and the development of nonspecific physiological (e.g., fever, pain, malaise, fatigue, anorexia) and behavioral adaptations (e.g., anhedonia, lethargy, social withdrawal, depressed mood, cognitive impairment) upon exposure to infection or inflammation collectively known as "sickness behavior" [31, 33, 35–42]. Recent immunological data suggest that cytokines (e.g., interleukin-1, tumor necrosis factor alpha) released by macrophages, dendritic cells, and mast cells act on the hypothalamus to provoke alterations in the normal homeostatic condition, including elevated body temperature, increased sleep, loss of appetite, and alterations in lipid and protein metabolism which appear directed toward enhancing the normal immune responses [38].

Animal studies have demonstrated that the administration of lipopolysaccharide (LPS) induces sickness behavior, which requires activation of proinflammatory cytokine signaling in the brain [32, 33]. Microglia are the primary recipients of peripheral inflammatory signals that reach the brain [43, 44]. Activated microglia, in turn, initiate an inflammatory cascade whereby release of relevant cytokines, chemokines, inflammatory mediators, reactive nitrogen species (RNS), and reactive oxygen species (ROS) induces mutual activation of astroglia, thereby amplifying inflammatory signals within the CNS. Cytokines, including IL-1, IL-6, and TNF-alpha, as well as IFN-alpha and IFN-gamma (from T cells), induce the enzyme indoleamine 2,3 dioxygenase (IDO), which breaks down tryptophan (TRP), the primary precursor of serotonin (5-hydroxytryptamine, 5-HT), into quinolinic acid (QUIN), a potent N-methyl-D-aspartate (NMDA) agonist and stimulator of glutamate (GLU) release. Excessive exposure to cytokines, QUIN, and RNS/ROS leads to a compromised of multiple astrocytic functions, ultimately leading to downregulation of glutamate transporters, impaired glutamate reuptake, and increased glutamate release, as well as decreased production of neurotrophic factors (Fig. 10.4) [24, 44].

Similarly, overactivation of the CNS inflammatory cascade, particularly overexposure to cytokines, leads to oligodendroglia neurotoxicity, potentially contributing to apoptosis and demyelination. The confluence of excessive astrocytic GLU release, inadequate GLU reuptake by astrocytes and oligodendroglia, activation of NMDA receptors by QUIN, increased GLU binding and activation of extrasynaptic NMDA receptors (accessible to glutamate released from glial elements and associated with inhibition of brain-derived neurotrophic factor [BDNF] expression), decline in neurotrophic support, and oxidative stress ultimately disrupt neural plasticity through excitotoxicity and apoptosis (Fig. 10.5) [24, 44–49]. Brain-derived neurotrophic factor (BDNF) is an important member of the neurotrophins family and has many effects on the nervous system plasticity, particularly on neuronal growth, differentiation, and repair [50].

Peripheral or systemic factors may elicit a central neuroinflammatory response by multiple potential pathways. These may include a variety of immune-brain communication pathways, namely, (a) the "neural pathway," (b) the "humoral pathway," (c) active transport systems across the BBB, and (d) a "leaky" BBB. In the neural pathway, peripherally produced pathogen-associated molecular patterns (PAMPs) and cytokines activate primary afferent nerves, such as the vagus nerve (Fig. 10.6a) [51–53]. The humoral pathway involves circulating PAMPs that reach the brain at the level of the choroid plexus (CP) and the circumventricular organs where PAMPs induce the production and release of proinflammatory cytokines by macrophage-like cells expressing Toll-like receptors (TLRs) (Fig. 10.6b) [51, 52]. Several studies have demonstrated that patients develop delirium during acute medical hospitalizations experienced elevation of CRP, IL-6, TNF-alpha, IL-1RA, IL-10, and IL-8, as compared with patients who did not have delirium, even after adjusting for infection, age, and cognitive impairment, suggesting an association between proinflammatory cytokines and the pathogenesis of delirium [16, 29, 54].

Several classes of influx and efflux transporters located on the luminal and abluminal sides of the brain endothelia regulate the transport of both endogenous and exogenous molecules in and out of brain parenchyma [55]. The BBB is a regulatory interface in response to cytokines. Functioning one way, the BBB can selectively transport several cytokines. This includes interleukin (IL)-1α and IL-1β [56–58],

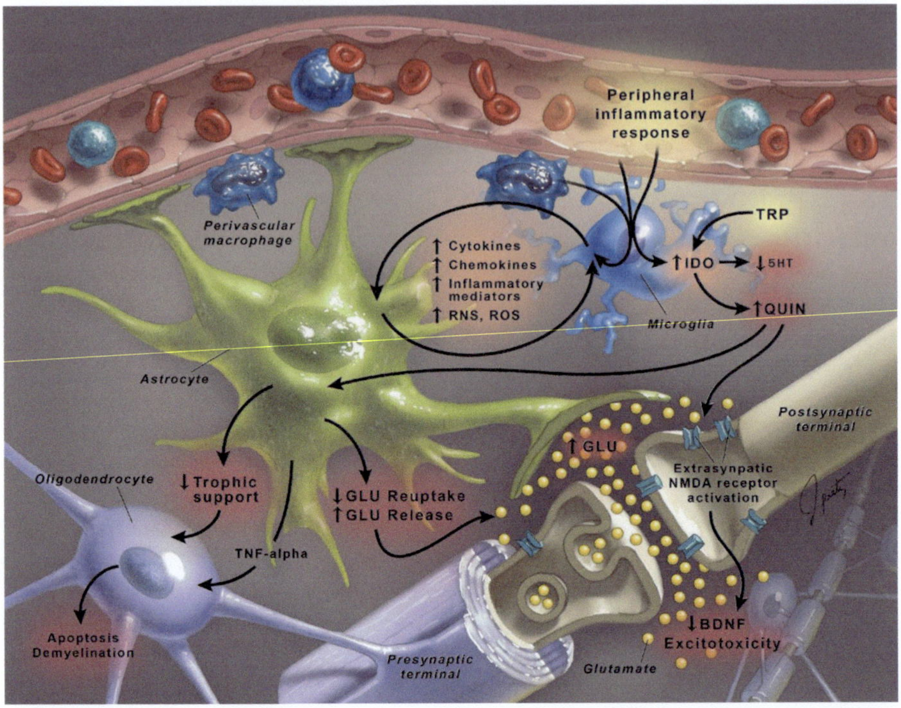

Fig. 10.4 Effects of the CNS inflammatory cascade on neural plasticity. As peripheral inflammatory signals reach the brain, activated microglia initiate the inflammatory cascade, whereby release of relevant cytokines (e.g., IL-1, IL-6, TNF-alpha, IFN-alpha, and IFN-gamma), chemokines, inflammatory mediators, and RNS and ROS has a number of negative effects on neural plasticity: (**a**) induces sickness behavior; (**b**) induces astroglia activation, thus amplifying inflammatory signals within the CNS; (**c**) enhances the activity of the ubiquitous indoleamine 2,3-dioxygenase (IDO), leading to deficient tryptophan (TRP) levels, thus a reduction in serotonin and melatonin production, and a shift to the production of kynurenine (KYN) and other neurotoxic tryptophan-derived metabolites; (**d**) excessive exposure to cytokines, QUIN, and RNS/ROS leading to compromise of astrocytic functions, ultimately leading to downregulation of glutamate transporters, impaired glutamate reuptake, and increased glutamate release, as well as decreased production of neurotrophic factors; and, finally, (**e**) oligodendroglia especially sensitive to the CNS inflammatory cascade. Cytokines overexposure (e.g., TNF-alpha) causes oligodendroglial neurotoxicity, which further contributes to apoptosis and demyelination. (Source: [44])

IL-1 receptor antagonist (IL-1ra) [59], IL-6 [60], tumor necrosis factor-α (TNF) [61–66], leukemia inhibitory factor (LIF) [61–64], ciliary neurotrophic factor [67], and many adipokines [68–70]. The transported cytokines play important roles in the physiological response to inflammation and neuroregeneration. The "leaky BBB" pathway is discussed in the next section.

Finally, many of delirium's precipitant factors (e.g., infections, intraoperative anesthesia, postoperative sedation) are themselves associated with potential BBB integrity compromise. For example, it has been found that the BBB is disrupted in cases of septic encephalopathy, which allows for increased blood-brain transport of neutral amino acids [71]. Similarly, systemic inflammation is common in liver fail-

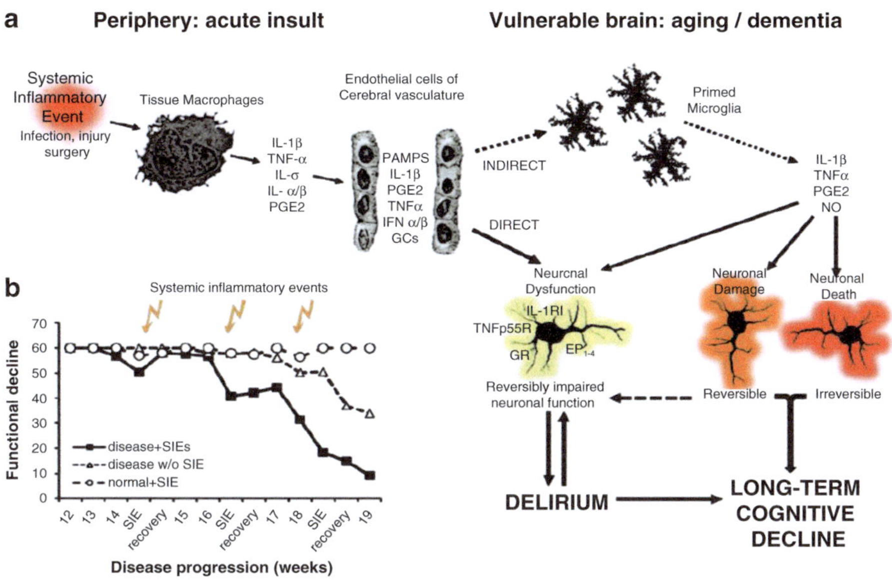

Fig. 10.5 Neuroinflammatory hypothesis *[NIH]*. (**a**) Systemic inflammatory events trigger the release of inflammatory mediators by tissue macrophages and brain vascular endothelial cells. These mediators may affect neuronal function directly or via the activation of microglial cells that have become primed by neurodegenerative disease or aging. Inflammatory mediators may cause reversible disruption of neuronal function as in the case of delirium, may be irreversible and contribute to long-term cognitive decline, or may bring about neuronal death and contribute to the accumulating damage and neuropathological burden. (**b**) Successive systemic inflammatory insults induce acute dysfunction, which is progressively less reversible each time but also contribute to the progression of permanent disability. *IL-1RI* interleukin-1 receptor type I, *TNFp55* TNFp55 receptor, *GCs* glucocorticoids, *GR* glucocorticoid receptor, *NO* nitric oxide, *EP1–4*, prostaglandin receptors 1–4, *PAMPs* pathogen-associated molecular patterns, *IFNα/β* interferon *α/β* SIEs, systemic inflammatory events. (Source: [24])

ure, and its acquisition is a predictor of hepatic encephalopathy (HE) severity. Studies provide convincing evidence for a role of neuroinflammation in liver failure; this evidence includes activation of microglia together with increased synthesis in situ of proinflammatory cytokines (i.e., TNF, IL-1beta, and IL-6). The proposed "liver-brain signaling mechanisms" in liver failure include direct effects of systemic proinflammatory molecules, recruitment of monocytes after microglial activation, brain accumulation of ammonia, lactate and manganese, and altered permeability of the BBB [72, 73]. This provides an intersection between the NIH and the neurotransmitter hypothesis (NTH), as the above changes may contribute to the alteration in neurotransmitter functioning in cases of HE (e.g., increased DA, 5HT, GABA).

There is mounting evidence that some of the same proinflammatory cytokines that induce sickness behavior also enhance activity of the ubiquitous indoleamine 2,3-dioxygenase (IDO) [74, 75]. Activation of IDO leads to a shift in the metabolism of tryptophan (TRP) away from the production of serotonin and melatonin (contributing to sleep disturbance and depressive-like behavior) but, instead, to an increased production of kynurenine (KYN) and other tryptophan-derived

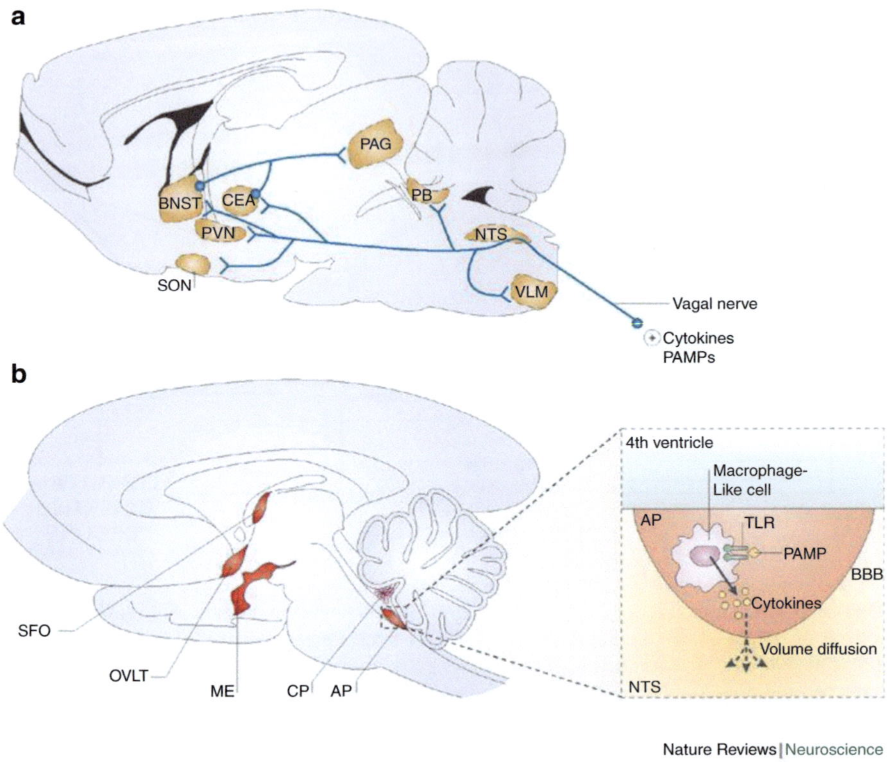

Fig. 10.6 Pathways that transduce immune signals from the periphery to the brain. **(a)** In the *neural pathway*, peripherally produced pathogen-associated molecular patterns (PAMPs) and cytokines activate primary afferent nerves (e.g., vagal nerve, trigeminal nerves). **(b)** The *humoral pathway* involves circulating PAMPs that reach the brain at the level of the choroid plexus (CP) and the circumventricular organs, where PAMPs induce the production and release of proinflammatory cytokines, likely reaching the brain by diffusion. (Source: [51])

metabolites that have neurotoxic effects [45, 46, 51, 76], providing an intersection between the NIH and sleep dysregulation patterns described among patients with delirium [13, 15]. In fact, cytokines may play a role in normal sleep regulation, by increasing non-REM sleep and decreasing REM sleep, and during inflammatory events, an increase in cytokine levels may intensify their impact on sleep regulation [77].

Blood-Brain Barrier Dysfunction and Delirium

CNS resident cells react to the presence of peripheral immune signals, leading to production of cytokines and other mediators in the brain, and promote cell proliferation and activation of the hypothalamus-pituitary-adrenal axis [NEH] through a complex system of interactions. These neuroinflammatory changes cause BBB permeability disruption, as suspected by elevations of S100 beta [S100B] (a calcium-binding protein with cytokine-like properties; is a dimeric calcium-binding protein with α and β subunits; the β subunit is highly specific to the brain and is synthesized in glial cells throughout the CNS) [78] and changes in synaptic transmission, neural excitability, and cerebral blood flow, leading to the neurobehavioral and cognitive symptoms characteristic of delirium (e.g., disruption in behavior and cognitive functions) [14]. Secreted mostly by astrocytes under conditions of metabolic stress, S100B is considered a putative biomarker of CNS damage; increased levels in cerebrospinal fluid (CSF) and serum have been linked with adverse CNS outcomes, specifically among delirious patients [79–82].

During various disease states, leukocytes adhere to the BBB's endothelial cells (EC) and become activated, leading to degranulation and the release of free oxygen radicals and enzymes. This, in turn, leads to EC membrane destruction, disruption of cell-cell adhesions, and increased endothelial permeability which is associated with extravascular fluid shifts and the development of perivascular edema in cerebral tissue, leading to decreased perfusion and longer diffusion distance for oxygen [14, 22, 83–85]. These processes may lead to such extensive perfusion impairment that the blood flow in individual capillaries becomes disrupted: thus, systemic inflammation as a response to trauma or illness leads to microcirculatory impairment and subsequent ischemic injury. Among the pertinent neurotransmitters, acetylcholine (ACh) synthesis and release may be the most sensitive to this type of hypoxic injury and other homeostatic changes in the brain [86]. Similarly, neuroinflammatory injuries have also been associated with imbalances in other neurotransmitters including dopamine, serotonin, and norepinephrine [12, 15, 87]; see also Fig. 10.2. In response to traumatic and systemic events, the systemic inflammatory response is activated causing monocytes and macrophages to produce neopterin, cytokines, and reactive oxygen species, which can be found in the plasma, urine, and cerebrospinal fluid of delirious patients [12, 14, 29, 54, 88–91]. Neopterin is produced by human monocytes/macrophages upon stimulation with the cytokine interferon-y and thus can serve as a maker for immune system activation [92]. In addition, disruptions of the EC may also lead to enhanced cytokine transport across the disrupted BBB and infiltration of leukocytes and cytokines into the CNS, producing ischemia and neuronal apoptosis [14, 93, 94].

More recently, studies have suggested that the use of various general anesthetics (e.g., sevoflurane, isoflurane) can cause marked flattening of the surfaces of brain vascular endothelial cells along with disruption of BBB-associated tight junctions at cell margins, leading to holes in the vascular endothelial lining and increased BBB permeability, thus facilitating plasma influx into the brain interstitium (Fig. 10.7) [95, 96]. The frequency and magnitude of this effect increases with age, thus potentially serving as a mechanism to mediate postoperative delirium and its increased occurrence among elderly patients.

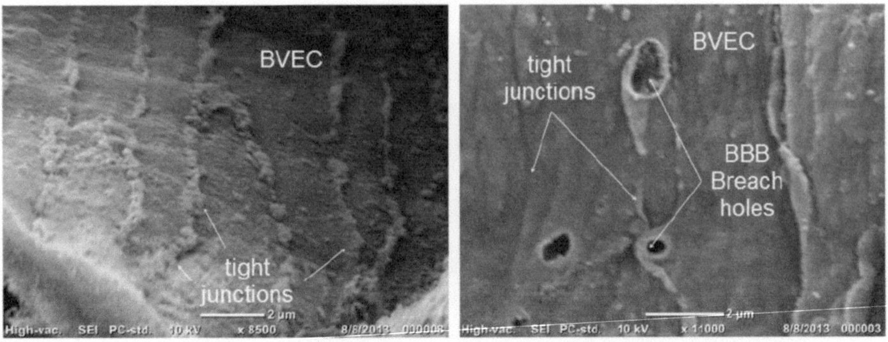

Control 3 hr anesthesia using sevoflurane

Fig. 10.7 Anesthesia may cause short-term BBB breakdown – possible mechanism of postoperative delirium. Anesthetic agents (e.g., sevoflurane, isoflurane) induce immediate changes in the surface of brain vascular endothelial cells, including a profound smoothing of surface membranes, visible "holes" in the BBB, and the leak of plasma components into the brain tissue. Older rats exhibited more anesthetic-induced BBB breakdown and less recovery at 24 h. (Source: [95])

Evidence in Support of Inflammation as Mediator of Delirium

In this section, we summarize the published data regarding the relationship between multiple inflammatory markers and delirium development. Studies are presented in chronological order of publication. See Table 10.1 for a summary of studied inflammatory biomarkers.

A study of adult patients admitted to inpatient medicine wards showed that those who developed delirium had significantly elevated levels (i.e., above the detection limit) of IL-6 (53% versus 31%) and IL-8 (45% versus 22%), compared with patients who did not develop delirium, even after adjusting for infection, age, and cognitive impairment [29]. This was the first study to show a relationship between peripherally measured cytokine levels and delirium as a symptom of sickness behavior in acutely admitted elderly. The study demonstrated that cognitive function can be impaired by a systemic infection in patients with a neurodegenerative disorder such as Alzheimer's disease. It also found that the cognitive decline was preceded by raised serum levels of IL-1H. Furthermore, aging and neurodegenerative disorders exaggerate microglial responses following stimulation by systemic immune stimuli such as peripheral inflammation and/or infection.

An observational study of acutely ill patients age ≥70 years ($n = 86$) at a university teaching hospital found a strong association between C-reactive protein (CRP) levels in serum and incident delirium (defined as occurring when the initial Confusion Assessment Method [CAM] assessment was negative and any subsequent one was positive). In a binary logistic analysis, including age, sex, initial Mini-Mental State Examination (MMSE), Acute Physiological Score of APACHE-II (APS) scale, disability score, and CRP, only the CRP level predicted the incidence of delirium ($P = 0.018$) [97].

Table 10.1 Inflammatory biomarkers linked to the development of delirium

Adiponectin [170]
Brain-derived neurotrophic factor (BDNF) [99, 143]
Cortisol [25, 90, 138, 169, 174, 176, 183, 239–247]
C-reactive protein (CRP) [16, 21, 29, 54, 91, 97, 131, 133, 134, 136, 139, 146, 148–150, 153, 155, 156, 180, 247–251]
Fas [158]
Galectin-3 [180]
Glial fibrillary acidic protein (GFAP) [26, 197]
High-mobility group box 1 (HMGB1) [160]
Interferon-gamma (IFN-γ) [137, 172, 181]
IL-1
IL-2 [131, 132, 157, 249, 252]
IL-5 [137]
IL-6 [16, 21, 26, 29, 90, 100, 137, 139, 148, 152, 155, 157, 158, 160, 171, 172, 174, 175, 177, 178, 246, 249, 253–256]
IL-8 [16, 25, 29, 137, 171, 175, 177, 256, 257]
IL-10 [16, 25, 29, 137, 147, 172–175, 175, 176]
IL-11 [158]
IL-17 [158]
Insulin-like growth factor-1 (IGF-1) [151, 176, 181, 254]
Leptin [106, 128, 129, 158]
Macrophage inflammatory protein (MIP)-1 alpha [137, 197]
Macrophage inflammatory protein-3 alpha (MIP-3alpha) [158]
Matrix metalloproteinase-9 (MMP-9) [179]
Methyl-accepting chemotaxis protein-1 (MCP-1) [25, 137]
Methyl-accepting chemotaxis protein-3 (MCP-3) [158]
Myeloid progenitor inhibitory factor-1 (MPIF-1) [158]
Neopterin [91, 147, 254]
Neuron-specific enolase (NSE) [82, 99, 143, 258]
Procalcitonin [25, 54, 138]
Protein C [179]
S100β [25, 80–82, 90, 99, 169, 172, 178, 180, 184–186, 197, 245, 259, 260]
Tumor necrosis factor (TNF) [16, 25, 29, 131, 132, 137, 170, 172, 177, 179, 181, 197, 255, 261]
Soluble tumor necrosis factor receptor-1 (sTNFR1) [170, 179]
Zinc alpha-2 glycoprotein (AZGP1) [249]
Inflammatory markers in delirium – meta-analyses [169, 262]

A study of elderly hip fracture patients ($n = 41$) prospectively followed after surgical repair found that those who developed postoperative delirium (POD) experienced elevations of CRP ($P = 0.008$) and IL-8 ($P = 0.08$) [16].

A study of patients aged ≥65 years acutely admitted after hip fracture ($n = 120$) found elevation in S100β levels when comparing samples obtained during delirium to samples of non-delirious patients ($P < 0.001$) [82]. Of note, there were no significant difference in S100β ($P = 0.43$) seen between the various motoric delirium subtypes. Similarly, a study of acutely admitted medical patients age ≥65 years ($n = 412$) found marked elevations in S100β levels between patients with delirium and those without ($P = 0.004$) [81]. As in the previous study, delirium motoric subtype and S100B level were not significantly correlated.

A study of older patients age ≥62 years with hip fracture and awaiting surgery assessed for delirium before and 3–4 days after surgery. CSF was obtained in all recruited patients at the onset of spinal anesthesia. The study found that patients who experienced delirium had higher CSF IL-8 levels than those without ($P = 0.003$). Similarly, patients experiencing delirium were also found to have higher serum IL-6 levels than those without delirium ($P = 0.01$) [98].

Among patients admitted to an intensive care unit, serum brain-derived neurotrophic factor (BDNF) levels and neuron-specific enolase (NSE; the γ-subunit of enolase present primarily in the cytoplasm of neurons) values were significantly higher in patients who became delirious than in those who did not ($P < 0.01$, for both) [99]. On the other hand, they found no significant differences in serum S100β levels between the delirious and non-delirious groups.

Similarly, a recent study found that high preoperative neopterin levels predicted delirium after cardiac surgery in older adults, thus suggesting that plasma neopterin levels may be a candidate biomarker for delirium among this patient population [91].

A prospective preliminary study of acute hip fracture in patients age ≥60 years ($n = 45$) found that the mean Log_{10} CSF S100B concentrations were significantly elevated in those with preoperative delirium compared to those without delirium ($P = 0.035$) [80]. Thus the authors suggest a link between S100B, a marker of astrocyte activation and potential CNS damage or dysfunction, leading to delirium.

A study of older patients age ≥75 years admitted for surgical repair of an acute hip fracture ($n = 61$) collected preoperative CSF samples and found that preoperative concentrations of FMS-like tyrosine kinase-3 ($P = 0.021$), interleukin-1 receptor antagonist ($P = 0.032$), and interleukin-6 ($P = 0.005$) were significantly lower in patients who developed delirium postoperatively, suggesting that delirium after surgery results from a dysfunctional neuroinflammatory response and stressing the role of reduced levels of anti-inflammatory mediators in delirium development [100].

Another study of acute hip fracture patients age ≥60 ($N = 43$), whose CSF samples were taken at induction of spinal anesthesia and examined with enzyme-linked immunosorbent assays (ELISA), assessed for delirium before and 3–4 days after surgery and found elevation in CSF IL-1β in patients with incident delirium as compared to those without delirium [101]. Similarly, CSF/serum IL-1β ratios and CSF IL-1 receptor antagonist (IL-1ra) were both higher in delirious than non-delirious patients.

Leptin is a hormone with broad effects on the CNS, including effects on several neurotransmitter systems [102, 103], influencing a number of neural functions [102, 104, 105], and modulating the immune response [14, 106]. In fact, low leptin levels have been associated with other neuropsychiatric disorders, such as depression [107–112], schizophrenia [113–117], narcolepsy [118–120], and both Alzheimer's disease and vascular types of dementias [121–127].

Among patients age ≥65 years admitted to a general hospital, leptin levels were significantly lower in patients with delirium compared with those without this disorder, and leptin levels were associated with the presence of delirium [128]. Additionally, there is a negative correlation between leptin levels and the number of comorbidities and number of medications. This suggests that there is a relationship between this hormone and the severity of the patient's clinical condition, which is related to these parameters. The association between leptin levels and the presence of delirium remained after adjustment for number of diagnoses and number of medications. Similarly, a study of patients ≥65 years old undergoing surgery ($n = 186$) for a femoral neck fracture or an intertrochanteric fracture, whose blood was drawn before administration of the anesthetic agent, found that lower plasma leptin levels (OR, 0.385; 95% CI, 0.286–0.517; $P < 0.001$) (and age; OR, 1.137; 95% CI, 1.073–1.205; $P < 0.001$) were highly associated with postoperative delirium after hip fracture surgery [129].

A multicenter study of patients age ≥65 years admitted to general medicine wards found that the mean change in blood natural killer (NK) cell activity was significantly greater in patients who developed delirium (89%) than in patients without delirium (40%) ($P = 0.045$), even after adjusting for age, the history of previous delirium, and the Clinical Dementia Rating score [130]. These findings suggest that the mean change in blood NK cell activity has a sensitivity of 89%, specificity 60%, positive predictive value 50%, negative predictive value 92%, positive likelihood ratio 2.22, and negative likelihood ratio 0.19 for distinguishing between the two groups.

A retrospective study of 710 patients >70 years old admitted to a medical acute admissions unit found a strong association between elevated CRP and delirium ($P < 0.001$), independent of other potential risk factors for delirium [131]. A prospective, observational cohort study of patients who underwent coronary artery bypass graft (CABG) surgery with cardiopulmonary bypass (CPB) ($n = 113$) found that raised levels of IL-2 and TNF-α measured in the postoperative period were associated with the development of delirium among CABG surgery patients (independent association for IL-2 [$p = 0.023$] and trend toward significance for TNF-α [$p = 0.056$]), independent of age, gender, cognitive status, psychiatric and physical comorbidity, duration of surgery, CPB time, and midazolam dose [132].

In addition, patients undergoing elective vascular surgery ($n = 277$) were prospectively evaluated for the diagnosis of POD, and it was found that those who developed delirium experienced postoperative elevated CRP levels ($P = 0.001$) [133]. Similarly, a study of patients admitted to the intensive care unit (ICU) ($n = 223$) found that patients with delirium had significantly higher CRP values than those without ($P = 0.0001$), even after adjusting for confounding variables (including age, sex, Acute Physiology and Chronic Health Evaluation II, intubation, living alone, physical restraint, alcohol drinking, smoking, type of medical condition, and hospital length of stay before ICU admission [134]. In addition, an increase in CRP greater than 8.1 mg/L within 24 h was associated with fourfold increase in the risk of delirium (odds ratio: 4.47, 95% confidence interval, 1.28–15.60).

A quantitative proteomic analysis of CSF obtained from hospitalized patients experiencing delirium provides confirmatory evidence that the inflammatory response is a component of delirium [135]. This quantitative proteomics analysis of CSF in delirium patients identified more than 270 proteins with a high level of confidence, about 10% of which had dysregulated protein expression levels in 50% or more of delirium subjects. A surprising outcome of this study was the level of similarity of CSF protein profiles among patients with delirium, given the diversity of causes (e.g., infections, metabolic problems, and adverse drug reactions) of the syndrome in this large patient sample. Of particular interest, there were several protein functional clusters (associated with inflammation, granins, apolipoproteins, clotting factors, protease inhibitors, and regulatory proteins) which have not been studied in the context of delirium.

A retrospective study investigating the multivariate relationships among the various risk factors for postoperative delirium in patients undergoing head and neck surgery for the treatment of oral cancer ($n = 110$) found that in univariate analysis, C-reactive protein (CRP) level of patients with delirium was significantly increased compared to that of the patients without delirium ($P < 0.05$) [136].

A study of patients age ≥55 years undergoing elective major knee surgery ($n = 10$) was very small in overall size, and it is difficult to know what the findings mean given that only one patient developed delirium, while six developed postoperative cognitive dysfunction (POCD) [137]. Despite the very small sample size, at different postoperative time points, statistically significant changes compared to baseline were present in IL-5, IL-6, I-8, IL-10, monocyte chemotactic protein (MCP)-1, macrophage inflammatory protein (MIP)-1α, IL-6/IL-10, and receptor for advanced glycation end products in plasma and in IFN-γ, IL-6, IL-8, IL-10, MCP-1, MIP-1α, MIP-1β, IL-8/IL-10, and TNF-α in CSF.

A study of older patients (≥65 years) undergoing oral surgery for cancer treatment ($n = 112$) demonstrated that although there were no baseline (i.e., preoperative state) differences in the levels of studied biomarkers studied, patients who developed POD experienced elevated levels of interleukin-6 ($P > 0.01$), C-reactive protein ($P > 0.01$), procalcitonin ($P > 0.01$), cortisol ($P > 0.01$), and Aβ1–40 ($P > 0.01$) as measured in plasma during the postoperative period [138]. A study of patients undergoing surgical repair following hip fracture ($n = 60$) found that in patients without prior cognitive impairment, CRP levels in the CSF were higher in participants with delirium than in those without delirium ($P = 0.01$) [139].

To study the effects of illness-induced neuropeptide release secondary to systemic illness over a CNS-specific inflammatory response, a group of researchers induced acute pancreatitis (by injecting 2.5% taurocholic acid directly into the pancreatic duct) in 8–10-week-old rats and collected brain tissue 12 and 24 h following pancreatic injury to measure neuropeptide and cytokine tissue levels [140]. They found that the tissue levels of β-endorphin, orexin, and oxytocin were significantly increased 12 h after induction of acute pancreatitis compared to the control group. Yet, only β-endorphin protein levels remained significantly increased at 24 h after the induction of acute pancreatitis. Meanwhile, they found no differences in the protein levels of α-MSH, neurotensin, substance P, and S100B in the study groups. Given the absence of an increase in the protein levels of TNFα, IL-6, or IL-10 in the prefrontal cortex of studied animals, the authors theorized that the differences in the protein levels of β-endorphin, orexin, and oxytocin occurred in the absence of significant microglia activation. These findings seem to confirm, as others have theorized, that the CNS exhibits clear features of immune activation in response to distant infectious processes [141]. In fact, others have demonstrated that multiple peripheral (e.g., sepsis and peripheral challenge with lipopolysaccharide) as well as localized injuries (e.g., ruptured aneurysms and cranioencephalic trauma) are able to induce a steep increase in brain TNFα levels and cause significant brain inflammation [142]. This may suggest that neuropeptides may serve as the pivotal alarm system, triggering an acute inflammatory CNS response in situations where the BBB remains intact and the microglial cells are not elicited [140].

Among acute ischemic stroke patients, the incidence of delirium was 18.3% (mostly hypoactive type, 72.7%), yet there was no significant statistical difference between delirious and non-delirious patients in respect of levels of TNF-alpha, IL-1 beta, IL-18, BDNF, and NSE [143].

On the other hand, among patients undergoing spine surgery, plasma BDNF was collected at baseline and at least hourly intraoperatively, and then patients were followed after surgery [144]. Results suggest that BDNF levels generally declined intraoperatively. While there was no difference in baseline BDNF levels by delirium status, the percent decline in BDNF was greater in patients who developed delirium (median 74% [IQR 51–82]) vs in those who did not develop delirium (median 50% [IQR 14–79]; $P = 0.03$). Each 1% decline in BDNF was associated with increased odds of delirium in unadjusted (odds ratio [OR] 1.02 [95% confidence interval (CI) 1.00–1.04]; $P = 0.01$), multivariable-adjusted (OR 1.02 [95% CI 1.00–1.03]; $P = 0.03$), and propensity score-adjusted models (OR 1.02 [95% CI 1.00–1.04]; $P = 0.03$).

A study of dementia-free adults ≥70 years old undergoing major scheduled noncardiac surgery ($n = 566$) found that compared to controls, patients with POD had significantly higher CRP levels ($P < 0.01$) during the immediate postoperative period [145]. Of interest, in this particular sample, elevated pre- and postoperative plasma levels of CRP were associated with delirium, suggesting that a pre-inflammatory state and heightened inflammatory response to surgery are potential pathophysiological mechanisms of delirium.

Similarly, a study of patients admitted to the intensive care unit ($n = 618$) found that an increased postoperative C-reactive protein (CRP) concentration was associated with higher odds of POD ($P < 0.001$) and was consistently predictive of longer duration of POD [146].

A study of biomarkers among ICU patients at risk for delirium (based on the PRE-DELIRIC model) was included in the dynamic light application to reduce ICU-acquired delirium (DLA) study ($n = 86$) [147]. The study found that there was no difference between patients with and without delirium in the studied inflammatory markers (i.e., IL-6, IL-10, MCP-1). When differentiating between clinical subtypes of delirium, levels of Tau protein and the ratio of Tau/Aβ1–42 were significantly higher in the hypoactive delirium group compared to the non-delirium group ($P = 0.009$ and $P = 0.003$, respectively). In addition, in the subgroup of patients with hypoactive delirium, levels of neopterin and IL-10 were significantly higher than in the mixed-type delirium group ($P = 0.001$).

A meta-analysis of 54 observational studies [148] found that levels of C-reactive protein (CRP) were significantly increased in POD [100, 139, 149–152] and in POCD [16, 153–156]. Similarly, interleukin (IL)-6 concentrations were also elevated in both POD [100, 139, 151, 152, 157] and POCD [16, 155, 158–160] patients.

Vulnerability States and Acute Brain Dysfunction

The degree and severity of the underlying disease process is also significantly correlated with the development of delirium [3, 161–165]. These facts suggest that either a low dose of precipitant in a vulnerable patient (e.g., elderly, immunocompromised, frail patients) or a high dose in the non-vulnerable individual may overwhelm the system and lead to delirium. Thus, it seems likely that more severe systemic inflammatory responses are more likely to induce delirium, but preexisting pathology in cognitive circuitry is a stronger predictor. Thus, the interaction between these two factors is key [166, 167].

In predisposed patients, even minor insults, such as a urinary tract infection or pneumonia, may trigger an acute confusional state. This out of proportion reaction, similar to an exaggerated sickness behavior, seems to be a response re-exposure to infectious agents, such as in the case of a CNS inflammatory responses to systemic challenge with bacterial LPS [168]. In fact, studies have demonstrated that microglia, the major macrophage population of the brain, seem to be primed by prior neurodegenerative pathology, thus triggering a more robust response to systemic inflammatory signals (Fig. 10.5) [169, 170]. Additionally, there appears to be a correlation between the severity of the patient's underlying medical problem and the development of delirium [161, 162].

In one of the most recent systematic reviews published [169], the most common inflammatory biomarkers in various studies of acutely ill patients include IL-6 [16, 25, 29, 90, 97, 137, 172–180], CRP [16, 25, 29, 54, 91, 97, 131, 134, 176, 181–183], IL-8 [16, 25, 90, 137, 171, 173, 177–179, 181], IL-10 [16, 25, 29, 137, 170, 171, 173, 175, 176], IL-1 [16, 25, 29, 101, 170, 175, 181], and TNF [16, 25, 29, 170, 172, 181] and S100β [25, 80–82, 90, 99, 172, 178, 180, 184–186]. In particular, S100β has been studied as a biomarker of brain damage in response to inflammation, ischemia, and metabolic stress [14, 185, 186].

Also, there is evidence that CD19-directed chimeric antigen receptor (CAR)-T cell therapy, although effective against B cell malignancies in children and adults

[187, 188], has been associated with a number of adverse side effects, including neurotoxicity occurring in approximately 40% of patents. Manifestations range from mild delirium to fatal cerebral edema [189], likely associated with cytokine release syndrome (CRS) [190, 191]. Evidence suggests that systemic inflammatory signaling during CAR-T cell expansion leads to disruption of the BBB [192, 193]. Some have suggested that monocyte-derived cytokines are required for the development of immune effector cell-associated neurotoxicity syndrome (ICANS) [194, 195]. Given the intimate involvement of astrocytes in the regulation of the BBB [196], some have hypothesized that glial dysfunction is part of the pathophysiology of ICANS [197].

In a recent study of acute lymphocytic leukemia (ALL) patients treated with CAR-T, 44% of subjects developed neurotoxicity, among which delirium was the most common symptom, affecting 79% [197]. While there was no difference in baseline CSF protein and cell counts among groups, neurotoxicity was associated with rise in CSF glial fibrillary acidic protein (GFAP; $P = 0.0037$) and S100β ($P = 0.0002$). There was also an association of elevated granulocyte macrophage colony-stimulating factor, granzyme B (GzB), interferon-γ (IFNγ), interleukin (IL)-6, interleukin (IL)-10, tumor necrosis factor (TNF)-α, and macrophage inflammatory protein (MIP)-1α levels with neurotoxicity [197]. These findings suggest that toxicity is primarily mediated by the inflammatory cytokine surge that accompanies CAR-T cell expansion in the marrow [197].

Studies among postpartum women admitted to the ICU have demonstrated that serum levels of galectin-3 (a proinflammatory protein involved in multiple aspects, including cell adhesion, proliferation, clearance, apoptosis, cell activation, cell migration, and phagocytosis [200–203]), S100β, and C-reactive protein were all independent predictors for delirium [180]. In fact, the area under the curve (AUC) of serum galectin-3 levels was similar to that of S100β levels and significantly exceeded those of C-reactive protein levels and APACHE II scores.

Relationship Between Inflammation and Neurotransmitter Abnormalities

The syndrome of delirium is essentially a neurobehavioral syndrome caused by an alteration in neurotransmitter synthesis, function, and/or availability and a dysregulation of neuronal activity secondary to systemic disturbances which mediates the complex phenotypic and neurocognitive changes observed in delirium [13]. While many neurotransmitter systems have been implicated in its development, the most commonly described changes associated with the development of delirium include *deficiencies* in acetylcholine (↓Ach) and/or melatonin (↓MEL) availability; *excess* in dopamine (↑DA), norepinephrine (↑NE), and/or glutamate (↑GLU) release; and *variable alterations* (e.g., either a decreased or increased activity, depending on delirium presentation and cause) in serotonin (↓↑5HT), histamine (↓↑H1&2), and/or gamma-aminobutyric acid (↓↑GABA). The manifestations of the specific delirium picture (i.e., phenotype) result from a combination of the alteration in neurotransmitter synthesis, function, and/or availability, and the variability in integration and appropriate processing of sensory information and motor responses, mediated by an acute breakdown in brain network connectivity. The presence of a CNS inflammatory process usually leads to alteration in neurotransmitter function or availability; in turn, the alteration of one neurotransmitter pathway invariably leads to dysregulation of others (see Fig. 10.8 [12, 13, 15]).

For example, acetylcholine (ACh) synthesis and release may be most sensitive to hypoxic brain insults and other homeostatic changes in the brain [86]. Inadequate oxidative metabolism may be one of the underlying causes of the basic metabolic problems initiating the cascade that leads to the development of delirium, namely, inability to maintain ionic gradients causing cortical spreading depression (i.e., spreading of a self-propagating wave of cellular depolarization in the cerebral cortex) [204–209]; abnormal neurotransmitter synthesis, metabolism, and release [210–218]; and a failure to effectively eliminate neurotoxic by-products [209, 210, 214]. Deficiencies in oxidative metabolism will lead to a failure of the ATPase pump system and an influx of Ca^{2+} which may lead to a dramatic release of various neurotransmitters, particularly glutamate (GLU) and dopamine (DA) [217, 218].

On the other hand, infectious, traumatic, and other systemic events may elicit an inflammatory response, causing monocytes and macrophages to produce neopterin, cytokines, and reactive oxygen species, which can be found in the plasma, urine, and CSF of delirious patients [12, 14, 29, 54, 88–91]. There is evidence that these neuroinflammatory reactions may lead to alterations in various neurotransmitter systems, including dopamine, serotonin, and norepinephrine [12, 15, 87]. In addition, disruptions of the EC may lead to enhanced cytokine transport across the disrupted BBB and infiltration of leukocytes and cytokines into the CNS, producing ischemia and neuronal apoptosis, with corresponding alterations in neurotransmitter production and utilization [14, 93, 94]. Furthermore, as previously mentioned, many of delirium's precipitant factors (e.g., infections, intraoperative anesthesia, postoperative sedation) may themselves be associated with potential BBB integrity compromise.

Delirious states are usually associated with impairment of central cholinergic transmission [12, 27, 221–223], and impaired cholinergic transmission is often considered "a common denominator" in delirium (or toxic-metabolic encephalopathies) [222]. The cholinergic system is one of the most important modulatory neurotransmitter systems in the brain, controlling activities that depend on selective attention, which themselves are an essential component of conscious awareness [223] (the two key components for diagnosing delirium). Adequate ACh levels are also essential for the regulation of multiple neuropsychiatric functions, including rapid eye movement (REM) sleep, memory, and synchronization of the electroencephalogram (EEG), all of which are impaired in delirium.

Glutamate (GLU) is the brain's principal excitatory neurotransmitter, and excessive excitotoxicity resulting from glutamate hypertransmission is one of the proposed theories to explain the abnormal neuronal responses to acute medical insults, such as delirium [226–230].

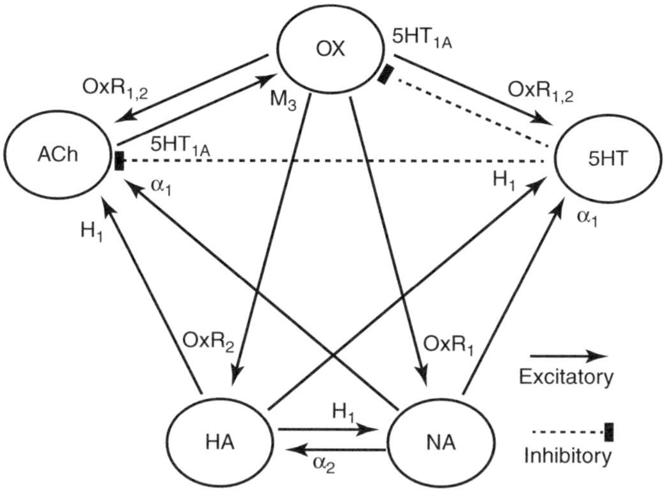

Fig. 10.8 Interrelationship of primary neurotransmitter systems regulating wakefulness and attention. *ACh* (one of the most important modulatory neurotransmitter systems in the brain, controlling activities that depend on selective attention, which themselves are an essential component of conscious awareness); adequate ACh levels are also essential for the regulation of multiple neuropsychiatric functions, including rapid eye movement (REM) sleep, memory, and synchronization of the electroencephalogram (EEG), all of which are somehow impaired in delirium. *DA* both regulates sleep-wake states and helps regulate melatonin; *MEL* helps regulate circadian rhythms in the body as a reaction to environmental lighting conditions; 5-HT helps to maintain arousal and cortical responsiveness as well as inhibiting REM sleep; *orexin* (hypocretin), produced in the hypothalamus, is responsible for regulating many different systems involved with sleep and stabilizing both awake and sleep states. The orexin system regulates DA, NA, histamine, and ACh systems. It is also responsible for integrating different metabolic demand, circadian rhythms, and sleep debt to decide what state the body should be in (asleep or awake). (Source: [263])

γ-aminobutyric acid (GABA) is the chief inhibitory neurotransmitter in the CNS and plays a role in regulating neuronal excitability throughout the nervous system, including regulation of muscle tone. There is evidence suggesting that GABA activity is increased [211, 229, 230] in some types of delirium while decreased in others – as in the case of ethanol or CNS-depressant withdrawal [231] and antibiotic-induced delirium [232].

Delirium has long been speculated to be associated with excess release of norepinephrine (NE) [15, 233, 234]. Excess norepinephrine release secondary to hypoxia or ischemia leads to further neuronal injury and the development or worsening of delirium [235]. Studies have found that increased epinephrine and norepinephrine urinary levels predicted the incidence of delirium among hospitalized, elderly patients [236].

Conclusions

Delirium is a neurobehavioral syndrome caused by the transient disruption of normal neuronal activity mediated by alterations in neurotransmitter and neuronal network functioning, secondary to systemic (metabolic) disturbances. To date, most of the existing theories on the etiology of delirium are complementary, rather than competing, and none of them fully explain the phenomenon of delirium.

Chief among them is the link between delirium and a broad array of infectious and inflammatory abnormalities, suggesting that the CNS and the peripheral immune system maintain a dynamic cross talk to tightly coordinate the innate immune response. In fact, there are multiple potential pathways by which peripheral or systemic factors may elicit a central neuroinflammatory response, including, but not limited to, actual disruptions in the integrity of the BBB.

The presence of infectious agents or inflammatory processes leads to the development of nonspecific physiological and behavioral, as in the case of "sickness behavior" and delirium. The Systems Integration Failure Hypothesis (SIFH) of delirium proposes that alterations in neurotransmitter function combined with a failure of the complex, highly organized, and interconnected brain systems lead to a failure in the CNS's functional integration and appropriate processing of information and response mechanisms. Thus, according to the SIFH, individuals have varying degrees of critical etiological factors and that this "load" will determine the basic fragility (e.g., aging, chronic illness, frailty) of the system in an inverse relationship with acute "precipitants and modifiable" factors (e.g., infection and inflammation, sleep deprivation, trauma, surgery, hypoxia, medication use, substances of abuse, organ failure, electrolyte imbalance, metabolic derangement).

The interplay between the alterations in neurotransmitter dysfunction and which network emerges as dominant or unchecked gives rise to the various clinical manifestations observed in the various delirial motoric phenotypes (e.g., hyperactive, hypoactive, mixed). Thus, the manifestations of the specific delirium picture (i.e., phenotype) result from a combination of the alteration in neurotransmitter function and availability, and the variability in integration and appropriate processing of sensory information and motor responses, mediated by an acute breakdown in brain network connectivity. In other words, the form of delirium that ensues will depend upon how and which networks breaks down, influenced by both the individual's baseline network connectivity and the degree of change in inhibitory tone produced. In addition, the presence of a number of physiological states (i.e., cognitive or physiological vulnerabilities) may further predispose individuals, allowing an inflammatory process to have an even greater detrimental effect, which may explain the relationship between experiencing delirium and subsequent episodes of cognitive impairment or even dementia.

References

1. Maldonado JR. Acute brain failure: pathophysiology, diagnosis, management, and sequelae of delirium. Crit Care Clin. 2017;33(3):461–519.
2. Maldonado JR. Delirium: neurobiology, characteristics and management. In: Fogel B, Greenberg D, editors. Psychiatric care of the medical patient. New York: Oxford University Press; 2015. p. 823–907.

3. Maldonado JR. Delirium in the acute care setting: characteristics, diagnosis and treatment. Crit Care Clin. 2008;24(4):657–722.
4. NICE. In: N.I.f.H.a.C. Excellence, editor. Delirium: diagnosis, prevention and management. Manchester: NICE; 2010.
5. Inouye SK. Delirium in hospitalized elderly patients: recognition, evaluation, and management. Conn Med. 1993;57(5):309–15.
6. Dyer CB, Ashton CM, Teasdale TA. Postoperative delirium. A review of 80 primary data-collection studies. Arch Intern Med. 1995;155(5):461–5.
7. Wiesel O, et al. Post-operative delirium of the elderly patient – an iceberg? Harefuah. 2011;150(3):260–3.. 303
8. Ely EW, et al. Evaluation of delirium in critically ill patients: validation of the confusion assessment method for the intensive care unit (CAM-ICU). Crit Care Med. 2001;29(7):1370–9.
9. Engel GL, Romano J. Delirium, a syndrome of cerebral insufficiency. J Chronic Dis. 1959;9(3):260–77.
10. Lipowski ZJ. Update on delirium. Psychiatr Clin North Am. 1992;15(2):335–46.
11. Brown, T.M., Basic mechanisms in the pathogenesis of delirium, The psychiatric care of the medical patient, F.B. Stoudemire, Greenberg DB. 2000, Oxford Press: New York. 571–580.
12. Maldonado JR. Pathoetiological model of delirium: a comprehensive understanding of the neurobiology of delirium and an evidence-based approach to prevention and treatment. Crit Care Clin. 2008;24(4):789–856.
13. Maldonado JR. Delirium pathophysiology: an updated hypothesis of the etiology of acute brain failure. Int J Geriatr Psychiatry. 2018;33(11):1428–57.
14. Cerejeira J, et al. The neuroinflammatory hypothesis of delirium. Acta Neuropathol. 2010;119(6):737–54.
15. Maldonado JR. Neuropathogenesis of delirium: review of current etiologic theories and common pathways. Am J Geriatr Psychiatry. 2013;21(12):1190–222.
16. Beloosesky Y, Hendel D, Weiss A, Hershkovitz A, Grinblat J, Pirotsky A, Barak V. Cytokines and C-reactive protein production in hip-fracture-operated elderly patients. J Gerontol A Biol Sci Med Sci. 2007;62(4):420–6.
17. Elie M, et al. Delirium risk factors in elderly hospitalized patients. J Gen Intern Med. 1998;13(3):204–12.
18. Zampieri FG, et al. Sepsis-associated encephalopathy: not just delirium. Clinics (Sao Paulo). 2011;66(10):1825–31.
19. van Gool WA, van de Beek D, Eikelenboom P. Systemic infection and delirium: when cytokines and acetylcholine collide. Lancet. 2010;375(9716):773–5.
20. Simone MJ, Tan ZS. The role of inflammation in the pathogenesis of delirium and dementia in older adults: a review. CNS Neurosci Ther. 2011;17(5):506–13.
21. Lemstra AW, et al. Pre-operative inflammatory markers and the risk of postoperative delirium in elderly patients. Int J Geriatr Psychiatry. 2008;23(9):943–8.
22. Hala M. Pathophysiology of postoperative delirium: systemic inflammation as a response to surgical trauma causes diffuse microcirculatory impairment. Med Hypotheses. 2007;68(1):194–6.
23. Frederiks JA. Inflammation of the mind. On the 300th anniversary of Gerard van Swieten. J Hist Neurosci. 2000;9(3):307–10.
24. Cunningham C. Systemic inflammation and delirium: important co-factors in the progression of dementia. Biochem Soc Trans. 2011;39(4):945–53.
25. van den Boogaard M, et al. Biomarkers associated with delirium in critically ill patients and their relation with long-term subjective cognitive dysfunction; indications for different pathways governing delirium in inflamed and noninflamed patients. Crit Care. 2011;15(6):R297.
26. van Munster BC, et al. Neuroinflammation in delirium: a postmortem case-control study. Rejuvenation Res. 2011;14(6):615–22.
27. Lipowski ZJ. Delirium: how its concept has developed. Int Psychogeriatr. 1991;3(2):115–20.
28. Sakai A. Phrenitis: inflammation of the mind and the body. Hist Psychiatry. 1991;2(6):193–205.

29. de Rooij SE, et al. Cytokines and acute phase response in delirium. J Psychosom Res. 2007;62(5):521–5.
30. Godbout JP, et al. Exaggerated neuroinflammation and sickness behavior in aged mice following activation of the peripheral innate immune system. FASEB J. 2005;19(10):1329–31.
31. Dantzer R. Cytokine-induced sickness behavior: mechanisms and implications. Ann N Y Acad Sci. 2001;933:222–34.
32. Dantzer R. Cytokine-induced sickness behaviour: a neuroimmune response to activation of innate immunity. Eur J Pharmacol. 2004;500(1–3):399–411.
33. Dantzer R, et al. Cytokines and sickness behavior. Ann N Y Acad Sci. 1998;840:586–90.
34. Cunningham C, et al. Systemic inflammation induces acute behavioral and cognitive changes and accelerates neurodegenerative disease. Biol Psychiatry. 2009;65(4):304–12.
35. Kronfol Z, Remick DG. Cytokines and the brain: implications for clinical psychiatry. Am J Psychiatry. 2000;157(5):683–94.
36. Shattuck EC, Muehlenbein MP. Human sickness behavior: ultimate and proximate explanations. Am J Phys Anthropol. 2015;157(1):1–18.
37. Eisenberger NI, et al. In sickness and in health: the co-regulation of inflammation and social behavior. Neuropsychopharmacology. 2017;42(1):242–53.
38. Tizard I. Sickness behavior, its mechanisms and significance. Anim Health Res Rev. 2008;9(1):87–99.
39. Dantzer R. Cytokine, sickness behavior, and depression. Neurol Clin. 2006;24(3):441–60.
40. De La Garza R 2nd. Endotoxin- or pro-inflammatory cytokine-induced sickness behavior as an animal model of depression: focus on anhedonia. Neurosci Biobehav Rev. 2005;29(4–5):761–70.
41. Kelley KW, et al. Cytokine-induced sickness behavior. Brain Behav Immun. 2003;17(Suppl 1):S112–8.
42. Hart BL. Biological basis of the behavior of sick animals. Neurosci Biobehav Rev. 1988;12(2):123–37.
43. Miller AH, et al. Cytokine targets in the brain: impact on neurotransmitters and neurocircuits. Depress Anxiety. 2013;30(4):297–306.
44. Miller AH, Maletic V, Raison CL. Inflammation and its discontents: the role of cytokines in the pathophysiology of major depression. Biol Psychiatry. 2009;65(9):732–41.
45. Behan WM, Stone TW. Role of kynurenines in the neurotoxic actions of kainic acid. Br J Pharmacol. 2000;129(8):1764–70.
46. Stone TW, et al. The role of kynurenines in the production of neuronal death, and the neuroprotective effect of purines. J Alzheimers Dis. 2001;3(4):355–66.
47. Stone TW, Forrest CM, Darlington LG. Kynurenine pathway inhibition as a therapeutic strategy for neuroprotection. FEBS J. 2012;279(8):1386–97.
48. Darlington LG, et al. On the biological importance of the 3-hydroxyanthranilic acid: anthranilic acid ratio. Int J Tryptophan Res. 2010;3:51–9.
49. Darlington LG, et al. Altered kynurenine metabolism correlates with infarct volume in stroke. Eur J Neurosci. 2007;26(8):2211–21.
50. Kochanek PM, et al. Biomarkers of primary and evolving damage in traumatic and ischemic brain injury: diagnosis, prognosis, probing mechanisms, and therapeutic decision making. Curr Opin Crit Care. 2008;14(2):135–41.
51. Dantzer R, et al. From inflammation to sickness and depression: when the immune system subjugates the brain. Nat Rev Neurosci. 2008;9(1):46–56.
52. Dantzer R, et al. Neural and humoral pathways of communication from the immune system to the brain: parallel or convergent? Auton Neurosci. 2000;85(1–3):60–5.
53. Piva S, McCreadie VA, Latronico N. Neuroinflammation in sepsis: sepsis associated delirium. Cardiovasc Hematol Disord Drug Targets. 2015;15(1):10–8.
54. McGrane S, et al. Procalcitonin and C-reactive protein levels at admission as predictors of duration of acute brain dysfunction in critically ill patients. Crit Care. 2011;15(2):R78.
55. Pan W, et al. Cytokine signaling modulates blood-brain barrier function. Curr Pharm Des. 2011;17(33):3729–40.

56. Banks WA, Kastin AJ, Durham DA. Bidirectional transport of interleukin-1 alpha across the blood-brain barrier. Brain Res Bull. 1989;23(6):433–7.
57. Banks WA, Kastin AJ. Blood to brain transport of interleukin links the immune and central nervous systems. Life Sci. 1991;48(25):PL117–21.
58. Banks RE, Patel PM, Selby PJ. Interleukin 12: a new clinical player in cytokine therapy. Br J Cancer. 1995;71(4):655–9.
59. Gutierrez EG, Banks WA, Kastin AJ. Blood-borne interleukin-1 receptor antagonist crosses the blood-brain barrier. J Neuroimmunol. 1994;55(2):153–60.
60. Banks WA, Kastin AJ, Gutierrez EG. Penetration of interleukin-6 across the murine blood-brain barrier. Neurosci Lett. 1994;179(1–2):53–6.
61. Pan W, et al. Neuroinflammation facilitates LIF entry into brain: role of TNF. Am J Physiol Cell Physiol. 2008;294(6):C1436–42.
62. Pan W, et al. Stroke upregulates TNFalpha transport across the blood-brain barrier. Exp Neurol. 2006;198(1):222–33.
63. Pan W, et al. Receptor-mediated transport of LIF across blood-spinal cord barrier is upregulated after spinal cord injury. J Neuroimmunol. 2006;174(1–2):119–25.
64. Pan W, Kastin AJ, Brennan JM. Saturable entry of leukemia inhibitory factor from blood to the central nervous system. J Neuroimmunol. 2000;106(1–2):172–80.
65. Osburg B, et al. Effect of endotoxin on expression of TNF receptors and transport of TNF-alpha at the blood-brain barrier of the rat. Am J Physiol Endocrinol Metab. 2002;283(5):E899–908.
66. Pan W, et al. Differential permeability of the BBB in acute EAE: enhanced transport of TNT-alpha. Am J Phys. 1996;271(4. Pt 1):E636–42.
67. Pan W, et al. Saturable entry of ciliary neurotrophic factor into brain. Neurosci Lett. 1999;263(1):69–71.
68. Pan W, Kastin AJ. Urocortin and the brain. Prog Neurobiol. 2008;84(2):148–56.
69. Pan W, Kastin AJ. Adipokines and the blood-brain barrier. Peptides. 2007;28(6):1317–30.
70. Kastin AJ, Pan W. Feeding peptides interact in several ways with the blood-brain barrier. Curr Pharm Des. 2003;9(10):789–94.
71. Jeppsson B, et al. Blood-brain barrier derangement in sepsis: cause of septic encephalopathy? Am J Surg. 1981;141(1):136–42.
72. Butterworth RF. The liver-brain axis in liver failure: neuroinflammation and encephalopathy. Nat Rev Gastroenterol Hepatol. 2013;10:522–8.
73. Bemeur C, Butterworth RF. Liver-brain proinflammatory signalling in acute liver failure: role in the pathogenesis of hepatic encephalopathy and brain edema. Metab Brain Dis. 2013;28(2):145–50.
74. Stone TW, Darlington LG. Endogenous kynurenines as targets for drug discovery and development. Nat Rev Drug Discov. 2002;1(8):609–20.
75. Stone TW, Darlington LG. The kynurenine pathway as a therapeutic target in cognitive and neurodegenerative disorders. Br J Pharmacol. 2013;169(6):1211–27.
76. Forrest CM, et al. Kynurenine metabolism predicts cognitive function in patients following cardiac bypass and thoracic surgery. J Neurochem. 2011;119(1):136–52.
77. Krueger JM, Majde JA. Humoral links between sleep and the immune system*: research issues*. Ann N Y Acad Sci. 2003;992:9–20.
78. Lewin GR, Barde YA. Physiology of the neurotrophins. Annu Rev Neurosci. 1996;19:289–317.
79. Bokesch PM, Izykenova GA, Justice JB, Easley KA, Dambinova SA. NMDA receptor antibodies predict adverse neurological outcome after cardiac surgery in high-risk patients. Stroke. 2006;37(6):1432–6.
80. Hall RJ, et al. Delirium and Cerebrospinal Fluid S100B in Hip Fracture Patients: a preliminary study. Am J Geriatr Psychiatry. 2013;21(12):1239–43.
81. van Munster BC, et al. Serum S100B in elderly patients with and without delirium. Int J Geriatr Psychiatry. 2010;25(3):234–9.
82. van Munster BC, et al. Markers of cerebral damage during delirium in elderly patients with hip fracture. BMC Neurol. 2009;9:21.

83. Bogatcheva NV, et al. Arachidonic acid cascade in endothelial pathobiology. Microvasc Res. 2005;69(3):107–27.
84. Uchikado H, et al. Activation of vascular endothelial cells and perivascular cells by systemic inflammation-an immunohistochemical study of postmortem human brain tissues. Acta Neuropathol. 2004;107(4):341–51.
85. He F, et al. Molecular mechanism for change in permeability in brain microvascular endothelial cells induced by LPS. Zhong Nan Da Xue Xue Bao Yi Xue Ban. 2010;35(11):1129–37.
86. Hirsch JA, Gibson GE. Selective alteration of neurotransmitter release by low oxygen in vitro. Neurochem Res. 1984;9(8):1039–49.
87. Hshieh TT, et al. Cholinergic deficiency hypothesis in delirium: a synthesis of current evidence. J Gerontol A Biol Sci Med Sci. 2008;63(7):764–72.
88. Dantzer R, et al. Identification and treatment of symptoms associated with inflammation in medically ill patients. Psychoneuroendocrinology. 2008;33(1):18–29.
89. Sorrells SF, et al. The stressed CNS: when glucocorticoids aggravate inflammation. Neuron. 2009;64(1):33–9.
90. van Munster BC, et al. Cortisol, interleukins and S100B in delirium in the elderly. Brain Cogn. 2010;74(1):18–23.
91. Osse RJ, et al. High preoperative plasma neopterin predicts delirium after cardiac surgery in older adults. J Am Geriatr Soc. 2012;60:661–8.
92. Murr C, et al. Neopterin as a marker for immune system activation. Curr Drug Metab. 2002;3(2):175–87.
93. Huber JD, et al. Blood-brain barrier tight junctions are altered during a 72-h exposure to lambda-carrageenan-induced inflammatory pain. Am J Physiol Heart Circ Physiol. 2002;283(4):H1531–7.
94. Brooks TA, et al. Chronic inflammatory pain leads to increased blood-brain barrier permeability and tight junction protein alterations. Am J Physiol Heart Circ Physiol. 2005;289(2):H738–43.
95. Forsberg M, et al. Breakdown of the blood-brain barrier by anesthetics: possible role in post-surgical delirium. Baltimore: American Delirium Society; 2014.
96. Varatharaj A, Galea I. The blood-brain barrier in systemic inflammation. Brain Behav Immun. 2016;60:1.
97. Macdonald A, et al. C-reactive protein levels predict the incidence of delirium and recovery from it. Age Ageing. 2007;36(2):222–5.
98. MacLullich AM, et al. Cerebrospinal fluid interleukin-8 levels are higher in people with hip fracture with perioperative delirium than in controls. J Am Geriatr Soc. 2011;59(6):1151–3.
99. Grandi C, et al. Brain-derived neurotrophic factor and neuron-specific enolase, but not S100beta, levels are associated to the occurrence of delirium in intensive care unit patients. J Crit Care. 2011;26(2):133–7.
100. Westhoff D, et al. Preoperative cerebrospinal fluid cytokine levels and the risk of postoperative delirium in elderly hip fracture patients. J Neuroinflammation. 2013;10:122.
101. Cape E, et al. Cerebrospinal fluid markers of neuroinflammation in delirium: a role for interleukin-1beta in delirium after hip fracture. J Psychosom Res. 2014;77(3):219–25.
102. Zupancic ML, Mahajan A. Leptin as a neuroactive agent. Psychosom Med. 2011;73(5):407–14.
103. Harvey J. Leptin regulation of neuronal excitability and cognitive function. Curr Opin Pharmacol. 2007;7(6):643–7.
104. Harvey J. Leptin: a diverse regulator of neuronal function. J Neurochem. 2007;100(2):307–13.
105. Stieg MR, et al. Leptin: a hormone linking activation of neuroendocrine axes with neuropathology. Psychoneuroendocrinology. 2015;51:47–57.
106. Quasim T, et al. The relationship between leptin concentrations, the systemic inflammatory response and illness severity in surgical patients admitted to ITU. Clin Nutr. 2004;23(2):233–8.
107. Zou X, et al. Role of leptin in mood disorder and neurodegenerative disease. Front Neurosci. 2019;13:378.
108. Ge T, et al. Leptin in depression: a potential therapeutic target. Cell Death Dis. 2018;9(11):1096.

109. Li YT, et al. The association between serum leptin and post stroke depression: results from a cohort study. PLoS One. 2014;9(7):e103137.
110. Hafner S, et al. Social isolation and depressed mood are associated with elevated serum leptin levels in men but not in women. Psychoneuroendocrinology. 2011;36(2):200–9.
111. Westling S, et al. Low CSF leptin in female suicide attempters with major depression. J Affect Disord. 2004;81(1):41–8.
112. Atmaca M, et al. Serum leptin and cholesterol values in suicide attempters. Neuropsychobiology. 2002;45(3):124–7.
113. Kraus T, et al. Low leptin levels but normal body mass indices in patients with depression or schizophrenia. Neuroendocrinology. 2001;73(4):243–7.
114. Venkatasubramanian G, et al. Neuropharmacology of schizophrenia: is there a role for leptin? Clin Chem Lab Med. 2010;48(6):895–6.
115. Nurjono M, Neelamekam S, Lee J. Serum leptin and its relationship with psychopathology in schizophrenia. Psychoneuroendocrinology. 2014;50:149–54.
116. Martorell L, et al. Increased levels of serum leptin in the early stages of psychosis. J Psychiatr Res. 2019;111:24–9.
117. Gohar SM, et al. Association between leptin levels and severity of suicidal behaviour in schizophrenia spectrum disorders. Acta Psychiatr Scand. 2019;139(5):464–71.
118. Schuld A, et al. Reduced leptin levels in human narcolepsy. Neuroendocrinology. 2000;72(4):195–8.
119. Kok SW, et al. Reduction of plasma leptin levels and loss of its circadian rhythmicity in hypocretin (orexin)-deficient narcoleptic humans. J Clin Endocrinol Metab. 2002;87(2):805–9.
120. Dahmen N, et al. Peripheral leptin levels in narcoleptic patients. Diabetes Technol Ther. 2007;9(4):348–53.
121. Paz-Filho G, Wong ML, Licinio J. Leptin levels and Alzheimer disease. JAMA. 2010;303(15):1478.. author reply 1478-9
122. Marwarha G, Ghribi O. Leptin signaling and Alzheimer's disease. Am J Neurodegener Dis. 2012;1(3):245–65.
123. Magalhaes CA, et al. Leptin in Alzheimer's disease. Clin Chim Acta. 2015;450:162–8.
124. Harvey J. Leptin: the missing link in Alzheimer disease? Clin Chem. 2010;56(5):696–7.
125. Carro EM. Therapeutic approaches of leptin in Alzheimer's disease. Recent Pat CNS Drug Discov. 2009;4(3):200–8.
126. Baranowska-Bik A, et al. Plasma leptin levels and free leptin index in women with Alzheimer's disease. Neuropeptides. 2015;52:73–8.
127. King A, et al. Disruption of leptin signalling in a mouse model of Alzheimer's disease. Metab Brain Dis. 2018;33(4):1097–110.
128. Sanchez JC, Ospina JP, Gonzalez MI. Association between leptin and delirium in elderly inpatients. Neuropsychiatr Dis Treat. 2013;9:659–66.
129. Chen XW, et al. Preoperative plasma leptin levels predict delirium in elderly patients after hip fracture surgery. Peptides. 2014;57:31–5.
130. Hatta K, et al. The predictive value of a change in natural killer cell activity for delirium. Prog Neuro-Psychopharmacol Biol Psychiatry. 2014;48:26–31.
131. Ritchie CW, et al. The association between C-reactive protein and delirium in 710 acute elderly hospital admissions. Int Psychogeriatr. 2014;26(5):717–24.
132. Kazmierski J, et al. Raised IL-2 and TNF-alpha concentrations are associated with postoperative delirium in patients undergoing coronary-artery bypass graft surgery. Int Psychogeriatr. 2014;26(5):845–55.
133. Pol RA, et al. C-reactive protein predicts postoperative delirium following vascular surgery. Ann Vasc Surg. 2014;28(8):1923–30.
134. Zhang Z, et al. Prediction of delirium in critically ill patients with elevated C-reactive protein. J Crit Care. 2014;29(1):88–92.
135. Poljak A, et al. Quantitative proteomics of delirium cerebrospinal fluid. Transl Psychiatry. 2014;4:e477.

136. Hasegawa T, et al. Risk factors associated with postoperative delirium after surgery for oral cancer. J Craniomaxillofac Surg. 2015;43(7):1094–8.
137. Hirsch J, et al. Perioperative cerebrospinal fluid and plasma inflammatory markers after orthopedic surgery. J Neuroinflammation. 2016;13(1):211.
138. Sun L, et al. Production of inflammatory cytokines, cortisol, and Abeta1-40 in elderly oral cancer patients with postoperative delirium. Neuropsychiatr Dis Treat. 2016;12:2789–95.
139. Neerland BE, et al. Associations between delirium and preoperative cerebrospinal fluid C-reactive protein, Interleukin-6, and Interleukin-6 receptor in individuals with acute hip fracture. J Am Geriatr Soc. 2016;64(7):1456–63.
140. Hamasaki MY, et al. Neuropeptides in the brain defense against distant organ damage. J Neuroimmunol. 2016;290:33–5.
141. Lucas SM, Rothwell NJ, Gibson RM. The role of inflammation in CNS injury and disease. Br J Pharmacol. 2006;147(Suppl 1):S232–40.
142. Hoogland IC, et al. Systemic inflammation and microglial activation: systematic review of animal experiments. J Neuroinflammation. 2015;12:114.
143. Kozak HH, et al. Delirium in patients with acute ischemic stroke admitted to the non-intensive stroke unit: incidence and association between clinical features and inflammatory markers. Neurol Neurochir Pol. 2017;51(1):38–44.
144. Wyrobek J, et al. Association of intraoperative changes in brain-derived neurotrophic factor and postoperative delirium in older adults. Br J Anaesth. 2017;119(2):324–32.
145. Dillon ST, et al. Higher C-reactive protein levels predict postoperative delirium in older patients undergoing major elective surgery: a longitudinal nested case-control study. Biol Psychiatry. 2017;81(2):145–53.
146. Cereghetti C, et al. Independent predictors of the duration and overall burden of postoperative delirium after cardiac surgery in adults: an observational cohort study. J Cardiothorac Vasc Anesth. 2017;31(6):1966–73.
147. Simons KS, et al. Temporal biomarker profiles and their association with ICU acquired delirium: a cohort study. Crit Care. 2018;22(1):137.
148. Liu X, Yu Y, Zhu S. Inflammatory markers in postoperative delirium (POD) and cognitive dysfunction (POCD): a meta-analysis of observational studies. PLoS One. 2018;13(4):e0195659.
149. Guenther U, et al. Predisposing and precipitating factors of delirium after cardiac surgery: a prospective observational cohort study. Ann Surg. 2013;257(6):1160–7.
150. Lee HJ, et al. Early assessment of delirium in elderly patients after hip surgery. Psychiatry Investig. 2011;8(4):340–7.
151. Shen H, et al. Insulin-like growth Factor-1, a potential predicative biomarker for postoperative delirium among elderly patients with open abdominal surgery. Curr Pharm Des. 2016;22(38):5879–83.
152. Liu P, et al. High serum interleukin-6 level is associated with increased risk of delirium in elderly patients after noncardiac surgery: a prospective cohort study. Chin Med J. 2013;126(19):3621–7.
153. Wu C, et al. Preoperative serum MicroRNA-155 expression independently predicts postoperative cognitive dysfunction after laparoscopic surgery for colon cancer. Med Sci Monit. 2016;22:4503–8.
154. Chen Y, et al. Relationship between hs-CRP, IL-6 and the cognitive function decrease of elderly after sevoflurane anesthesia. Chin J Health Labratory Technol. 2011;10:2431–3.
155. Li Y, et al. Correlation between postoperative cognitive dysfunction and peri-operative inflammation in elderly patients undergoing total hip-replacement surgery. Shanghai Med J. 2011;34(4):249–52.
156. Burkhart CS, et al. Postoperative cognitive dysfunction (POCD), markers of brain damage and systemic inflammation in elderly patients. Eur J Anaesthesiol. 2011;28:223.
157. Capri M, et al. Pre-operative, high-IL-6 blood level is a risk factor of post-operative delirium onset in old patients. Front Endocrinol (Lausanne). 2014;5:173.
158. Zhang Y, et al. Differential expressions of serum cytokines in cognitive dysfunction patients after colorectal surgery. Xi Bao Yu Fen Zi Mian Yi Xue Za Zhi. 2015;31(2):231–4.

159. F Z, J Z, L Y. Relativity research of expression of S-100β protein, IL-1β, IL-6 and α-TNF to recognition after Total knee arthroplasty. J Zhejiang Univ Tradit Chin Med. 2012;12:1290–2.
160. Lin GX, et al. Serum high-mobility group box 1 protein correlates with cognitive decline after gastrointestinal surgery. Acta Anaesthesiol Scand. 2014;58(6):668–74.
161. Ouimet S, et al. Incidence, risk factors and consequences of ICU delirium. Intensive Care Med. 2007;33(1):66–73.
162. Pandharipande P, et al. Lorazepam is an independent risk factor for transitioning to delirium in intensive care unit patients. Anesthesiology. 2006;104(1):21–6.
163. Girard TD, et al. Efficacy and safety of a paired sedation and ventilator weaning protocol for mechanically ventilated patients in intensive care (awakening and breathing controlled trial): a randomised controlled trial. Lancet. 2008;371(9607):126–34.
164. Ryan DJ, et al. Delirium in an adult acute hospital population: predictors, prevalence and detection. BMJ Open. 2013;3:1.
165. Srinonprasert V, et al. Risk factors for developing delirium in older patients admitted to general medical wards. J Med Assoc Thail. 2011;94(Suppl 1):S99–104.
166. Maclullich AM, et al. Unravelling the pathophysiology of delirium: a focus on the role of aberrant stress responses. J Psychosom Res. 2008;65(3):229–38.
167. Cunningham C, Maclullich AM. At the extreme end of the psychoneuroimmunological spectrum: delirium as a maladaptive sickness behaviour response. Brain Behav Immun. 2013;28:1–13.
168. Combrinck MI, Perry VH, Cunningham C. Peripheral infection evokes exaggerated sickness behaviour in pre-clinical murine prion disease. Neuroscience. 2002;112(1):7–11.
169. Cunningham C, Wilcockson DC, Campion S, Lunnon K, Perry VH. Central and systemic endotoxin challenges exacerbate the local inflammatory response and increase neuronal death during chronic neurodegeneration. J Neurosci. 2005;25(40):9275–84.
170. Murray C, Sanderson DJ, Barkus C, et al. Systemic inflammation induces acute working memory deficits in the primed brain: relevance for delirium. Neurobiol Aging. 2012;33(3):603–16.
171. Michels M, et al. Biomarker predictors of delirium in acutely ill patients: a systematic review. J Geriatr Psychiatry Neurol. 2019;32(3):119–36.
172. Ritter C, et al. Inflammation biomarkers and delirium in critically ill patients. Crit Care. 2014;18(3):R106.
173. Alexander SA, et al. Interleukin 6 and apolipoprotein E as predictors of acute brain dysfunction and survival in critical care patients. Am J Crit Care. 2014;23(1):49–57.
174. Jorge-Ripper C, et al. Prognostic value of acute delirium recovery in older adults. Geriatr Gerontol Int. 2017;17(8):1161–7.
175. Tomasi CD, et al. Baseline acetylcholinesterase activity and serotonin plasma levels are not associated with delirium in critically ill patients. Rev Bras Ter Intensiva. 2015;27(2):170–7.
176. Plaschke K, et al. Early postoperative delirium after open-heart cardiac surgery is associated with decreased bispectral EEG and increased cortisol and interleukin-6. Intensive Care Med. 2010;36(12):2081–9.
177. Rudolph JL, et al. Chemokines are associated with delirium after cardiac surgery. J Gerontol A Biol Sci Med Sci. 2008;63(2):184–9.
178. Cerejeira J, et al. The stress response to surgery and postoperative delirium: evidence of hypothalamic-pituitary-adrenal axis hyperresponsiveness and decreased suppression of the GH/IGF-1 Axis. J Geriatr Psychiatry Neurol. 2013;26(3):185–94.
179. van Munster BC, et al. Time-course of cytokines during delirium in elderly patients with hip fractures. J Am Geriatr Soc. 2008;56(9):1704–9.
180. Erikson K, et al. Elevated serum S-100beta in patients with septic shock is associated with delirium. Acta Anaesthesiol Scand. 2019;63(1):69–73.
181. Girard TD, et al. Associations of markers of inflammation and coagulation with delirium during critical illness. Intensive Care Med. 2012;38(12):1965–73.
182. Zhu Y, et al. Serum galectin-3 levels and delirium among postpartum intensive care unit women. Brain Behav. 2017;7(8):e00773.

183. Adamis D, Treloar A, Martin FC, Gregson N, Hamilton G, Macdonald AJ. APOE and cytokines as biological markers for recovery of prevalent delirium in elderly medical inpatients. Int J Geriatr Psychiatry. 2007;22(7):688–94.
184. Khan BA, et al. S100 calcium binding protein B as a biomarker of delirium duration in the intensive care unit – an exploratory analysis. Int J Gen Med. 2013;6:855–61.
185. Nguyen DN, et al. Cortisol is an associated-risk factor of brain dysfunction in patients with severe sepsis and septic shock. Biomed Res Int. 2014;2014:712742.
186. Hughes CG, et al. Endothelial activation and blood-brain barrier injury as risk factors for delirium in critically ill patients. Crit Care Med. 2016;44(9):e809–17.
187. Porter JT, McCarthy KD. Astrocytic neurotransmitter receptors in situ and in vivo. Prog Neurobiol. 1997;51(4):439–55.
188. Pinto SS, et al. Immunocontent and secretion of S100B in astrocyte cultures from different brain regions in relation to morphology. FEBS Lett. 2000;486(3):203–7.
189. Annesley CE, et al. The evolution and future of CAR T cells for B-cell acute lymphoblastic leukemia. Clin Pharmacol Ther. 2018;103(4):591–8.
190. Brudno JN, Kochenderfer JN. Chimeric antigen receptor T-cell therapies for lymphoma. Nat Rev Clin Oncol. 2018;15(1):31–46.
191. Gust J, Taraseviciute A, Turtle CJ. Neurotoxicity associated with CD19-targeted CAR-T cell therapies. CNS Drugs. 2018;32(12):1091–101.
192. Le RQ, et al. FDA approval summary: tocilizumab for treatment of chimeric antigen receptor T cell-induced severe or life-threatening cytokine release syndrome. Oncologist. 2018;23(8):943–7.
193. Teachey DT, et al. Identification of predictive biomarkers for cytokine release syndrome after chimeric antigen receptor T-cell therapy for acute lymphoblastic leukemia. Cancer Discov. 2016;6(6):664–79.
194. Gust J, et al. Endothelial activation and blood-brain barrier disruption in neurotoxicity after adoptive immunotherapy with CD19 CAR-T cells. Cancer Discov. 2017;7(12):1404–19.
195. Taraseviciute A, et al. Chimeric antigen receptor T cell-mediated neurotoxicity in nonhuman primates. Cancer Discov. 2018;8(6):750–63.
196. Lee DW, et al. ASTCT consensus grading for cytokine release syndrome and neurologic toxicity associated with immune effector cells. Biol Blood Marrow Transplant. 2019;25(4):625–38.
197. Norelli M, et al. Monocyte-derived IL-1 and IL-6 are differentially required for cytokine-release syndrome and neurotoxicity due to CAR T cells. Nat Med. 2018;24(6):739–48.
198. Sofroniew MV. Astrocyte barriers to neurotoxic inflammation. Nat Rev Neurosci. 2015;16(5):249–63.
199. Gust J, et al. Glial injury in neurotoxicity after pediatric CD19-directed chimeric antigen receptor T cell therapy. Ann Neurol. 2019;86:42–54.
200. Zhang H, et al. Galectin-3 as a marker and potential therapeutic target in breast cancer. PLoS One. 2014;9(9):e103482.
201. Liang N, et al. Effect of galectin-3 on the behavior of Eca109 human esophageal cancer cells. Mol Med Rep. 2015;11(2):896–902.
202. Li LC, Li J, Gao J. Functions of galectin-3 and its role in fibrotic diseases. J Pharmacol Exp Ther. 2014;351(2):336–43.
203. Jiang SS, et al. Galectin-3 is associated with a poor prognosis in primary hepatocellular carcinoma. J Transl Med. 2014;12:273.
204. Basarsky TA, Feighan D, MacVicar BA. Glutamate release through volume-activated channels during spreading depression. J Neurosci. 1999;19(15):6439–45.
205. Iijima T, Shimase C, Iwao Y, Sankawa H. Relationships between glutamate release, blood flow and spreading depression: real-time monitoring using an electroenzymatic dialysis electrode. Neurosci Res. 1998;32(3):201–7.
206. Moghaddam B, Schenk JO, Stewart WB, Hansen AJ. Temporal relationship between neurotransmitter release and ion flux during spreading depression and anoxia. Can J Physiol Pharmacol. 1987;65(5):1105–10.

207. Shimizu-Sasamata M, Bosque-Hamilton P, Huang PL, Moskowitz MA, Lo EH. Attenuated neurotransmitter release and spreading depression-like depolarizations after focal ischemia in mutant mice with disrupted type I nitric oxide synthase gene. J Neurosci. 1998;18(22):9564–71.
208. Somjen GG, Aitken PG, Balestrino M, et al. Extracellular ions, hypoxic irreversible loss of function and delayed postischemic neuron degeneration studied in vitro. Acta Physiol Scand Suppl. 1989;582:58.
209. Somjen GG, et al. Spreading depression-like depolarization and selective vulnerability of neurons. A brief review. Stroke. 1990;21(11 Suppl):III179–83.
210. Busto R, et al. Extracellular release of serotonin following fluid-percussion brain injury in rats. J Neurotrauma. 1997;14(1):35–42.
211. Busto R, et al. Effect of mild hypothermia on ischemia-induced release of neurotransmitters and free fatty acids in rat brain. Stroke. 1989;20(7):904–10.
212. Globus MY, et al. Glutamate release and free radical production following brain injury: effects of posttraumatic hypothermia. J Neurochem. 1995;65(4):1704–11.
213. Globus MY, Busto R, Dietrich WD, et al. Effect of ischemia on the in vivo release of striatal dopamine, glutamate, and gamma-aminobutyric acid studied by intracerebral microdialysis. J Neurochem. 1988;51(5):1455–64.
214. Globus MY, et al. Intra-ischemic extracellular release of dopamine and glutamate is associated with striatal vulnerability to ischemia. Neurosci Lett. 1988;91(1):36–40.
215. Globus MY, et al. Direct evidence for acute and massive norepinephrine release in the hippocampus during transient ischemia. J Cereb Blood Flow Metab. 1989;9(6):892–6.
216. Globus MY, et al. Ischemia induces release of glutamate in regions spared from histopathologic damage in the rat. Stroke. 1990;21(11 Suppl):III43–6.
217. Globus MY, et al. Ischemia-induced extracellular release of serotonin plays a role in CA1 neuronal cell death in rats. Stroke. 1992;23(11):1595–601.
218. Takagi K, et al. Effect of hyperthermia on glutamate release in ischemic penumbra after middle cerebral artery occlusion in rats. Am J Phys. 1994;267(5 Pt 2):H1770–6.
219. Kirsch JR, Diringer MN, Borel CO, Hart GK, Hanley DF Jr. Brain resuscitation. Medical management and innovations. Crit Care Nurs Clin North Am. 1989;1(1):143–54.
220. Siesjo BK. Cerebral circulation and metabolism. J Neurosurg. 1984;60(5):883–908.
221. Flacker JM, Cummings V, Mach JR Jr, et al. The association of serum anticholinergic activity with delirium in elderly medical patients. Am J Geriatr Psychiatry. 1998;6(1):31–41.
222. Flacker JM, Lipsitz LA. Neural mechanisms of delirium: current hypotheses and evolving concepts. J Gerontol A Biol Sci Med Sci. 1999;54(6):B239–46.
223. Trzepacz PT. Anticholinergic model for delirium. Semin Clin Neuropsychiatry. 1996;1(4):294–303.
224. Blass J, Gibson G, Duffy T, et al. Cholinergic dysfunction: a common denominator in metabolic encephalopathies. In: Pepeu G, Ladinsky H, editors. Cholinergic mechanisms. New York: Plenum Publishing Corp; 1981. p. 921–8.
225. Perry E, et al. Acetylcholine in mind: a neurotransmitter correlate of consciousness? Trends Neurosci. 1999;22(6):273–80.
226. Choi DW, Rothman SM. The role of glutamate neurotoxicity in hypoxic-ischemic neuronal death. Annu Rev Neurosci. 1990;13:171–82.
227. Obrenovitch TP, Urenjak J, Zilkha E. Intracerebral microdialysis combined with recording of extracellular field potential: a novel method for investigation of depolarizing drugs in vivo. Br J Pharmacol. 1994;113(4):1295–302.
228. Wahl F, et al. Extracellular glutamate during focal cerebral ischaemia in rats: time course and calcium dependency. J Neurochem. 1994;63(3):1003–11.
229. Rennie MJ, et al. Skeletal muscle glutamine transport, intramuscular glutamine concentration, and muscle-protein turnover. Metabolism. 1989;38(8 Suppl 1):47–51.
230. Haussinger D, et al. Cellular hydration state: an important determinant of protein catabolism in health and disease. Lancet. 1993;341(8856):1330–2.

231. Ferenci P, Schafer DF, Kleinberger G, Hoofnagle JH, Jones EA. Serum levels of gamma-aminobutyric-acid-like activity in acute and chronic hepatocellular disease. Lancet. 1983;2(8354):811–4.
232. Ross CA. CNS arousal systems: possible role in delirium. Int Psychogeriatr. 1991;3(2):353–71.
233. Maldonado J. An approach to the patient with substance use and abuse. Med Clin North Am. 2010;94(6):1169–205.. x-i
234. Akaike N, Shirasaki T, Yakushiji T. Quinolones and fenbufen interact with GABAA receptor in dissociated hippocampal cells of rat. J Neurophysiol. 1991;66(2):497–504.
235. van der Mast RC. Pathophysiology of delirium. J Geriatr Psychiatry Neurol. 1998;11(3):138–45.. discussion 157-8
236. van der Mast RC, et al. Is delirium after cardiac surgery related to plasma amino acids and physical condition? J Neuropsychiatry Clin Neurosci. 2000;12(1):57–63.
237. Bhardwaj A, et al. Ischemia in the dorsal hippocampus is associated with acute extracellular release of dopamine and norepinephrine. J Neural Transm Gen Sect. 1990;80(3):195–201.
238. Rigney T. Allostatic load and delirium in the hospitalized older adult. Nurs Res. 2010;59(5):322–30.
239. Basavaraju N, Phillips SL. Cortisol deficient state. A cause of reversible cognitive impairment and delirium in the elderly. J Am Geriatr Soc. 1989;37(1):49–51.
240. Bisschop PH, et al. Cortisol, insulin, and glucose and the risk of delirium in older adults with hip fracture. J Am Geriatr Soc. 2011;59(9):1692–6.
241. Kazmierski J, et al. Cortisol levels and neuropsychiatric diagnosis as markers of postoperative delirium: a prospective cohort study. Crit Care. 2013;17(2):R38.
242. Manenschijn L, et al. Glucocorticoid receptor haplotype is associated with a decreased risk of delirium in the elderly. Am J Med Genet B Neuropsychiatr Genet. 2011;156B(3):316–21.
243. McIntosh TK, Bush HL, Yeston NS, et al. Beta-endorphin, cortisol and postoperative delirium: a preliminary report. Psychoneuroendocrinology. 1985;10(3):303–13.
244. O'Keeffe ST, Devlin JG. Delirium and the dexamethasone suppression test in the elderly. Neuropsychobiology. 1994;30(4):153–6.
245. Pearson A, et al. Cerebrospinal fluid cortisol levels are higher in patients with delirium versus controls. BMC Res Notes. 2010;3:33.
246. Kazmierski J, et al. Mild cognitive impairment with associated inflammatory and cortisol alterations as independent risk factor for postoperative delirium. Dement Geriatr Cogn Disord. 2014;38(1–2):65–78.
247. Pfister D, et al. Cerebral perfusion in sepsis-associated delirium. Crit Care. 2008;12(3):R63.
248. Cerejeira J, et al. The cholinergic system and inflammation: common pathways in delirium pathophysiology. J Am Geriatr Soc. 2012;60(4):669–75.
249. Vasunilashorn SM, et al. High C-reactive protein predicts delirium incidence, duration, and feature severity after major noncardiac surgery. J Am Geriatr Soc. 2017;65(8):e109–16.
250. Vasunilashorn SM, et al. The association between C-reactive protein and postoperative delirium differs by catechol-O-methyltransferase genotype. Am J Geriatr Psychiatry. 2019;27(1):1–8.
251. Vasunilashorn SM, et al. Development of a dynamic multi-protein signature of postoperative delirium. J Gerontol A Biol Sci Med Sci. 2019;74(2):261–8.
252. Baranyi A, Rothenhausler HB. The impact of soluble interleukin-2 receptor as a biomarker of delirium. Psychosomatics. 2014;55(1):51–60.
253. Skrobik Y, et al. Factors predisposing to coma and delirium: fentanyl and midazolam exposure; CYP3A5, ABCB1, and ABCG2 genetic polymorphisms; and inflammatory factors. Crit Care Med. 2013;41(4):999–1008.
254. Egberts A, et al. Neopterin: a potential biomarker for delirium in elderly patients. Dement Geriatr Cogn Disord. 2015;39(1–2):116–24.
255. Liu L, et al. Effects of dexmedetomidine combined with sufentanil on postoperative delirium in young patients after general anesthesia. Med Sci Monit. 2018;24:8925–32.

256. van Munster BC, Zwinderman AH, de Rooij SE. Genetic variations in the interleukin-6 and interleukin-8 genes and the interleukin-6 receptor gene in delirium. Rejuvenation Res. 2011;14(4):425–8.
257. Zhang ZY, et al. Impact of length of red blood cells transfusion on postoperative delirium in elderly patients undergoing hip fracture surgery: a cohort study. Injury. 2016;47(2):408–12.
258. Caplan GA, et al. Cerebrospinal fluid in long-lasting delirium compared with Alzheimer's dementia. J Gerontol A Biol Sci Med Sci. 2010;65(10):1130–6.
259. Beishuizen SJ, et al. Timing is critical in determining the association between delirium and S100 calcium-binding protein B. J Am Geriatr Soc. 2015;63(10):2212–4.
260. Liu J, et al. Predictive value of serum S100B levels in patients with multiple trauma combined delirium for their outcome at intensive care unit discharge. Zhonghua Yi Xue Za Zhi. 2018;98(9):692–5.
261. Sun Y, et al. Effects of dexmedetomidine on emergence delirium in pediatric cardiac surgery. Minerva Pediatr. 2017;69(3):165–73.
262. Schreuder L, et al. Pathophysiological and behavioral effects of systemic inflammation in aged and diseased rodents with relevance to delirium: a systematic review. Brain Behav Immun. 2017;62:362–81.
263. Brown RE, et al. Control of sleep and wakefulness. Physiol Rev. 2012;92(3):1087–187.

Chapter 11
The Electroencephalogram and Delirium

Suzanne C. A. Hut, Frans S. Leijten, and Arjen J. C. Slooter

Introduction

Delirium has been recognized since ancient times as an acute brain dysfunction associated with illness. Electroencephalography (EEG) is one of the oldest techniques for studying brain function. Despite this long history, the scientific literature on EEG in delirium is limited. One of the reasons for this lack of progress may be inconsistent terminology across medical disciplines to describe neuropsychiatric changes in acute systemic illness. Whereas most geriatricians, psychiatrists, anesthesiologists, and intensivists appear to prefer the term "delirium," neurologists, neurointensivists, and clinical neurophysiologists would describe the same entity as "encephalopathy." In this chapter, we will use the term "delirium" to refer to a clinical state characterized by a combination of features defined by diagnostic systems such as the fifth edition of the *Diagnostic and Statistical Manual of Mental Disorders* (DSM-5) [1] or the tenth revision of the *International Statistical Classification of Diseases and Related Health Problems* (ICD-10) [2]. The term "acute encephalopathy" in this chapter will refer to a rapidly developing (over less than 4 weeks, but usually within hours to a few days) pathobiological process in the brain that can lead to a clinical presentation of delirium or, in case of a severely decreased level of consciousness, to coma. In this chapter we will preferentially use the term

S. C. A. Hut (✉) · A. J. C. Slooter
Department of Intensive Care Medicine, University Medical Center Utrecht, Utrecht University, Utrecht, The Netherlands

UMC Utrecht Brain Center, Utrecht, The Netherlands
e-mail: s.c.a.hut@umcutrecht.nl

F. S. Leijten
UMC Utrecht Brain Center, Utrecht, The Netherlands

Department of Neurology and Neurosurgery, University Medical Center Utrecht, Utrecht University, Utrecht, The Netherlands

C. G. Hughes et al. (eds.), *Delirium*, https://doi.org/10.1007/978-3-030-25751-4_11

"delirium," and we will review the EEG literature on both delirium and (acute) encephalopathy.

Despite the fact that delirium can be precipitated by a range of pathophysiologically diverse conditions, its clinical presentation is relatively homogeneous leading some to suggest there is a final common pathway. However, the substrate of this presumed common pathway is unclear. Studies on different etiologies of delirium are difficult to perform as it is usually impossible to assign one specific cause for delirium [3]. Studies on encephalopathy are more often focused on one specific etiology (e.g., septic encephalopathy) usually neglecting concomitant pathology (e.g., organ dysfunction or medication use).

EEG in Normal Adults

There may be some misconceptions regarding the interpretation of EEG. We therefore start with a brief introduction on basic concepts of EEG to provide non-neurological clinicians and non-neuroscience researchers an appreciation of its scope and limitations.

EEG signals are voltage potentials mainly generated by neurons in the cerebral cortex (gray matter). However, action potentials of individual neurons are too weak and too brief to be recorded on an EEG. EEG recordings from a single electrode reflect the postsynaptic activity of thousands or even millions of cortical neurons. The EEG signal predominantly originates from neurons that are aligned radially to the recording surface (such that their excitatory and inhibitory postsynaptic potentials can be summated). These compound potentials generate currents flowing in the extracellular space that can be detected at the surface of the brain. Yet electrical activity recorded at the brain's surface does not only reflect the spontaneous activity of large populations of cortical neurons but also depends on important input from subcortical structures, in particular the thalamus and brainstem reticular formation. EEG abnormalities may therefore result from disruption of cortical networks or from modification of subcortical input on cortical neurons. It should be noted that activity generated in the lateral surfaces of the brain is recorded more precisely than is activity arising from interhemispheric, mesial, or basal areas [4]. Further, not all potentials that may be recorded at the cortical surface are detectable at the scalp. Summated potentials from the cerebral cortex are attenuated or distorted by overlying structures, such as the pia mater, the subarachnoid space that is filled with cerebrospinal fluid, the dura mater, and the skull. For these reasons, spatial resolution of regular, low-density EEG is poor, which hampers anatomical inferences. Another limitation of EEG is its low specificity – widely disparate diseases and conditions may produce similar changes in EEG. By contrast, temporal resolution is excellent, so that changes in milliseconds may be visible in EEG. In addition, EEG is relatively cheap and applicable at the bedside in patients with delirium, in contrast with other neuroimaging techniques such as magnetic resonance imaging (MRI) or positron emission tomography (PET).

A basic EEG array usually consists of up to 25 electrodes distributed over the scalp, covering a large part of the underlying cortex. The electrodes are typically placed proportionally to the head size in the so-called International 10–20 system [5], so that in each individual the electrodes carry names that reflect the sub-lobar area that is sampled. Odd numbers indicate left hemisphere locations, and even numbers are on the right (e.g., F3 is over the left lateral frontal cortex).

In clinical use, the EEG signal is typically displayed as a tracing of voltage changes over time and can be regarded as composed of oscillatory activity in various frequency ranges, or *bands*. These oscillations may result from the synchronized, rhythmic induction of postsynaptic potentials by populations of neurons that are interconnected with feedback loops. A frequently used measure is *EEG power*, the square of the average of the amplitude of the EEG signal, across the time sampled. EEG power spectrum analysis allows for the calculation of the distribution of signal power across frequency bands in a certain time frame. Distinct frequency bands can often be observed and may all be present in a healthy EEG, depending on the state of the individual or ongoing cognitive processes.

Delta activity (<4 Hz) appears during slow-wave sleep and is not normally present in adults when they are awake. Healthy adults may show some theta activity (4–8 Hz) over the temporal regions during drowsiness. During wakefulness, activity in the 8–13 Hz range is present in occipital regions while the eyes are closed (alpha rhythm) and in pericentral regions while the hands are at rest (mu rhythm), and beta activity (13–30 Hz) is normally present over the frontal areas. Slow activity (in theta bands) slightly increases with aging [6], whereas the use of certain medications such as benzodiazepines or barbiturates may increase the amount of beta activity [7]. In general, the slower the activity, the higher the amplitude, with beta usually below 30 μV, alpha around 70 μV, and delta often over 150 μV. The overall picture of an awake EEG with these frequency characteristics is called the background activity.

Moreover, an EEG in healthy awake individuals shows an *anterior to posterior gradient*, that is, the increase of amplitudes and decrease of predominant frequencies from anterior to posterior sites. In the awake person, the frontal lobe is dominated by beta activity of low amplitude, whereas a prominent alpha rhythm will dominate the posterior regions after eye closure. *EEG reactivity* in healthy individuals refers to the attenuation of the alpha rhythm upon fixation or opening of the eyes and the mu rhythm that disappears with contralateral hand movement. An example is provided in Fig. 11.1a. In summary, EEG rhythms in awake, healthy adults commonly manifest as relatively low in amplitude, while the frequencies of these oscillations may be mixed [8] and the lowest, delta activity, being absent or rare.

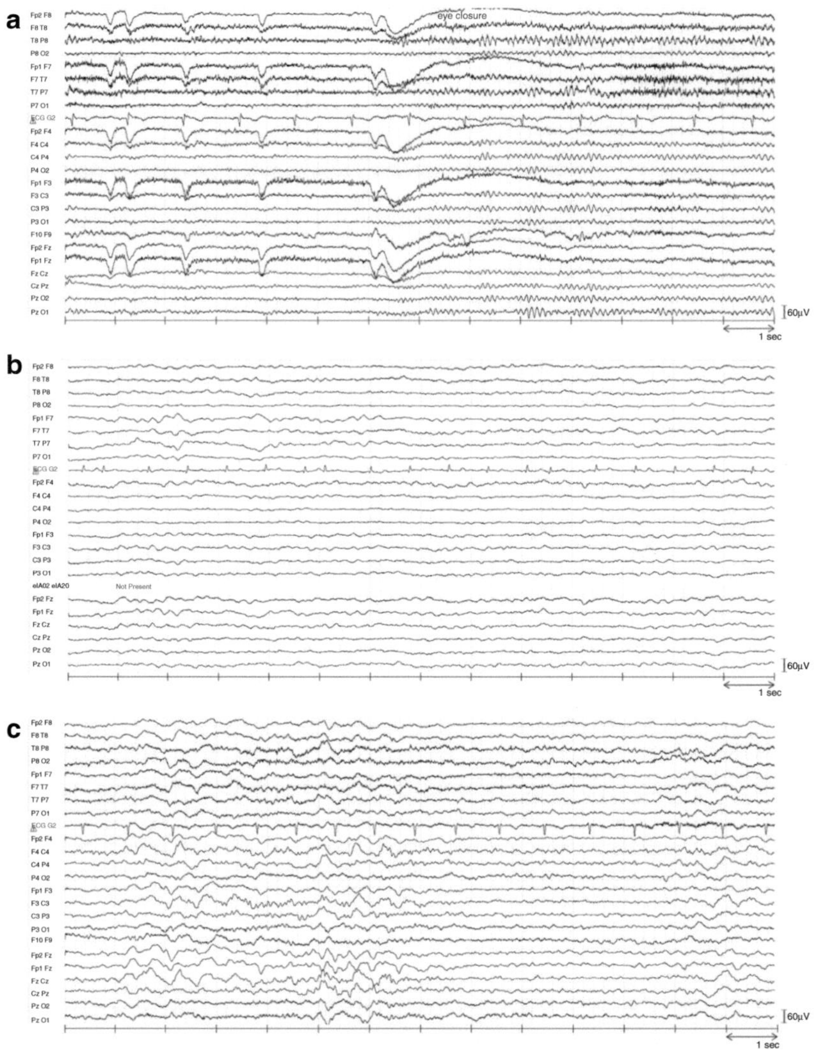

Fig. 11.1 Examples of 14 s of EEG recordings. EEGs are represented in a bipolar montage. The first four lines represent the most lateral part of the right hemisphere, the next four the corresponding part on the left. Under the ECG, lines represent the lateral part more cranially, halfway over the side of the skull, again the first four over the right and then four over the left. The last six channels are over the cranial midline. Filter settings 0.16–70 Hz. (**a**) 45-year-old male, 3 days after cardiac surgery, without complications. He is awake and oriented. The EEG shows eyeblink artifacts in the frontopolar leads and muscle artifacts (dense blackening of the curve, especially in the second four lines at the end). After eye closure, halfway the page, an alpha rhythm arises over the posterior leads. Conclusion: normal EEG. (**b**) 80-year-old female, heart and kidney failure. She is slightly obtunded and confused. The EEG shows no anterior to posterior gradient and is dominated by polymorphous slow (delta) rhythms. There is no background differentiation; the eyes are closed. Conclusion: delirium. (**c**) 60-year-old male with cerebral aspergillosis after stem cell transplant for multiple myeloma. Clinical delirium. The EEG shows periods of high-amplitude polymorphous delta activity, interspersed with periods of attenuation. There are no features of stage 2–3 sleep such as spindles or K-complexes. Conclusion: delirium

EEG Characteristics of Delirium

In delirium, the EEG is characterized by a diffuse increase of theta and delta oscillations. This pathological slowing is typically more prominent over frontal regions where low-amplitude beta normally reigns. Increased power in the delta band may consist of polymorphous (i.e., irregularly shaped) delta activity, frontal intermittent rhythmic delta activity (FIRDA), and triphasic waves (TWs) [9].

The presence of diffuse polymorphous delta activity during the awake state is typical in the delirium EEG. Polymorphous delta activity when restricted to lateralized or focal regions is also seen with focal brain pathology such as stroke or brain tumors [10–12]. Thus, it is important that the delta activity is bilateral and diffuse to indicate delirium. However, diffuse polymorphous delta activity is also a characteristic of stage 2–3 non-rapid eye movement (NREM) sleep [9]. This delta activity will be more continuous during sleep and not intermittent such as in most cases of delirium. Normal stage 2–3 NREM sleep can further be distinguished because of special features (sleep spindles, vertex waves, K-complexes) that are absent in the EEG of an awake delirious patient. Still, an EEG suggestion of delirium is best taken from an awake EEG. In a way, one might speculate that delirium is the intrusion of bouts of NREM sleep in the awake state. Indeed, extreme sleep deprivation may cause delirium as well as produce such EEG sleep intrusion in the healthy adult [13].

Polymorphous delta activity in delirium may be continuous (Fig. 11.1b) but is usually intermittent (Fig. 11.1c). Intermittent delta activity may appear in a rhythmical (i.e., monomorphic and repetitive) fashion as short, moderate- to high-amplitude runs that last between 2 and 6 s over the frontal areas, alternated by episodes of faster frequencies or even a normal background pattern. Frontal intermittent rhythmical delta activity (FIRDA), also referred to as generalized rhythmic delta activity (GRDA) with frontal predominance, is associated with various pathological processes such as increased intracranial pressure, intoxication, posterior fossa pathology, and certain diseases such as Lewy body dementia, as well as with hyperventilation in normal individuals [14]. Due to its non-specificity, it may not be surprising that FIRDA may also manifest with delirium of various etiologies, such as sepsis [15], hyperglycemia, and uremia [16].

Triphasic waves may also occur in the delta frequency band and can be recognized by their large, frontally predominant positive peak (>70 μV), flanked by two negative deflections (i.e., plotted upward, in accordance with the EEG polarity convention for surface negative waveforms). They typically occur in prolonged runs approximately once per second and attenuate during sleep. In the American Clinical Neurophysiology Society standardized ICU EEG nomenclature, these are referred to as generalized periodic discharges (GPDs) with triphasic morphology. TWs are associated with delirium due to a variety of causes and with increased risk of unfavorable outcomes such as mortality [17, 18]. Akin to FIRDA, TWs may be a reflection of a number of conditions but have historically been described in hepatic failure [19], which frequently results in delirium [20]. An example of TWs is provided in Fig. 11.2a.

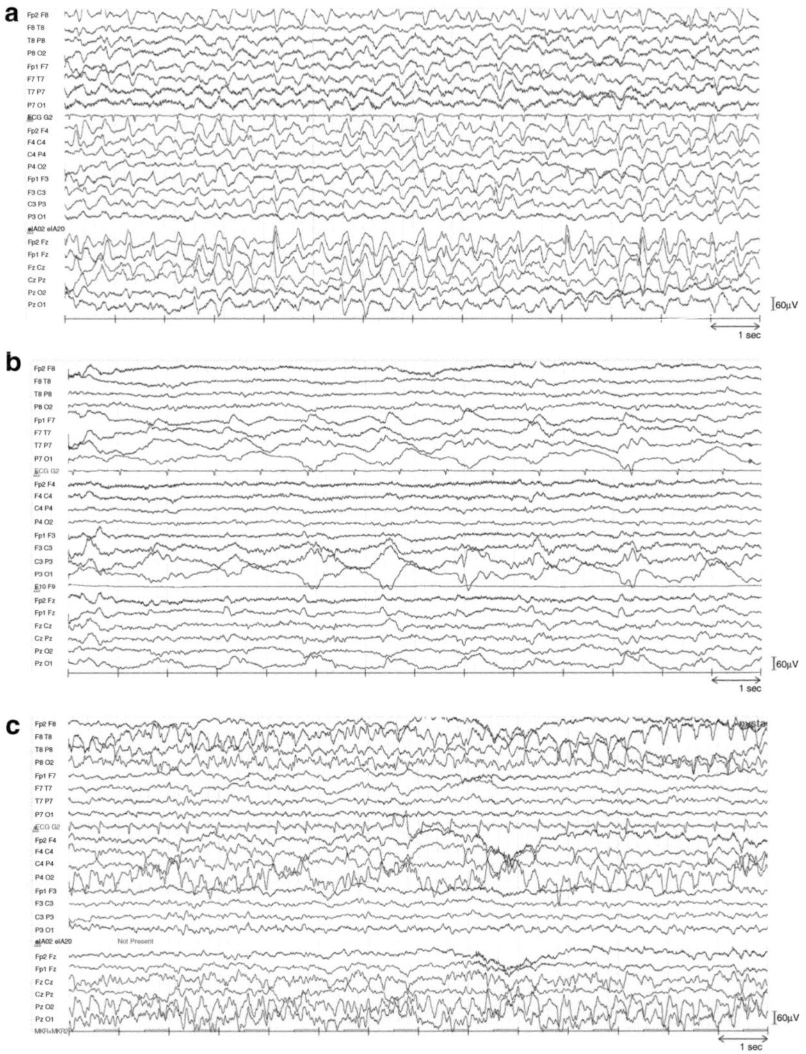

Fig. 11.2 Some specific examples of 14 s EEG recordings. Filter settings 0.16–70 Hz. (**a**) 43-year-old female, hepatic failure with high ammonia serum levels due to valproic acid intoxication. Clinical delirium with periodic unrest; also asterixis and confusion. The shown episode is during a short period of relaxation. The EEG shows high-amplitude delta with prominent frontal-predominant sharp waves at leads, so-called triphasic waves in delirium associated with hepatic failure. (**b**) 58-year-old male, glioblastoma in the left hemisphere, after he suffered a generalized tonic-clonic seizure. He has dysphasia, but is responsive, no unrest. The EEG shows relatively normal background activity over the right hemisphere, but a highly abnormal pattern over the left hemisphere with so-called periodic lateralized discharges, which in this case reflects a postictal and tumor-related focal phenomenon. (**c**) 66-year-old male, glioblastoma in the right hemisphere with focal seizures with jerking of the left arm. He was found at home and brought to the ICU with respiratory problems and unresponsiveness, but no jerking. The EEG shows an evolving rhythmical pattern over the right hemisphere that waxes and wanes and polymorphous delta activity over the left hemisphere. Conclusion: non-convulsive status epilepticus

The occurrence of various features of the EEG thus sometimes allows for the detection of underlying causes of delirium. Nevertheless, quantitative spectral patterns may vary between individuals, and more research is needed to associate certain spectral features with clinical phenotypes, e.g., hypoactive or hyperactive delirium [21]. For now, general slowing and disorganization of the background EEG appear to be shared features of the delirium EEG.

The increase of power in the theta and delta band is inseparably paired with a reduction of power in the alpha and beta frequency band. While EEG reactivity with appearance of a posterior alpha rhythm upon eye closure is observed in healthy adults, during delirium the EEG often shows an abnormal lack of posterior alpha rhythm. The relative alpha power is thus reduced in delirium, while relative power in the theta and delta band typically increases. Consequently, the ratio of fast-to-slow band power is reduced in delirium. Interestingly, upon recovery, a shift from predominant delta power back into theta, alpha, and higher frequency bands may be observed [21]. EEG manifestations of delirium are thus reversible, following the clinical symptoms.

In clinical practice, EEG may be helpful in detecting delirium in certain populations [21], and the amount of relative delta power in spectral analysis might provide a tool for quantification and follow-up [22].

Delirium Due to Non-convulsive Seizures

Non-convulsive seizures can be thought of as abnormal excessive or synchronous neuronal activity without obvious motor activity [23, 24]. In case of persistence or recurrence without interictal return to baseline, the term non-convulsive status epilepticus is used. Criteria for non-convulsive seizures include the presence of epileptic activity as detected with EEG (e.g., Figure 11.2b, c) and clinical or EEG improvement after the administration of a rapidly acting anti-epileptic drug [25, 26]. Non-convulsive seizures can present with a variety of symptoms and signs that may be nonspecific, including a decreased level of consciousness, confusion, psychosis, eye deviation, nystagmus, subtle convulsions, rigidity, automatisms, chewing, tachycardia, sweating, or an increase in intracranial pressure [27].

Some symptoms and signs of non-convulsive seizures therefore show overlap with features of delirium, and their persistence could point to non-convulsive status epilepticus. Causes of non-convulsive status epilepticus overlap with causes of delirium. These include metabolic alterations (such as hepatic and renal failure, electrolyte abnormalities), drug intoxications, and acute withdrawal of certain drugs [28]. Not only can delirium manifest during seizures (in the ictal period), delirium can also persist after or between electrographic seizures (postictal confusion) [29]. The issue whether non-convulsive status epilepticus leads to delirium is relevant, as status epilepticus should be treated with anti-epileptic drugs, which might be withheld in case of a mistaken diagnosis of delirious state due to other causes. Sometimes, non-convulsive status epilepticus may consist of intermittent seizures that can be missed with a conventional 30-min EEG recording. To definitely rule out non-convulsive status epilepticus, prolonged or continuous EEG recording is advised [30], which may be logistically challenging.

It may not come as a surprise that the literature on delirium due to non-convulsive status epilepticus is limited. In three studies on non-neurological intensive care unit (ICU) patients who underwent continuous EEG monitoring for evaluation of altered consciousness, non-convulsive status epilepticus was detected in 0% ($n = 62$ patients with sepsis), 6% ($n = 154$ surgical ICU patients), and 10% ($n = 201$ medical ICU patients) [15, 31, 32]. Another study in patients presenting with delirium found a much higher proportion of patients with non-convulsive status epilepticus using continuous EEG (28%) or conventional 20-min EEG (6%) [33]. However, the selection of study participants was unclear, as well as the required quantity of certain EEG features to classify as epileptic. Furthermore, the majority of patients classified with non-convulsive status epilepticus showed an EEG feature of generalized periodic discharges, which most experts do not consider typically epileptic.

Non-convulsive status epilepticus is an important but relatively rare underlying cause of delirium, especially in the patient without primary (focal) brain disease and without a history of seizures. Clues to non-convulsive status epilepticus may include subtle motor movements, such as gaze deviation, nystagmus, subtle limb twitches, rigidity, and oral and manual automatisms, particularly in cases with a (hyper)acute onset of delirium and a prior history of seizures. The single most helpful test to detect non-convulsive status epilepticus is EEG [28].

During a 30-min EEG recording, brief episodes of non-convulsive seizures may be missed. However, if electrographic seizure activity does not occur during apparent behavioral phenomena, this argues against an epileptic origin of these features. Diagnosis of non-convulsive status epilepticus is supported when the administration of a rapidly acting anti-epileptic drug results in both clinical and EEG recovery.

Applications of EEG in Delirium Research and Management

The EEG has the potential to contribute to various areas of delirium research and management.

Firstly, it may provide insight in the pathophysiology of delirium. In the last two decades, there appears to be a renaissance of interest in EEG among neuroscientists fueled by rapid developments in network science. Network science has introduced new opportunities for understanding the brain as a complex system of interacting units [34]. Networks consist of nodes (vertices) that are connected to edges. When a neural network is constructed from EEG, the EEG electrodes can be considered the nodes of the network and the strength of the phase coupling between the EEG channels as edges. Using this network construct, EEG is usually analyzed within the commonly accepted EEG frequency bands (i.e., delta, theta, alpha, and beta). A variety of network characteristics can thus be computed, including the average connectivity strength and measures of network topology. It appears that network alterations during delirium are characterized by loss of functional connectivity in the alpha band and changes toward a more random and less integrated network [35, 36]. With these analyses, hypoactive delirium could be distinguished from a similar state which occurs during recovery from anesthesia [36].

Network analyses can also be used to study whether delirium due to different causes results in similar alterations in connectivity and topology, strengthening the argument for a final common pathophysiologic pathway. This could be investigated by comparing delirium due to a different etiology (e.g., postoperative, infectious, metabolic) with regard to various EEG characteristics. It is however difficult to classify delirium into etiological subgroups because of its multifactorial nature.

Another interesting approach is to build computational models that represent populations of interconnected inhibitory and excitatory neurons, resulting in an artificial EEG signal. By modifying the components of these so-called neural mass models, such as ion channel thresholds, this EEG signal acquires or loses certain characteristics and features, which can be compared with an EEG signal during delirium. Neural mass *in silico* models can thus fundamentally increase our understanding of EEG disturbances in delirium [37].

Secondly, EEG may be applied in routine diagnosis and monitoring of delirium. Delirium is often not recognized in daily clinical practice by non-delirium experts, such as ICU physicians [38]. To improve recognition, delirium screening tools have been developed. While clinical tests suffice in a research setting with a limited number of research assistants administering the test [39, 40], they appear insensitive in daily routine practice with numerous nurses in day-to-day care [41, 42]. There is therefore a need for an objective delirium detection tool which is easy to use. A conventional 30-min 25-channel EEG recording is not practical for large-scale, routine monitoring. Fortunately, quantitative analysis of 1-min, two-channel EEG could reliably distinguish patients with "definite delirium" from those with "definite no delirium" after cardiac surgery [43]. These results were validated in an independent cohort of postoperative patients (n = 159, area under the receiver operating characteristic curve 0.75 based on the relative delta power, and 0.78 based on explorative analysis of relative power from 1 to 6 Hz) [44]. Another recent study also showed high specificity and sensitivity when a bispectral EEG device was used, even with the inclusion of patients with dementia [45]. Before brief EEG recordings can be introduced in daily clinical practice, usability needs to be optimized.

Thirdly, EEG could be used to assess prognosis of delirium. Quantification of slowing of EEG background activity over time might provide a more accurate measure of monitoring the resolution of delirium than clinical monitoring with scores such as the Glasgow Coma Scale. However, although associations have been described between different grades of slowing of EEG background activity and outcome, prognosis seems to be predominantly determined by etiology [46]. EEG reactivity, e.g., modulation of background activity in response to stimulation, is related with a more favorable prognosis. Further more, presence of physiological EEG elements during NREM sleep appears to have prognostic value. These include vertex waves, sleep spindles, and K-complexes. Particularly the presence of K-complexes was found to be associated with favorable outcomes [47]. In summary, EEG is a sensitive tool, and various EEG features seem to have prognostic value in delirium. It is still unclear which EEG characteristics are optimal in predicting delirium outcome [48].

Conclusions

The EEG in delirium is characterized by slowing of background activity, resulting in increased power in the theta and especially delta frequency range. Several other features may also be present in the EEG of delirious patients, such as FIRDA and TWs. The use of EEG in detection and monitoring of delirium seems promising, and the sensitivity of EEG for delirium is high. Certain EEG elements may also have prognostic value, which could be of clinical relevance. Moreover, network analyses and *in silico* models offer opportunities to study the presence of common pathways due to different causes. Lastly, EEG is a useful tool in further investigation of non-convulsive seizures and their link to delirium. EEG, even when a limited number of electrodes is used, is thus a valid method that could aid prediction, detection, and monitoring of delirium.

Declaration of Interests Authors AJCS and FSL are advisors for Prolira, a start-up company that is working on the development of an EEG-based delirium monitor. Any (future) profits from EEG-based delirium monitoring will be used for future scientific research only.

References

1. American Psychiatric Association. Diagnostic and statistical manual of mental disorders, 5th Edition (DSM-5). Diagnostic Stat Man Ment Disord 4th Ed TR. 2013.
2. World Health Organisation. ICD-10 version: 2010. World Health Organisation. 2010.
3. Ely E, Gautam S, Margolin R, Francis J, May L, Speroff T, et al. The impact of delirium in the intensive care unit on hospital length of stay. Intensive Care Med. 2001;27(12):1892–900.
4. Hahn CD, Emerson RG. Electroencephalography and evoked potentials. In: Daroff RB, Jankovic J, Mazziotta JC, Pomeroy SL, editors. Bradley's neurology in clinical practice. 7th ed. Philadelphia: Elsevier Saunders; 2016.. chap 34.
5. Seeck M, Koessler L, Bast T, Leijten F, Michel C, Baumgartner C, et al. The standardized EEG electrode array of the IFCN. Clin Neurophysiol. 2017;128(10):2070–7.
6. Klimesch W. EEG alpha and theta oscillations reflect cognitive and memory performance: a review and analysis. Brain Res Rev. 1999;29(2–3):169–95.
7. Van Lier H, Drinkenburg WHI, Van Eeten YJ, Coenen AM. Effects of diazepam and zolpidem on EEG beta frequencies are behavior-specific in rats. Neuropharmacology. 2004;47(2):163–74.
8. Britton JW, Hopp JL, Korb P, Lievens WE, Pestana-Knight EM, Frey LC. The normal EEG. In: Louis EK, Frey LC, editors. Electroencephalography (EEG): an introductory text and atlas of normal and abnormal findings in adults, children, and infants. Chicago: American Epilepsy Society; 2016.

9. Niedermeyer E, Lopes da Silva FH, editors. Electroencephalography: basic principles, clinical applications, and related fields. London: Lippincott Williams and Wilkins; 2005. p. 441.
10. Fernandez-Bouzas A, Harmony T, Fernandez T, Silva-Pereyra J, Valdes P, Bosch J, et al. Sources of abnormal EEG activity in brain infarctions. Clin Electroencephalogr. 2000;31(4):165–9.
11. Hess R. Localized abnormalities. In: Rémond A, editor. Handbook of electroencephalography and clinical neurophysiology, vol. 11. Amsterdam: Elsevier; 1976. p. 11B88–11B1116.
12. Goldensohn ES. In: Klass DW, Daly DD, editors. Use of the EEG for evaluation of focal intracranial lesions. New York: Raven Press; 1979. p. 307–41.
13. Watson PL, Ceriana P, Fanfulla F. Delirium: is sleep important? Best Pract Res Clin Anaesthesiol. 2012;26(3):355–66.
14. Accolla EA, Kaplan PW, Maeder-Ingvar M, Jukopila S, Rossetti AO. Clinical correlates of frontal intermittent rhythmic delta activity (FIRDA). Clin Neurophysiol. 2011;122(1):27–31.
15. Young GB, Bolton CF, Archibald YM, Austin TW, Wells GA. The electroencephalogram in sepsis-associated encephalopathy. J Clin Neurophysiol. 1992;9(1):145–52.
16. Watemberg N, Alehan F, Dabby R, Lerman-Sagie T, Pavot P, Towne A. Clinical and radiologic correlates of frontal intermittent rhythmic delta activity. J Clin Neurophysiol. 2002;19(6):535–9.
17. Sutter R, Kaplan PW. Clinical and electroencephalographic correlates of acute encephalopathy. J Clin Neurophysiol. 2013;30(5):443–53.
18. Kaplan PW, Sutter R. Affair with triphasic waves – their striking presence, mysterious significance, and cryptic origins: what are they? J Clin Neurophysiol. 2015;32(5):401–5.
19. Amodio P, Montagnese S. Clinical neurophysiology of hepatic encephalopathy. J Clin Exp Hepatol. 2015;5:S60–8.
20. Coggins CC, Curtiss CP. Assessment and management of delirium: a focus on hepatic encephalopathy. Palliat Support Care. 11.4. 2013;11.4:341–52.
21. Palanca BJA, Wildes TS, Ju YS, Ching S, Avidan MS. Electroencephalography and delirium in the postoperative period. Br J Anaesth. 2017;119(2):294–307.
22. Fleischmann R, Tränkner S, Bathe-Peters R, Rönnefarth M, Schmidt S, Schreiber SJ, et al. Diagnostic performance and utility of quantitative EEG analyses in delirium: confirmatory results from a large retrospective case-control study. Clin EEG Neurosci. 2018;50(2):111–20.
23. Fisher RS, Van Emde Boas W, Elger C, Genton P, Lee P, Engel J Jr. Epileptic seizures and epilepsy: definitions proposed by the international league against epilepsy (ILAE) and the International Bureau for Epilepsy (IBE). Epilepsia. 2005;46(4):470–2.
24. Fisher RS, Cross JH, French JA, Higurashi N, Hirsch E, Jansen FE, et al. Operational classification of seizure types by the international league against epilepsy: position paper of the ILAE Commission for Classification and Terminology. Epilepsia. 2017;58(4):522–30.
25. Sutter R, Semmlack S, Kaplan PW. Nonconvulsive status epilepticus in adults — insights into the invisible. Nat Rev Neurol. 2016;12(5):281–93.
26. Kaplan PW. EEG criteria for nonconvulsive status epilepticus. Epilepsia. 2007;48:39–41.
27. Kaplan PW. Behavioral manifestations of nonconvulsive status epilepticus. Epilepsy Behav. 2002;3(2):122–39.
28. Kaplan PW. Delirium and epilepsy. Dialogues Clin Neurosci. 2003;5(2):187.
29. Shorvon S, Trinka E. Nonconvulsive status epilepticus and the postictal state. Epilepsy Behav. 2010;19(2):172–5.
30. Claassen J, Mayer SA, Kowalski RG, Emerson RG, Hirsch LJ. Detection of electrographic seizures with continuous EEG monitoring in critically ill patients. Neurology. 2004;62(10):1743–8.
31. Kurtz P, Gaspard N, Wahl AS, Bauer RM, Hirsch LJ, Wunsch H, et al. Continuous electroencephalography in a surgical intensive care unit. Intensive Care Med. 2014;40(2):228–34.
32. Oddo M, Carrera E, Claassen J, Mayer SA, Hirsch LJ. Continuous electroencephalography in the medical intensive care unit. Crit Care Med. 2009;37(6):2051–6.

33. Naeije G, Depondt C, Meeus C, Korpak K, Pepersack T, Legros B. EEG patterns compatible with nonconvulsive status epilepticus are common in elderly patients with delirium: a prospective study with continuous EEG monitoring. Epilepsy Behav. 2014;36:18–21.
34. Stam CJ. Modern network science of neurological disorders. Nat Rev Neurosci. 2014;15(10):683.
35. Van Dellen E, Van Der Kooi AW, Numan T, Koek HL, Klijn FAM, Buijsrogge MP, et al. Decreased functional connectivity and disturbed directionality of information flow in the electroencephalography of intensive care unit patients with delirium after cardiac surgery. Anesthesiology. 2014;121(2):328–35.
36. Numan T, Slooter AJC, van der Kooi AW, Hoekman AML, Suyker WJL, Stam CJ, et al. Functional connectivity and network analysis during hypoactive delirium and recovery from anesthesia. Clin Neurophysiol. 2017;128(6):914–92.
37. Ponten SC, Tewarie P, Slooter AJC, Stam CJ, van Dellen E. Neural network modeling of EEG patterns in encephalopathy. J Clin Neurophysiol. 2013;30(5):545–52.
38. Van Eijk MMJ, Van Marum RJ, Klijn IAM, De Wit N, Kesecioglu J, Slooter AJC. Comparison of delirium assessment tools in a mixed intensive care unit. Crit Care Med. 2009;37(6):1881–5.
39. Inouye SK, Van Dyck CH, Alessi CA, Balkin S, Siegal AP, Horwitz RI. Clarifying confusion: the confusion assessment method: a new method for detection of delirium. Ann Intern Med. 1990;113(12):941–8.
40. Ely EW, Inouye SK, Bernard GR, Gordon S, Francis J, May L, et al. Delirium in mechanically ventilated patients: validity and reliability of the confusion assessment method for the intensive care unit (CAM-ICU). JAMA. 2001;286(21):2703–10.
41. Van Eijk MM, Van Den Boogaard M, Van Marum RJ, Benner P, Eikelenboom P, Honing ML, et al. Routine use of the confusion assessment method for the intensive care unit: a multicenter study. Am J Respir Crit Care Med. 2011;184(3):340–4.
42. Rice KL, Bennett MJ, Gomez M, Theall KP, Knight M, Foreman MD. Nurses' recognition of delirium in the hospitalized older adult. Clin Nurse Spec. 2011;25(6):299–311.
43. Van Der Kooi AW, Zaal IJ, Klijn FA, Koek HL, Meijer RC, Leijten FS, et al. Delirium detection using EEG: what and how to measure. Chest. 2015;147(1):94–101.
44. Numan T, Van den Boogaard M, Kamper AM, Rood PJT, Peelen LM, Slooter, AJC on behalf of the Dutch Delirium Detection Study Group, et al. Br J Anaesth. 2019;122.1:60–8.
45. Shinozaki G, Chan A, Sparr N, Zarei K, Gaul L, Heinzman J, et al. Delirium detection by a novel bispectral EEG device in general hospital. Psychiatry Clin Neurosci. 2018;72(12):856–63.
46. Sutter R, Kaplan PW, Valença M, De Marchis GM. EEG for diagnosis and prognosis of acute nonhypoxic encephalopathy: history and current evidence. J Clin Neurophysiol. 2015;32(6):456–64.
47. Sutter R, Barnes B, Leyva A, Kaplan PW, Geocadin RG, Basel H. Electroencephalographic sleep elements and outcome in acute encephalopathic patients: a 4-year cohort study. Eur J Neurol. 2014;21(10):1268–75.
48. Claassen J, Taccone FS, Horn P, Holtkamp M, Stocchetti N, Oddo M. Recommendations on the use of EEG monitoring in critically ill patients: consensus statement from the neurointensive care section of the ESICM. Intensive Care Med. 2013;39(8):1337–51.

Chapter 12
Endothelial Health and Delirium

Marcos G. Lopez and Christopher G. Hughes

The endothelium comprises a surface area in the range of 4000–7000 m^2 in an adult human and plays an integral role in the regulation of perfusion, immune cell activation and inflammation, coagulation, and maintenance of the blood-brain barrier [1–3]. Each of these processes may potentially contribute to the development of delirium in critically ill patients (Fig. 12.1). This chapter will examine the potential

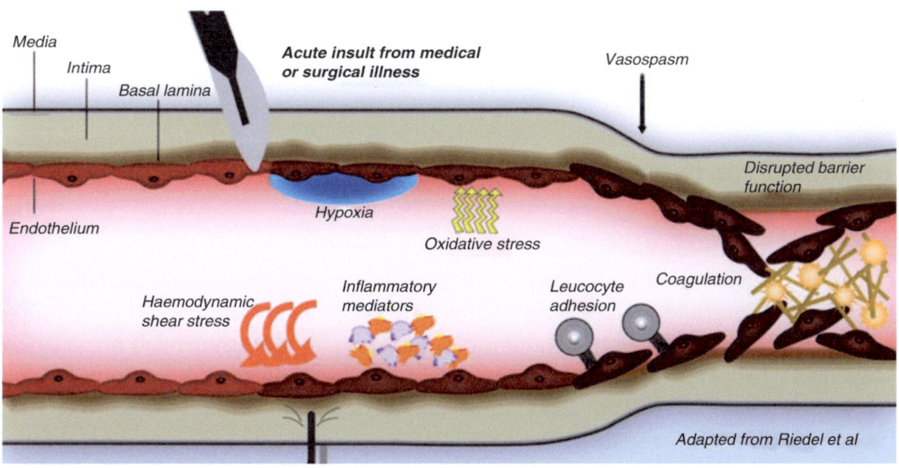

Fig. 12.1 Endothelial injury from acute illness. (Adapted from Riedel et al. [55])

M. G. Lopez (✉)
Division of Anesthesiology Critical Care Medicine, Department of Anesthesiology, Vanderbilt University Medical Center, Nashville, TN, USA
e-mail: marcos.g.lopez@vumc.org

C. G. Hughes
Critical Illness, Brain Dysfunction, and Survivorship Center and the Division of Anesthesiology Critical Care Medicine, Vanderbilt University Medical Center, Nashville, TN, USA

C. G. Hughes et al. (eds.), *Delirium*, https://doi.org/10.1007/978-3-030-25751-4_12

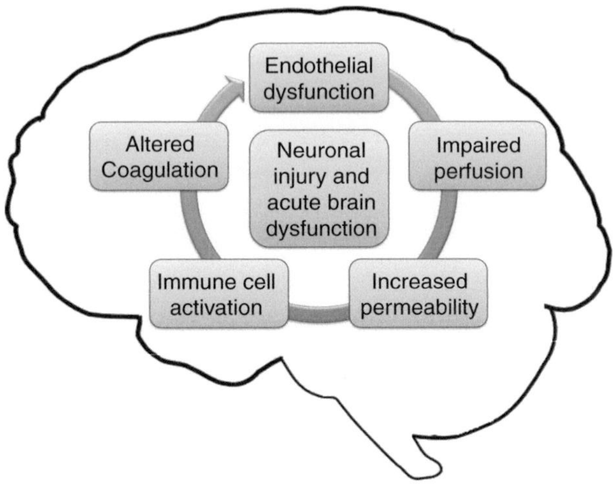

Fig. 12.2 Brain organ injury from endothelial dysfunction

contributions of these endothelial processes to delirium and acute brain dysfunction. While several associations between markers of endothelial function and delirium are consistent with biologically plausible pathophysiology and provide clues to the mechanisms underlying delirium (Fig. 12.2), there remains a large knowledge gap in understanding the specific mechanisms linking endothelial dysfunction to delirium.

Endothelium-Regulated Perfusion

A primary role of the endothelium is to regulate vascular tone and, thus, perfusion of tissues. Major endothelium-mediated vasodilators include nitric oxide (NO), acetylcholine, adenosine, and prostaglandins [4]. Vasoconstriction can be induced by endogenous or exogenous catecholamines, vasopressin, dopamine, and nitric oxide scavengers [5]. The balance of these signals is integrated by endothelium-derived mechanisms and can lead to differential perfusion across different organ vascular beds, including the cerebral circulation.

The endothelium plays an essential role in the modulation of cerebral blood flow. Large cerebral vessels exhibit flow-mediated dilation, an increase in the luminal diameter of the blood vessel in response to increased shear stress that is largely mediated by nitric oxide generated by endothelial nitric oxide synthase [6, 7]. Nitric oxide can freely diffuse to smooth muscle cells where it binds and activates guanylate cyclase. Guanylate cyclase generates guanosine 3′,5′-cyclic monophosphate (cGMP) which activates myosin light chain phosphatase leading to smooth muscle relaxation and resultant vasodilation [8]. In humans, endothelium-dependent (and nitric oxide-mediated) vasodilation is present in cerebral arteries [9]. Regional cerebral blood flow decreases while patients have delirium and returns to normal after delirium resolves, indicating that there is a possibility for a direct role for altered cerebral blood flow in the pathogenesis of delirium [10]. Endothelial modulation of cerebral blood flow may affect or underlie the observed association between altered cerebral blood flow and delirium.

Delirium and acute brain dysfunction might be precipitated by hypoperfusion, hyperperfusion, ischemia-reperfusion events, or altered cerebral autoregulation. In patients undergoing cardiac surgery, cerebral hyperoxia and hyperoxic cerebral reperfusion measured with near-infrared spectroscopy are independently associated with increased odds of postoperative delirium [11]. Dysregulation of cerebral blood flow by the endothelium or an impaired ability of the endothelium to modulate blood flow in this setting may contribute to the development of delirium in patients with cerebral hyperoxia or hyperoxic cerebral reperfusion. This is further supported by findings that disturbed cerebral autoregulation is associated with delirium in patients with sepsis [12].

Impaired perfusion of small arterioles and capillaries, termed microvascular dysfunction or microvascular disease, may be particularly affected by endothelium-dependent mechanisms. Microvascular dysfunction has long been hypothesized as a contributor to organ dysfunction in patients with sepsis and may be a contributor to brain dysfunction in other disease states [13], and microvascular dysfunction is associated with long-term cognitive decline [14]. Structural and functional alterations of brain capillary endothelial cells are associated with impaired microcirculation [15]. Decreased reactive hyperemia index, a measurement of endothelium-dependent reactive hyperemia in the digital vascular bed elicited in response to an ischemic stimulus, is associated with increased delirium duration and decreased delirium/coma-free days in medical and surgical ICU patients [16]. Thus, worse endothelium-mediated vascular reactivity in a peripheral microvascular tissue bed is associated with increased delirium. Interestingly, this association was not mediated by blood-brain barrier function in a subsequent study, suggesting an independent contribution of endothelium-dependent perfusion [17]. The direct causal pathway underlying this association, however, is not known, nor is the correlation between peripheral and cerebral measurements of endothelial reactivity. Associations between delirium and endothelium-mediated vascular reactivity responses in larger conduit (e.g., brachial) arteries and direct assessment of endothelial function in resistance arterioles using wire myography are currently being examined in ongoing studies [18]. It remains unknown (1) if there are therapies that improve microvascular or conduit artery vascular reactivity in the acute phase and (2) what effects these therapies have on the development of delirium in patients. One pilot study, however, has demonstrated that early physical therapy during critical illness can improve endothelial vascular reactivity and that improvement in endothelial vascular reactivity is associated with decreased delirium [19].

Current evidence supports that microcirculatory blood flow abnormalities from endothelial dysfunction contribute to delirium. The direct influence of the endothelium on regional blood flow appears important in achieving the metabolic balance needed by brain tissue for normal functioning, but other contributing factors of the endothelium also likely influence brain activity such as selective permeability or barrier function.

Endothelium and the Blood-Brain Barrier

The blood-brain barrier is a selectively permeable layer made of specialized endothelial cells and astrocytes that regulate the flow of substances across the central nervous system (CNS) capillary bed based on size and polarity in the absence of other specific para- and transcellular transport mechanisms [20, 21]. Blood-brain barrier permeability is primarily affected by the tight and adherens junctions between endothelial cells in the CNS capillary bed. Tight junctions seal the cleft between individual endothelial cells, and adherens junctions facilitate contact between endothelial cells [22]. The blood-brain barrier protects central neurons and brain function via this selective permeability. Blood-brain barrier disruption has the potential to allow injurious molecules such as reactive oxygen species or inflammatory mediators from the periphery to directly damage tissue or alter neurotransmission by brain neurons.

Multiple models of sepsis or brain ischemia have demonstrated an increased interactions between the endothelium and blood-brain barrier permeability. Structural alterations correlating with altered permeability are seen in blood-brain barrier endothelial cells [23], and hypoxia leads to blood-brain barrier endothelial cell permeability changes via tight junction protein phosphorylation [24]. Upregulation of inducible nitric oxide synthase and superoxide production is seen in brains of septic mice [15]. In vitro and animal investigations observed that cytokines such as tumor necrosis factor-alpha, interleukin-1B, and vascular endothelial growth factor-A increase permeability of the blood-brain barrier [25–27]. Proinflammatory cytokines can also modulate astrocytes' energy metabolism and cellular stress defenses, which may contribute to altered blood-brain barrier function and neuronal vulnerability [28]. Meta-analyses have identified that increasing age is associated with increased blood-brain barrier permeability in patients [29]. Further, blood-brain barrier breakdown is one of the earliest predictors of cognitive impairment [30] and is commonly seen after cardiac surgery [31]. Interestingly, advanced age, structural changes on brain imaging, prior cognitive impairment, and cardiac surgery are some of the strongest risk factors for the development of delirium. Thus, it is possible that increased blood-brain barrier permeability is a major contributing factor to the increased risk of delirium.

Measuring the permeability of the blood-brain barrier in patients with acute illness, however, is challenging. Calcium-binding protein S100 beta (S100B) is a marker of blood-brain barrier disruption and astrocyte injury after central nervous system injury or ischemia [32–34]. By comparing the quotient of S100B in cerebrospinal fluid to the concentration in serum in patients with severe traumatic brain injury, Blyth et al. identified that circulating S100B concentrations accurately reflect blood-brain barrier dysfunction in patients. Subsequently, it was noted that plasma concentrations of S100B are associated with delirium in elderly patients with hip fractures [35], septic patients [36], and patients in shock or with respiratory failure [17] and with neuropsychiatric disorders after cardiac surgery [37, 38]. Thus, S100B is a well-validated peripheral marker of blood-brain barrier disruption that is independently associated with delirium in critically ill patients. The exact nature of injury (or vulnerability) that is precipitated by blood-brain barrier disruption is not yet known, but evidence suggests that changes in the blood-brain barrier act separately and in addition to changes in the microcirculation with regard to delirium [17].

The blood-brain barrier functions to reduce toxin exposure, prevent neuronal injury, and maintain electrochemical gradients necessary for normal CNS cellular function. Current evidence highlights that disruption of the blood-brain barrier likely contributes to the development of delirium in patients. Potential mechanisms leading to acute cognitive dysfunction in this setting are direct damage to tissue or cells, disruption of neurochemical signaling, and alterations of the extracellular milieu including electrochemical gradients. It is unclear what therapies, interventions, or clinical practices can reduce blood-brain barrier disruption during acute illness and if doing so will make a clinically important impact for patients.

Endothelial Activation and Modulation of Immune Responses

Systemic inflammation is seen in pathologic states such as sepsis, trauma, and use of mechanical circulatory support and is associated with delirium [39–42]. Inflammatory stimuli such as pathogens or trauma induce leukocytes to release cytokines that activate endothelial cells to express surface ligands called endothelial-leukocyte adhesion molecules [43]. These adhesion molecules facilitate endothelium and leukocyte interactions that initiate leukocyte rolling. Activated endothelial cells also express additional chemokines that increase contact area between leukocytes and endothelium, cluster surface integrins for firm attachment, and stimulate chemokinesis – all necessary steps for leukocyte extravasation into tissue [44]. This process is obligatory for normal responses to injuries or pathogens. Neuroinflammation is thought to contribute to neurodegenerative pathologies such as Alzheimer's disease and Parkinson's disease, and systemic inflammation causes acute neurocognitive dysfunction from impaired synaptic transmission. The endothelium is an integral modulator and activator of inflammatory cascades that likely elicits brain dysfunction. Furthermore, inflammation has been tied to endothelial dysfunction in chronic disease states such as hypertension, obesity, and diabetes mellitus [45, 46].

E-selectin, ICAM-1, and VCAM-1 are surface endothelial-leukocyte adhesion molecules expressed by endothelial cells after tissue injury or in the presence of inflammatory cytokines and mediate endothelial cell-immunocyte interaction [47]. Excess endothelial activation is a possible inflammation-mediated mechanism for neuronal dysfunction and delirium. A postmortem examination of human brain tissue identified associations between the systemic marker of inflammation and acute-phase reactant C-reactive protein and endothelial activation markers including intercellular adhesion molecule-1, CD40, and cyclooxygenase-2 in perivascular brain tissue [48]. Endothelial activation markers are associated with blood-brain barrier leukocyte adhesion and dysfunction [49]. Additionally, isolated brain endothelial cells have been noted to express Toll-like receptors 3 and 4, which are important for myeloid cell differentiation during inflammation, and that activation of these receptors leads to increased intercellular endothelial leak [50]. These preclinical studies support the hypothesis that systemic inflammation affects brain tissue through activation of endothelial cells and increased blood-brain barrier permeability.

In critically ill patients with delirium, increased plasma concentration of E-selectin is associated with increased odds of delirium, further supporting the idea that excess endothelial activation is a likely contributor to the development of delirium [17]. Additionally, E-selectin concentration during hospitalization for critical illness is associated with long-term cognitive decline indicating that endothelial activation in the acute phase may play an important role in the neurocognitive health of patients in the long term [51].

Endothelial activation of immune cells induces inflammatory cascades, increased endothelial leak, and potentially neurologic dysfunction and injury. Future investigations will need to more directly quantify the effects of endothelial activation and to determine if there are other contributing factors to the development of delirium such as direct-activated immune cell-mediated damage to neurons.

The Endothelium, Coagulation, and Delirium

The endothelium is directly involved in the control of anticoagulation, platelet adhesion and activation, and fibrinolysis, but it is unclear if these processes contribute to the development of delirium. Impaired microvascular perfusion from dysregulated coagulation as is seen in disseminated intravascular coagulation has long been hypothesized to underlie cerebral dysfunction in patients [52], and experimental models have noted that endothelial activation is a necessary component of thrombus-related microvascular dysfunction in sepsis [53]. Lower plasma concentrations of protein C (suggesting increased coagulation) are significantly associated with increased probability of delirium in the ICU [54]. Hughes et al. noted that higher levels of plasminogen activator inhibitor-1 (PAI-1) are independently associated with fewer delirium- and coma-free days in critically ill patients. Furthermore, higher PAI-1 (suggesting suppressed fibrinolysis) concentration was associated with a longer duration of delirium adjusted for potential confounders of this association [17]. The mechanisms underlying this association remain incompletely defined, but the idea that increased activation of coagulant pathways could impair cerebral microvascular circulation and lead to a clinical presentation of delirium is plausible and supported by initial studies.

Summary

The vascular endothelium directly contributes to the control of perfusion, maintenance of the blood-brain barrier, activation of immune and inflammatory processes, and coagulation. Each of these endothelial functions has the potential to contribute to the development of delirium in patients, and while multiple investigations have identified associations between endothelial dysfunction or injury and delirium (Table 12.1), there remains a large gap in the knowledge surrounding the direct

Table 12.1 Summary of evidence for individual endothelial functions and associations with delirium or altered neurocognitive function

Endothelial function	Reference
Perfusion and vascular reactivity	
• Regional cerebral blood flow is decreased during delirium	[10]
• Intraoperative hyperoxic cerebral reperfusion is associated with increased odds of delirium after cardiac surgery	[11]
• Disturbed cerebral autoregulation is associated with delirium in septic patients	[12]
• Microvascular dysfunction is associated with long-term cognitive decline	[14]
• ↓ Digital vascular reactivity is associated with ↑ duration of delirium and ↓ delirium-/coma-free days in ICU patients	[16]
• Early physical therapy improves vascular reactivity and is associated with decreased delirium in critically ill patients	[19]
Endothelial barrier function	
• Blood-brain barrier breakdown is an early predictor of cognitive impairment	[30]
• Increased plasma concentrations of S100B are associated with delirium in patients with hip fractures	[35]
• Increased plasma S100B is associated with delirium in patients with sepsis	[36]
• Increased plasma S100B is associated with delirium in patients with shock or with respiratory failure	[17]
• Increased plasma S100B in critically ill patients is associated with long-term cognitive decline	[48]
Immune cell activation and inflammation	
• Systemic inflammation in sepsis, trauma, and use of mechanical circulatory support is associated with delirium/neurocognitive dysfunction	[39–42]
• Increased plasma E-selectin concentration is associated with increased odds of delirium in critically ill patients	[17]
• Increased plasma E-selectin concentration in critically ill patients is associated with long-term cognitive decline	[48]
Coagulation	
• Lower concentrations of protein C are significantly associated with increased probability of delirium in critically patients	[51]
• Increased PAI-1 plasma concentration is associated with ↑ duration of delirium and ↓ delirium-/coma-free days in ICU patients	[17]

pathophysiologic relationship between endothelial health and delirium. Potential treatments for endothelial dysfunction should be studied to determine if they reduce the incidence of delirium.

References

1. Moncada S, Radomski MW, Palmer RM. Endothelium-derived relaxing factor. Identification as nitric oxide and role in the control of vascular tone and platelet function. Biochem Pharmacol. 1988;37:2495–501.
2. De Caterina R, Libby P, Peng HB, et al. Nitric oxide decreases cytokine-induced endothelial activation. Nitric oxide selectively reduces endothelial expression of adhesion molecules and proinflammatory cytokines. J Clin Invest. 1995;96:60–8.
3. Janzer RC, Raff MC. Astrocytes induce blood-brain barrier properties in endothelial cells. Nature. 1987;325:253–7.
4. Radomski MW, Palmer RM, Moncada S. Comparative pharmacology of endothelium-derived relaxing factor, nitric oxide and prostacyclin in platelets. Br J Pharmacol. 1987;92:181–7.
5. Furchgott RF, Vanhoutte PM. Endothelium-derived relaxing and contracting factors. FASEB J. 1989;3:2007–18.
6. Yang ST, Mayhan WG, Faraci FM, Heistad DD. Endothelium-dependent responses of cerebral blood vessels during chronic hypertension. Hypertension. 1991;17:612–8.
7. Faraci FM, Heistad DD. Regulation of the cerebral circulation: role of endothelium and potassium channels. Physiol Rev. 1998;78:53–97.
8. Murad F. Shattuck Lecture. Nitric oxide and cyclic GMP in cell signaling and drug development. N Engl J Med. 2006;355:2003–11.
9. Aldasoro M, Martinez C, Vila JM, Medina P, Lluch S. Influence of endothelial nitric oxide on adrenergic contractile responses of human cerebral arteries. J Cereb Blood Flow Metab. 1996;16:623–8.
10. Yokota H, Ogawa S, Kurokawa A, Yamamoto Y. Regional cerebral blood flow in delirium patients. Psychiatry Clin Neurosci. 2003;57:337–9.
11. Lopez MG, Pandharipande P, Morse J, et al. Intraoperative cerebral oxygenation, oxidative injury, and delirium following cardiac surgery. Free Radic Biol Med. 2017;103:192–8.
12. Pfister D, Siegemund M, Dell-Kuster S, et al. Cerebral perfusion in sepsis-associated delirium. Crit Care. 2008;12:R63.
13. Vincent JL, De Backer D. Microvascular dysfunction as a cause of organ dysfunction in severe sepsis. Crit Care. 2005;9(Suppl 4):S9–12.
14. Scuteri A, Nilsson PM, Tzourio C, Redon J, Laurent S. Microvascular brain damage with aging and hypertension: pathophysiological consideration and clinical implications. J Hypertens. 2011;29:1469–77.
15. Yokoo H, Chiba S, Tomita K, et al. Neurodegenerative evidence in mice brains with cecal ligation and puncture-induced sepsis: preventive effect of the free radical scavenger edaravone. PLoS One. 2012;7:e51539.
16. Hughes CG, Morandi A, Girard TD, et al. Association between endothelial dysfunction and acute brain dysfunction during critical illness. Anesthesiology. 2013;118:631–9.
17. Hughes CG, Pandharipande PP, Thompson JL, et al. Endothelial activation and blood-brain barrier injury as risk factors for delirium in critically ill patients. Crit Care Med. 2016;44:e809–17.
18. Lopez MG, Pretorius M, Shotwell MS, et al. The risk of oxygen during cardiac surgery (ROCS) trial: study protocol for a randomized clinical trial. Trials. 2017;18:295.
19. Hughes CG, Brummel NE, Girard TD, Graves AJ, Ely EW, Pandharipande PP. Change in endothelial vascular reactivity and acute brain dysfunction during critical illness. Br J Anaesth. 2015;115:794–5.

20. Stamatovic SM, Keep RF, Andjelkovic AV. Brain endothelial cell-cell junctions: how to "open" the blood brain barrier. Curr Neuropharmacol. 2008;6:179–92.
21. Reese TS, Karnovsky MJ. Fine structural localization of a blood-brain barrier to exogenous peroxidase. J Cell Biol. 1967;34:207–17.
22. Rubin LL, Staddon JM. The cell biology of the blood-brain barrier. Annu Rev Neurosci. 1999;22:11–28.
23. Vajtr D, Benada O, Kukacka J, et al. Correlation of ultrastructural changes of endothelial cells and astrocytes occurring during blood brain barrier damage after traumatic brain injury with biochemical markers of BBB leakage and inflammatory response. Physiol Res. 2009;58:263–8.
24. Fleegal MA, Hom S, Borg LK, Davis TP. Activation of PKC modulates blood-brain barrier endothelial cell permeability changes induced by hypoxia and posthypoxic reoxygenation. Am J Physiol Heart Circ Physiol. 2005;289:H2012–9.
25. Argaw AT, Zhang Y, Snyder BJ, et al. IL-1beta regulates blood-brain barrier permeability via reactivation of the hypoxia-angiogenesis program. J Immunol. 2006;177:5574–84.
26. Tsao N, Hsu HP, Wu CM, Liu CC, Lei HY. Tumour necrosis factor-alpha causes an increase in blood-brain barrier permeability during sepsis. J Med Microbiol. 2001;50:812–21.
27. Zhang ZG, Zhang L, Tsang W, et al. Correlation of VEGF and angiopoietin expression with disruption of blood-brain barrier and angiogenesis after focal cerebral ischemia. J Cereb Blood Flow Metab. 2002;22:379–92.
28. Gavillet M, Allaman I, Magistretti PJ. Modulation of astrocytic metabolic phenotype by proinflammatory cytokines. Glia. 2008;56:975–89.
29. Farrall AJ, Wardlaw JM. Blood-brain barrier: ageing and microvascular disease – systematic review and meta-analysis. Neurobiol Aging. 2009;30:337–52.
30. Montagne A, Barnes SR, Sweeney MD, et al. Blood-brain barrier breakdown in the aging human hippocampus. Neuron. 2015;85:296–302.
31. Merino JG, Latour LL, Tso A, et al. Blood-brain barrier disruption after cardiac surgery. AJNR Am J Neuroradiol. 2013;34:518–23.
32. Blyth BJ, Farhavar A, Gee C, et al. Validation of serum markers for blood-brain barrier disruption in traumatic brain injury. J Neurotrauma. 2009;26:1497–507.
33. Kanner AA, Marchi N, Fazio V, et al. Serum S100beta: a noninvasive marker of blood-brain barrier function and brain lesions. Cancer. 2003;97:2806–13.
34. Kochanek PM, Berger RP, Bayir H, Wagner AK, Jenkins LW, Clark RS. Biomarkers of primary and evolving damage in traumatic and ischemic brain injury: diagnosis, prognosis, probing mechanisms, and therapeutic decision making. Curr Opin Crit Care. 2008;14:135–41.
35. van Munster BC, Korse CM, de Rooij SE, Bonfrer JM, Zwinderman AH, Korevaar JC. Markers of cerebral damage during delirium in elderly patients with hip fracture. BMC Neurol. 2009;9:21.
36. Nguyen DN, Spapen H, Su F, et al. Elevated serum levels of S-100beta protein and neuron-specific enolase are associated with brain injury in patients with severe sepsis and septic shock. Crit Care Med. 2006;34:1967–74.
37. Herrmann M, Ebert AD, Galazky I, Wunderlich MT, Kunz WS, Huth C. Neurobehavioral outcome prediction after cardiac surgery: role of neurobiochemical markers of damage to neuronal and glial brain tissue. Stroke. 2000;31:645–50.
38. Kilminster S, Treasure T, McMillan T, Holt DW. Neuropsychological change and S-100 protein release in 130 unselected patients undergoing cardiac surgery. Stroke. 1999;30:1869–74.
39. Cerejeira J, Firmino H, Vaz-Serra A, Mukaetova-Ladinska EB. The neuroinflammatory hypothesis of delirium. Acta Neuropathol. 2010;119:737–54.
40. Rudolph JL, Ramlawi B, Kuchel GA, et al. Chemokines are associated with delirium after cardiac surgery. J Gerontol A Biol Sci Med Sci. 2008;63:184–9.
41. Ritter C, Tomasi CD, Dal-Pizzol F, et al. Inflammation biomarkers and delirium in critically ill patients. Crit Care. 2014;18:R106.
42. Luo T, Wu J, Kabadi SV, et al. Propofol limits microglial activation after experimental brain trauma through inhibition of nicotinamide adenine dinucleotide phosphate oxidase. Anesthesiology. 2013;119:1370–88.

43. Bevilacqua MP, Pober JS, Mendrick DL, Cotran RS, Gimbrone MA Jr. Identification of an inducible endothelial-leukocyte adhesion molecule. Proc Natl Acad Sci U S A. 1987;84:9238–42.
44. Middleton J, Patterson AM, Gardner L, Schmutz C, Ashton BA. Leukocyte extravasation: chemokine transport and presentation by the endothelium. Blood. 2002;100:3853–60.
45. Yudkin JS, Stehouwer CD, Emeis JJ, Coppack SW. C-reactive protein in healthy subjects: associations with obesity, insulin resistance, and endothelial dysfunction: a potential role for cytokines originating from adipose tissue? Arterioscler Thromb Vasc Biol. 1999;19:972–8.
46. Bautista LE. Inflammation, endothelial dysfunction, and the risk of high blood pressure: epidemiologic and biological evidence. J Hum Hypertens. 2003;17:223–30.
47. Pigott R, Dillon LP, Hemingway IH, Gearing AJ. Soluble forms of E-selectin, ICAM-1 and VCAM-1 are present in the supernatants of cytokine activated cultured endothelial cells. Biochem Biophys Res Commun. 1992;187:584–9.
48. Uchikado H, Akiyama H, Kondo H, et al. Activation of vascular endothelial cells and perivascular cells by systemic inflammation-an immunohistochemical study of postmortem human brain tissues. Acta Neuropathol. 2004;107:341–51.
49. Vachharajani V, Cunningham C, Yoza B, Carson J Jr, Vachharajani TJ, McCall C. Adiponectin-deficiency exaggerates sepsis-induced microvascular dysfunction in the mouse brain. Obesity (Silver Spring). 2012;20:498–504.
50. Johnson RH, Kho DT, O'Carroll SJ, Angel CE, Graham ES. The functional and inflammatory response of brain endothelial cells to toll-like receptor agonists. Sci Rep. 2018;8:10102.
51. Hughes CG, Patel MB, Brummel NE, et al. Relationships between markers of neurologic and endothelial injury during critical illness and long-term cognitive impairment and disability. Intensive Care Med. 2018;44:345–55.
52. Ryan FP, Timperley WR, Preston FE, Holdsworth CD. Cerebral involvement with disseminated intravascular coagulation in intestinal disease. J Clin Pathol. 1977;30:551–5.
53. Secor D, Li F, Ellis CG, et al. Impaired microvascular perfusion in sepsis requires activated coagulation and P-selectin-mediated platelet adhesion in capillaries. Intensive Care Med. 2010;36:1928–34.
54. Girard TD, Ware LB, Bernard GR, et al. Associations of markers of inflammation and coagulation with delirium during critical illness. Intensive Care Med. 2012;38:1965–73.
55. Riedel BN, Browne K, Burbury K, Schier R. Perioperative implications of vascular endothelial dysfunction: current understanding of this critical sensor-effector organ. Curr Anesthesiol Rep. 2013;3:10.

Chapter 13
Preventive Strategies to Reduce Intensive Care Unit Delirium

Laura Beth Kalvas, Mary Ann Barnes-Daly, E. Wesley Ely, and Michele C. Balas

Introduction

Evidence-based interventions that aim to prevent the occurrence and/or reduce the duration of intensive care unit (ICU) delirium have the potential to dramatically improve both short- and long-term patient and family-centered outcomes. Unfortunately, studies evaluating pharmacologic and nonpharmacologic delirium prevention and reduction strategies in the ICU are few and generally methodologically weak. The most recent 2018 Clinical Practice Guidelines for the Prevention and Management of Pain, Agitation/Sedation, Delirium, Immobility, and Sleep Disruption (PADIS) Guidelines [1] acknowledge that this area of research is particularly challenging as any well-designed delirium prevention study would require a baseline evaluation of patients who are delirium-free at the time of ICU admission. This is challenging due to the high rates of delirium and/or coma present at the time of ICU admission and the unplanned nature of many critical care admissions. Nevertheless, the evidence to date suggests that it is possible to reduce the incidence and duration of ICU delirium through a number of nonpharmacologic, multicomponent, interprofessional approaches. The purpose of this chapter is to review the evidence for the effectiveness of interventions to prevent ICU delirium.

L. B. Kalvas (✉) · M. C. Balas
The Ohio State University, College of Nursing, Columbus, OH, USA
e-mail: kalvas.4@buckeyemail.osu.edu

M. A. Barnes-Daly
Sutter Health, Sacramento, CA, USA

E. W. Ely
Critical Illness, Brain Dysfunction, and Survivorship (CIBS) Center, Department of Medicine, Pulmonary and Critical Care, Vanderbilt University School of Medicine and the Tennessee Valley Veteran's Affairs Geriatric Research Education Clinical Center (GRECC), Nashville, TN, USA

C. G. Hughes et al. (eds.), *Delirium*, https://doi.org/10.1007/978-3-030-25751-4_13

Importance of Identifying and Removing Risk Factors

The first step toward preventing and reducing the duration of ICU delirium is to identify and remove, if possible, any underlying risk factors (see also Chap. 4). The development of delirium typically depends upon a complex interaction of multiple risk factors that are present prior to and during an ICU stay. These risk factors are generally divided into two broad categories: non-modifiable and modifiable.

Non-modifiable Risk Factors

The new PADIS Guidelines outline the non-modifiable risk factors with the strongest evidence for an association with ICU delirium. These include older age, preexisting dementia, prior coma, pre-ICU emergency surgery or trauma, and greater severity of illness [1]. There is also moderate evidence suggesting that a history of hypertension, current neurologic or trauma admission, and prior use of antipsychotics and anticonvulsants increase the risk of delirium. While non-modifiable risk factors cannot be changed, clinicians need to be aware of the relationship between these factors and the likelihood of delirium in order to better employ prevention and mitigation strategies early in the ICU stay in these high-risk patients.

Modifiable Risk Factors

The PADIS guidelines identify two modifiable risk factors for delirium: the administration of blood transfusions and the use of benzodiazepines [1]. Restricting blood transfusions to a threshold of hemoglobin level less than 7.0 g/dl for chronic ICU-related anemia may reduce the incidence of blood administration; however, transfusion often remains a necessary component of treatment for acute blood loss anemia, and therefore not modifiable in many cases. Psychoactive medications, including benzodiazepines and other sedatives, are widely understood to play an associative role in the development of delirium [2]. Other modifiable risk factors for the development of delirium identified in the literature include the practice of sedating patients more than clinically necessary [3–6], use of physical restraints with resulting immobility [7–9], social isolation [7], sleep deprivation [10, 11], and environmental factors such as excessive light and noise [7, 12]. Finally, the maintenance of clinical parameters such as serum glucose [13], electrolytes [14, 15], and other measures of homeostasis within normal limits has been shown to reduce the likelihood of the development of delirium. Clinicians should initiate preventative strategies that focus on these modifiable risk factors early in the ICU stay to decrease the incidence and duration of delirium in high-risk patients.

Pharmacologic Prevention of Delirium

A recent international survey found that 93% of intensive care unit (ICU) clinicians were using haloperidol in the treatment and prevention of delirium, while 53% were using antipsychotics for delirium-associated agitation [16]. This is concerning as the best evidence to date suggests that most pharmacological agents do not consistently aid in the prevention of ICU delirium [17–20]. Based upon this evidence, the PADIS guidelines do *not* recommend the use of antipsychotics (typical or atypical), dexmedetomidine, HMG-CoA reductase inhibitors, or ketamine to prevent delirium in critically ill adults [1].

Antipsychotics

A recent systematic review and meta-analysis of seven studies comprising 1970 ICU and non-ICU patients found no association between the use of preventative antipsychotics (haloperidol or atypical antipsychotics) and delirium incidence, duration, or severity [17]. A large, randomized, placebo-controlled trial of ICU patients at high risk for delirium (n = 1789) found that compared to controls, patients who received prophylactic haloperidol were no more likely to survive to 28 days [21]. Furthermore, no differences were noted in delirium incidence, delirium-free or coma-free days, duration of mechanical ventilation, or length of stay (LOS) between the two groups. While antipsychotics are not recommended for routine prevention or treatment of delirium, short-term doses of these medications may be necessary for patients who experience distressing symptoms (i.e., hallucinations, severe agitation) or are at risk for self-harm. Clinicians must be sure to discontinue these medications once the patient stops experiencing these symptoms, as many patients mistakenly remain on long-term antipsychotic therapy after discharge from the ICU [22, 23].

Dexmedetomidine

In a meta-analysis of 14 studies including both ICU and cardiac patients (n = 3029), dexmedetomidine was found to decrease the risk for delirium, agitation, and/or confusion [24]. Studies comparing the use of dexmedetomidine to propofol or benzodiazepines have also found statistically significant reductions in the incidence or duration of delirium and decreased duration of mechanical ventilation, but no impact on ICU LOS [25–28]. In a recent systematic review of pharmacologic prevention, the authors considered these studies to be of generally high quality with large sample sizes [29]. Conversely, another systematic review published in the same year examined three of these studies and found that issues with study design prohibited the ability to conclude that dexmedetomidine prevents delirium [30]. A key limitation to all of these studies was the comparison of dexmedetomidine to benzodiazepines (known risk factor for delirium) or propofol rather than to a placebo. Further, many of these studies are not strictly preventive trials since some patients already had delirium at the time of randomization into the studies.

Although the use of dexmedetomidine can decrease the need for benzodiazepines and allow for light levels of sedation without suppressing respiratory drive, the PADIS guidelines do *not* currently recommend dexmedetomidine for the prevention of delirium. This recommendation is based on the results of a recent randomized, double-blind, placebo-controlled study of 700 non-cardiac surgical ICU patients [18]. While this study did find a statistically significant reduction in delirium incidence in those who received prophylactic dexmedetomidine, no other improvement in clinical outcomes (i.e., duration of mechanical ventilation, ICU LOS, or mortality) was demonstrated. In addition, subjects in this study had a lower severity of illness than a typical ICU population, which inherently decreased the risk of delirium for those studied. More studies are needed to better understand the relationship between the use of dexmedetomidine and prevention of delirium and other clinical outcomes.

HMG-CoA Reductase Inhibitors

A recent systematic review and meta-analysis of six studies comprised of ICU and cardiac surgery patients (n = 289,773) found no significant difference in risk for delirium between patients who did and did not take statins prior to hospitalization [19]. However, in a prospective cohort study of 763 medical and surgical ICU patients, the initiation of statins during ICU stay, while controlling for prehospital statin use, was found to significantly reduce the odds of delirium [31]. Further, although prehospital statin use was not associated with delirium in this cohort, the longer a prehospital statin user's statin medication was held in the ICU, the higher their odds of delirium. The presence of sepsis and stage of ICU stay were significant moderators of these relationships.

Ketamine

In a recent multicenter, double-blind, randomized control trial (RCT), 672 patients undergoing major surgery were given preoperative ketamine at varying doses, or a placebo. Rates of postoperative delirium did not differ across groups, but patients who received ketamine were more likely to experience hallucinations and nightmares [20], suggesting that the use of ketamine is contraindicated.

Multicomponent Delirium Prevention Strategies

ABCDEF Bundle

The ABCDEF bundle [32–39] (Fig. 13.1) is a group of interprofessional, evidence-based interventions designed to limit the profound physical, cognitive, and/or mental health impairments associated with an ICU admission [40]. The bundle targets many modifiable risk factors for delirium and has been shown to limit the development and duration of delirium, duration of mechanical ventilation, and hospital mortality even when delivered incompletely (Table 13.1) [39, 41, 42]. Implementation of the ABCDEF bundle in 150 ICU patients resulted in an increase of 3 additional days spent breathing without mechanical ventilation and a decrease in the incidence of delirium by nearly half compared to the pre-implementation sample [42]. Another study including more than 6000 ICU patients demonstrated that *each* 10% increase in the *dose* of the ABCDEF bundle was associated with a statistically significant increase in both hospital survival and days free of delirium and coma [39]. Large-scale implementation of the ABCDEF bundle in 68 ICUs (n = 15,226 patients) demonstrated that the greater the proportion of ABCDEF bundle components a patient received per day, the better their clinical outcomes, including a higher likelihood of discharge and a lower likelihood of mortality, next-day mechanical ventilation, coma, delirium, or physical restraint [41, 43]. The multicomponent interventions that comprise the bundle are summarized below.

Assess, Prevent, and Manage Pain

Pain is defined as "an unpleasant sensory and emotional experience associated with actual or potential tissue damage, or described in terms of such damage"[44] (p475). It is not surprising that many ICU patients experience pain, both at rest and during procedures [45, 46]. Self-report is considered the gold standard for pain measurement, with pain being whatever the patient says it is, occurring wherever the patient says it does [47]. However, critically ill and mechanically ventilated patients are often unable to self-report; therefore the Behavioral Pain Scale (BPS) [48] and Critical-Care Pain Observation Tool (CPOT) [49] are considered valid and reliable alternatives. Health-care providers should not use vital sign alone to determine pain in non-communicative patients but rather use the BPS and CPOT in conjunction with these biological parameters [1].

In contrast to the common practice of initiating both an analgesic and sedation simultaneously at the time of intubation, the PADIS guidelines recommend routine pain assessment using a validated tool and protocol-driven management that allows for the assessment of the effectiveness of analgesia for pain relief, comfort, and sedation before adding a sedative agent [1]. This is referred to as the "pain-first approach." The use of pain management protocols has been found to decrease the

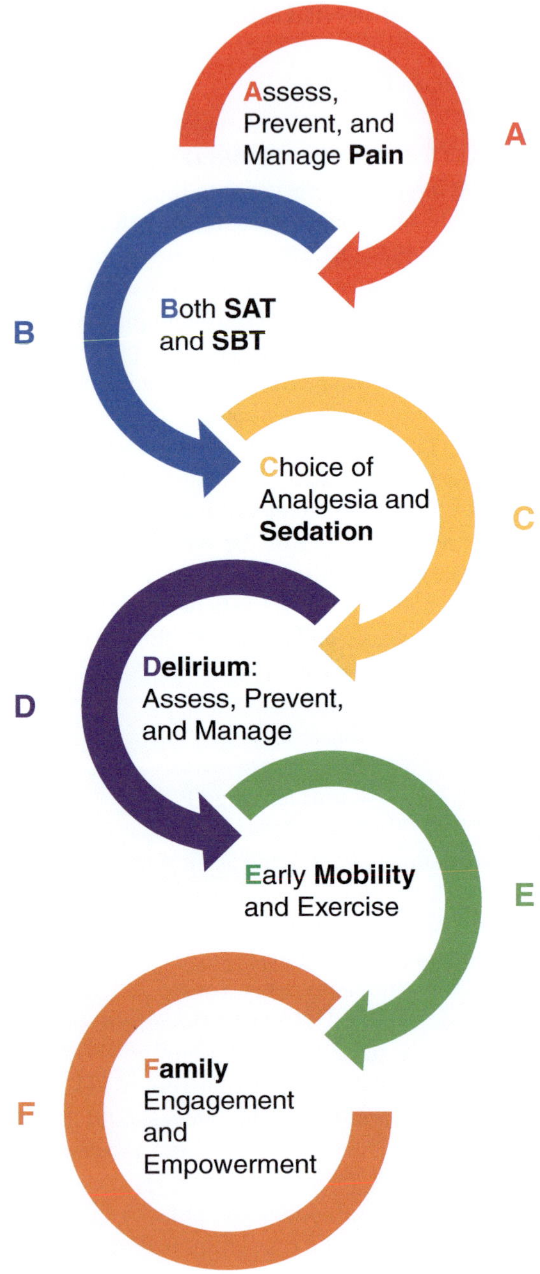

Fig. 13.1 ABCDEF bundle components

Table 13.1 ABCDEF implementation studies

Study	Balas et al. 2014 [42]	Barnes-Daly et al. 2016 [39]	Pun et al. 2019 [41]
Sample *n*	296	6064	15,226
Setting	5 ICUs	7 hospitals	68 ICUs
	1 step-down unit	Medical and surgical ICUs	
	1 hematology/oncology unit		
Intervention	**A**wakening and **b**reathing **c**oordination	**A**ssess, prevent, and manage pain	**A**ssess, prevent, and manage pain
	Delirium monitoring/ management	**B**oth SAT and SBT	**B**oth SAT and SBT
	Early exercise/mobility	**C**hoice of sedation/ analgesia	**C**hoice of sedation/ analgesia
		Delirium monitoring/ management	**D**elirium monitoring/ management
		Early mobility/exercise	**E**arly mobility/exercise
		Family engagement/ empowerment	**F**amily engagement/ empowerment
Outcomes	↑ SAT/SBT	89.1% Total compliance	↓ Next-day mechanical ventilation
	↑ Ventilator-free days	95.2% partial compliance	
	↑ ICU mobilization	↑ Delirium and coma-free days	↓ Next-day physical restraint
	↓ Delirium incidence	↓ Hospital mortality	↓ Next-day coma
	↓ Hospital mortality		↓ Next-day delirium
			↑ Pain
			↓ ICU readmission
			↓ Hospital mortality
			↑ ICU and hospital discharge
			↓ Discharge to facility

Green arrow = good outcome. Red arrow = bad outcome

use of analgesics and sedatives, reduce ICU LOS, and reduce time spent on mechanical ventilation [1, 48, 50]. Additional evidence suggests that untreated pain disrupts sleep quality and prevents early mobility in ICU patients [51, 52], both factors that can influence delirium risk.

Both SATs and SBTs

A spontaneous awakening trial (SAT) is a period of time each day during which all sedatives and opioids are discontinued and patients are allowed to wake up spontaneously to achieve a lighter level of arousal. Depending on patient response, sedatives and narcotics may remain off, or if needed, be restarted at a reduced rate (i.e., half of the original dose) and titrated as needed. When delivering the ABCDEF bundle, the interprofessional ICU team schedules the SAT at a time that precedes the performance of a spontaneous breathing trial (SBT). This coordinated practice, commonly called "Wake Up and Breathe," has been found to increase the number of days ICU patients spend breathing without assistance, decrease sedation use and coma duration, shorten ICU and hospital LOS, and decrease 1-year mortality rates [5, 53]. When performed in conjunction with other bundle components, SAT and SBT can help decrease delirium incidence and duration [39, 42].

Choice of Analgesia and Sedation

Maintaining a light level of sedation is recommended for all critically ill, mechanically ventilated patients unless (in rare situations) deep sedation is clinically indicated. Light sedation is associated with shorter time to extubation and a reduced tracheostomy rate and has not been found to increase rates of self-extubation [1, 6].

Imperative to the effective administration and titration of sedatives is the use of a validated assessment tool as well as an evidence-informed, provider-ordered, sedation target. Both the Sedation Agitation Scale (SAS) [54] and the Richmond Agitation and Sedation Scale (RASS) [55, 56] are recommended by the PADIS guidelines as valid and reliable tools for the assessment of patients' level of arousal. The correct use of these assessment tools requires targeted nursing education and ongoing audits to ensure that values are valid and used appropriately for analgesia and sedative titration. The sedation order should reflect a target for patient responsiveness that is as light as possible with consideration for the patient's clinical condition. The order should clearly direct sedation assessment after analgesia is administered, with the addition of a sedative agent only if the sedation target is not achieved.

The PADIS guidelines recommend the use of propofol or dexmedetomidine over benzodiazepines as both dexmedetomidine and propofol have shown decreased time required to lighten sedation as compared to benzodiazepine (i.e., midazolam, lorazepam) alternatives [1]. Despite conflicting evidence concerning the relationship between dexmedetomidine and delirium [24, 29, 30, 57], the use of light sedation with dexmedetomidine or propofol is thought to improve ICU patient outcomes such as time to extubation, which may in turn decrease the risk for delirium. Supporting this proposed relationship, a recent study of 703 patients across 42 ICUs found that increased depth of sedation in the first 48 h of mechanical ventilation predicted risk for prolonged intubation, delirium, and death [6]. However, the use of dexmedetomidine as the primary sedative agent in an RCT of 3904 ICU patients demonstrated no difference in 90-day mortality compared to those who received usual care, though patients receiving dexmedetomidine had more days alive and free of delirium and coma [58, 59]. Further studies are needed to understand the relationship between sedation with dexmedetomidine and clinical outcomes.

Delirium: Assess, Prevent, and Manage

Delirium screening with the Confusion Assessment Method for the ICU (CAM-ICU) [60, 61] or the Intensive Care Delirium Screening Checklist (ICDSC) [62] should be regularly performed [1]. Studies evaluating the benefit of delirium screening have had mixed results, with some finding no difference in time to diagnosis, ICU LOS, or duration of mechanical ventilation [63, 64], while others have found decreased antipsychotic use and decreased incidence and duration of delirium [65, 66]. Nevertheless, routine screening is recommended, as nurses and physicians often fail to recognize and diagnose delirium [66–70]. For more information related to the assessment and management of delirium, please refer to Chaps. 3 and 16.

Early Mobility and Exercise

Early mobility programs in the ICU can lead to decreased incidence and duration of delirium, mechanical ventilation, and ICU LOS, as well as improved functional outcomes at discharge [42, 71–73]. Studies are underway to determine what role mobility plays in long-term cognitive and functional outcomes of ICU patients [74]. Patients who experience delirium or receive opioid boluses or continuous sedation are less likely to participate in physical therapy [51]. Therefore, coordination of other bundle components such as SAT, SBT, and pain management is necessary for successful mobilization.

Providers are often hesitant to mobilize critically ill intubated patients due to safety concerns; however, as noted in the PADIS guidelines, across 12,200 physical therapy sessions reported in 13 studies, only 15 adverse events were reported [1]. These events included desaturations, unplanned extubation, and musculoskeletal injuries. Useful guidelines for when to initiate and terminate physical rehabilitation are provided in the PADIS guidelines. In patients for whom out-of-bed mobility is contraindicated, the use of in-bed cycling equipment is emerging as an alternative that can improve functional outcomes and reduce delirium incidence [75, 76].

Family Engagement and Empowerment

Family involvement in the care of their critically ill loved one is important. Increased family visitation is associated with decreased cardiovascular complications, mortality, and anxiety scores [77] as well as decreased duration of delirium, coma, and ICU LOS [78]. A recent pilot RCT of 30 ICU patients found that patients who received daily recorded orientation messages from a family member had more delirium-free days than those receiving automated orientation messages and significantly more delirium-free days than controls receiving usual care [79]. Family members can also benefit from involvement in delirium prevention, as witnessing unfamiliar behavior in a loved one can be psychologically distressing [80].

Doctors, nurses, and family members agree that family involvement in preventative delirium care in the ICU is important; however, communication among these groups can be difficult. Family members highlight the need for better delirium education from providers, and clinicians recognize the need to improve the accuracy and consistency of their communication [81, 82]. Clear and reliable communication with family members regarding delirium and its prevention can empower families to become active participants in bundled care.

Sleep Promotion

After discharge, ICU patients frequently identify sleep deprivation as one of the most distressing elements of their stay [83], and both objective and subjective measures have shown that ICU patients experience sleep fragmentation [84–86]. Patients cite many reasons for the poor quality of their sleep including pain, dyspnea, anxiety, noise, light, and nursing care [1, 87]. Associations have been found between decreased rapid eye movement sleep and delirium [88], as well as between high levels of patient reported subjective sleep quality and decreased delirium incidence [89]. Disruptions of circadian rhythms are frequently reported in delirious patients, and sleep deprivation is considered a likely precipitating factor for delirium [11, 52, 90]. The PADIS guidelines recommend the use of a multicomponent sleep promotion bundle to aid in the prevention of delirium [1].

Multicomponent Sleep Promotion Bundles

Sleep promotion protocols typically include interventions to decrease light and noise levels, as well as the clustering of nocturnal care, frequent orientation, and utilization of the ABCDEF bundle. A recent study of 421 ICU patients found that the reduction of nocturnal noise levels significantly reduced delirium incidence [91], while a systematic review and meta-analysis of five studies comprising 832 ICU patients found that earplug placement at night was associated with a decreased risk for delirium [92]. Studies of sleep promotion bundle implementation have found statistically significant reductions in the incidence and duration of delirium [86, 93–95], as well as decreased duration of mechanical ventilation and LOS [94].

Melatonin

Disruptions of the circadian levels of melatonin have been identified in delirious patients, indicating the possibility that supplementation may decrease the risk of delirium [93, 96, 97]. However, while one recent study of 500 postoperative cardiac surgery patients found a reduction in delirium incidence with prophylactic melatonin [98], a meta-analysis of 4 RCTs comprising 669 elderly patients found no significant difference in delirium incidence between those who received melatonin and those who received placebo [99]. Due to this conflicting evidence, the PADIS guidelines give no recommendation regarding the use of melatonin [1]. Multiple current studies are further investigating the effects of melatonin on delirium [100–102].

Light Application Therapy

To date, three studies have investigated the use of light therapy in critically ill patients to induce normal circadian rhythm; however, none have found a significant decrease in the incidence, duration, or severity of delirium [103–105]. The PADIS guidelines [1] do not recommend the use of bright light therapy due to limited evidence of utility and potential patient aversion [103].

Challenges to Delirium Prevention

While studies of the ABCDEF bundle suggest it is safe and effective, adoption of this intervention into everyday care on a wide scale basis remains limited. A recent international survey of 1521 ICU clinicians identified multiple barriers to bundle implementation [16]. Thirty percent of those surveyed worked in settings that did not monitor for delirium, and 58% had no specific screening tool. Additionally, while most clinicians endorsed the importance of early mobility (82%), few seemed to have the necessary resources; 69% had no dedicated mobility team. Only 35% of clinicians worked on units that had open visitation policies. Just over half of the clinicians in this sample reported use of either the 2013 Clinical Practice Guidelines for the Management of Pain, Agitation, and Delirium [106] (56.2%) or the ABCDEF bundle (56.6%). Two thirds of the sample reported use of bundle components for pain (62%), sedation (65%), SAT (66%), or SBT (67%).

Facilitators of bundle implementation include the presence of a preexisting organizational and ICU-based culture of patient safety and quality improvement, interdisciplinary collaboration, the use of multiple implementation strategies and educational methods, EMR optimization for documentation and prompts, engagement of key leaders, and consideration for both individual and organizational change [107–110]. Common barriers include staff and provider knowledge deficit or unwillingness to adopt evidence-based practice, workload burden or a perceived lack of resources, excessive turnover of the project implementation team and/or ICU leadership, and the use of registry staff who may lack training or engagement [107, 109, 111]. Without adequate recognition of delirium, or the resources and policies to prevent it, delirium will continue to be a major contributor to poor ICU outcomes.

Conclusion

Pharmacological efforts to mitigate delirium have not been successful. However, interventions that aim to maintain clinical parameters within normal limits, avoid patient exposure to benzodiazepines, deep sedation, prolonged mechanical ventilation, and excessive light and noise while increasing time spent out of bed and with family has the potential to decrease the incidence of delirium. Implementation of these measures is important for all ICU patients, but especially those most at risk for delirium (i.e., older patients with dementia receiving benzodiazepines who have a high severity of illness). Utilization of the ABCDEF bundle requires interdisciplinary collaboration and adequate resources and must address key barriers (i.e., staff knowledge deficits, patient safety concerns, out-of-date practice patterns) with multifaceted educational strategies, support from key leaders, and a focus on organizational change.

References

1. Devlin JW, Skrobik Y, Gélinas C, et al. Clinical practice guidelines for the prevention and management of pain, agitation/sedation, delirium, immobility, and sleep disruption in adult patients in the ICU. Crit Care Med. 2018;46(9):e825–73. https://doi.org/10.1097/CCM.0000000000003299.
2. Zaal IJ, Devlin JW, Hazelbag M, et al. Benzodiazepine-associated delirium in critically ill adults. Intensive Care Med. 2015;41(12):2130–7. https://doi.org/10.1007/s00134-015-4063-z.
3. Kress JP, Pohlman AS, O'Connor MF, Hall JB. Daily interruption of sedative infusions in critically ill patients undergoing mechanical ventilation. N Engl J Med. 2000;342(20):1471–7. https://doi.org/10.1056/NEJM200005183422002.
4. Reade MC, Finfer S. Sedation and delirium in the intensive care unit. N Engl J Med. 2014;370(5):444–54. https://doi.org/10.1056/NEJMra1208705.
5. Girard TD, Kress JP, Fuchs BD, et al. Efficacy and safety of a paired sedation and ventilator weaning protocol for mechanically ventilated patients in intensive care (awakening and breathing controlled trial): a randomised controlled trial. Lancet (London, England). 2008;371(9607):126–34. https://doi.org/10.1016/S0140-6736(08)60105-1.
6. Shehabi Y, Bellomo R, Kadiman S, et al. Sedation intensity in the first 48 hours of mechanical ventilation and 180-day mortality. Crit Care Med. 2018;46(6):850–9. https://doi.org/10.1097/CCM.0000000000003071.
7. Van Rompaey B, Elseviers MM, Schuurmans MJ, Shortridge-Baggett LM, Truijen S, Bossaert L. Risk factors for delirium in intensive care patients: a prospective cohort study. Crit Care. 2009;13(3):R77. https://doi.org/10.1186/cc7892.
8. Girard TD, Pandharipande PP, Ely EW. Delirium in the intensive care unit. Crit Care. 2008;12(Suppl 3):S3. https://doi.org/10.1186/cc6149.
9. Inouye SK, Charpentier PA. Precipitating factors for delirium in hospitalized elderly persons. Predictive model and interrelationship with baseline vulnerability. JAMA. 1996;275(11):852–7.
10. Figueroa-Ramos MI, Arroyo-Novoa CM, Lee KA, Padilla G, Puntillo KA. Sleep and delirium in ICU patients: a review of mechanisms and manifestations. Intensive Care Med. 2009;35(5):781–95. https://doi.org/10.1007/s00134-009-1397-4.

11. Weinhouse GL, Schwab RJ, Watson PL, et al. Bench-to-bedside review: delirium in ICU patients - importance of sleep deprivation. Crit Care. 2009;13(6):234. https://doi.org/10.1186/cc8131.
12. Wilson LM. Intensive care delirium. The effect of outside deprivation in a windowless unit. Arch Intern Med. 1972;130(2):225–6.
13. van Keulen K, Knol W, Belitser SV, et al. Diabetes and glucose dysregulation and transition to delirium in ICU patients. Crit Care Med. 2018; https://doi.org/10.1097/CCM.0000000000003285.
14. Wang L-H, Xu D-J, Wei X-J, Chang H-T, Xu G-H. Electrolyte disorders and aging: risk factors for delirium in patients undergoing orthopedic surgeries. BMC Psychiatry. 2016;16(1):418. https://doi.org/10.1186/s12888-016-1130-0.
15. Ahmed S, Leurent B, Sampson EL. Risk factors for incident delirium among older people in acute hospital medical units: a systematic review and meta-analysis. Age Ageing. 2014;43(3):326–33. https://doi.org/10.1093/ageing/afu022.
16. Morandi A, Piva S, Ely EW, et al. Worldwide survey of the "assessing pain, both spontaneous awakening and breathing trials, choice of drugs, delirium monitoring/management, early exercise/mobility, and family empowerment" (ABCDEF) bundle. Crit Care Med. 2017;45(11):e1111–22. https://doi.org/10.1097/CCM.0000000000002640.
17. Neufeld KJ, Yue J, Robinson TN, Inouye SK, Needham DM. Antipsychotic medication for prevention and treatment of delirium in hospitalized adults: a systematic review and meta-analysis. J Am Geriatr Soc. 2016;64(4):705–14. https://doi.org/10.1111/jgs.14076.
18. Su X, Meng Z-T, Wu X-H, et al. Dexmedetomidine for prevention of delirium in elderly patients after non-cardiac surgery: a randomised, double-blind, placebo-controlled trial. Lancet. 2016;388(10054):1893–902. https://doi.org/10.1016/S0140-6736(16)30580-3.
19. Vallabhajosyula S, Kanmanthareddy A, Erwin PJ, Esterbrooks DJ, Morrow LE. Role of statins in delirium prevention in critical ill and cardiac surgery patients: a systematic review and meta-analysis. J Crit Care. 2017;37:189–96. https://doi.org/10.1016/J.JCRC.2016.09.025.
20. Avidan MS, Maybrier HR, Abdallah AB, et al. Intraoperative ketamine for prevention of postoperative delirium or pain after major surgery in older adults: an international, multi-centre, double-blind, randomised clinical trial. Lancet. 2017;390(10091):267–75. https://doi.org/10.1016/S0140-6736(17)31467-8.
21. van den Boogaard M, Slooter AJC, Brüggemann RJM, et al. Effect of haloperidol on survival among critically ill adults with a high risk of delirium: the REDUCE randomized clinical trial. JAMA. 2018;319(7):680–90. https://doi.org/10.1001/jama.2018.0160.
22. Marshall J, Herzig SJ, Howell MD, et al. Antipsychotic utilization in the intensive care unit and in transitions of care. J Crit Care. 2016;33:119–24. https://doi.org/10.1016/j.jcrc.2015.12.017.
23. Tomichek JE, Stollings JL, Pandharipande PP, Chandrasekhar R, Ely EW, Girard TD. Antipsychotic prescribing patterns during and after critical illness: a prospective cohort study. Crit Care. 2016;20(1):378. https://doi.org/10.1186/s13054-016-1557-1.
24. Pasin L, Landoni G, Nardelli P, et al. Dexmedetomidine reduces the risk of delirium, agitation and confusion in critically ill patients: a meta-analysis of randomized controlled trials. J Cardiothorac Vasc Anesth. 2014;28(6):1459–66. https://doi.org/10.1053/j.jvca.2014.03.010.
25. Maldonado JR, Wysong A, van der Starre PJA, Block T, Miller C, Reitz BA. Dexmedetomidine and the reduction of postoperative delirium after cardiac surgery. Psychosomatics. 2009;50(3):206–17. https://doi.org/10.1176/appi.psy.50.3.206.
26. Pandharipande PP, Pun BT, Herr DL, et al. Effect of sedation with dexmedetomidine vs lorazepam on acute brain dysfunction in mechanically ventilated patients: the MENDS randomized controlled trial. JAMA. 2007;298(22):2644–53. https://doi.org/10.1001/jama.298.22.2644.
27. Riker RR, Shehabi Y, Bokesch PM, et al. Dexmedetomidine vs midazolam for sedation of critically ill patients: a randomized trial. JAMA. 2009;301(5):489. https://doi.org/10.1001/jama.2009.56.

28. Shehabi Y, Grant P, Wolfenden H, et al. Prevalence of delirium with dexmedetomidine compared with morphine based therapy after cardiac surgery: a randomized controlled trial (DEXmedetomidine COmpared to Morphine-DEXCOM study). Anesthesiology. 2009;111(5):1075–84. https://doi.org/10.1097/ALN.0b013e3181b6a783.
29. Serafim RB, Bozza FA, Soares M, et al. Pharmacologic prevention and treatment of delirium in intensive care patients: a systematic review. J Crit Care. 2015;30(4):799–807. https://doi.org/10.1016/J.JCRC.2015.04.005.
30. Nelson S, Muzyk AJ, Bucklin MH, Brudney S, Gagliardi JP. Defining the role of dexmedetomidine in the prevention of delirium in the intensive care unit. Biomed Res Int. 2015;2015(635737):1–7. https://doi.org/10.1155/2015/635737.
31. Morandi A, Hughes CG, Thompson JL, et al. Statins and delirium during critical illness: a multicenter, prospective cohort study. Crit Care Med. 2014;42(8):1899–909. https://doi.org/10.1097/CCM.0000000000000398.
32. Vasilevskis EE, Ely EW, Speroff T, Pun BT, Boehm L, Dittus RS. Reducing iatrogenic risks: ICU-acquired delirium and weakness--crossing the quality chasm. Chest. 2010;138(5):1224–33. https://doi.org/10.1378/chest.10-0466.
33. Pandharipande P, Banerjee A, McGrane S, Ely EW. Liberation and animation for ventilated ICU patients: the ABCDE bundle for the back-end of critical care. Crit Care. 2010;14(3):157. https://doi.org/10.1186/cc8999.
34. Taito S, Yasuda H. To what extent does ABCDEF bundle improve hospital survival and reduce brain dysfunction of 1,438 patients with mechanical ventilation in seven California community hospitals? Crit Care Med. 2017;45(6):e617. https://doi.org/10.1097/CCM.0000000000002339.
35. Marra A, Ely EW, Pandharipande PP, Patel MB. The ABCDEF bundle in critical care. Crit Care Clin. 2017;33(2):225–43. https://doi.org/10.1016/j.ccc.2016.12.005.
36. Ely EW. The ABCDEF bundle: science and philosophy of how ICU liberation serves patients and families. Crit Care Med. 2017;45(2):321–30. https://doi.org/10.1097/CCM.0000000000002175.
37. Miller MA, Govindan S, Watson SR, Hyzy RC, Iwashyna TJ. ABCDE, but in that order? A cross-sectional survey of Michigan intensive care unit sedation, delirium, and early mobility practices. Ann Am Thorac Soc. 2015;12(7):1066–71. https://doi.org/10.1513/AnnalsATS.201501-066OC.
38. Balas MC, Vasilevskis EE, Burke WJ, et al. Critical care nurses' role in implementing the "ABCDE bundle" into practice. Crit Care Nurse. 2012;32(2):35–8., 40–47; quiz 48. https://doi.org/10.4037/ccn2012229.
39. Barnes-Daly MA, Phillips G, Ely EW. Improving hospital survival and reducing brain dysfunction at seven California community hospitals. Crit Care Med. 2017;45(2):171–8. https://doi.org/10.1097/CCM.0000000000002149.
40. Needham DM, Davidson J, Cohen H, et al. Improving long-term outcomes after discharge from intensive care unit: report from a stakeholders' conference. Crit Care Med. 2012;40(2):502–9. https://doi.org/10.1097/CCM.0b013e318232da75.
41. Pun BT, Balas MC, Barnes-Daly MA, et al. Caring for critically ill patients with the ABCDEF bundle: results of the ICU liberation collaborative in over 15,000 adults. Crit Care Med. 2019;47(1):3–14. https://doi.org/10.1097/CCM.0000000000003482.
42. Balas MC, Vasilevskis EE, Olsen KM, et al. Effectiveness and safety of the awakening and breathing coordination, delirium monitoring/management, and early exercise/mobility bundle. Crit Care Med. 2014;42(5):1024–36. https://doi.org/10.1097/CCM.0000000000000129.
43. Barnes-Daly MA, Pun BT, Harmon LA, et al. Improving health care for critically ill patients using an evidence-based collaborative approach to ABCDEF bundle dissemination and implementation. Worldviews Evid-Based Nurs. 2018;15(3):206–16. https://doi.org/10.1111/wvn.12290.
44. Loeser JD, Treede R-D. The Kyoto protocol of IASP basic pain terminology. Pain. 2008;137(3):473–7. https://doi.org/10.1016/j.pain.2008.04.025.

45. Chanques G, Sebbane M, Barbotte E, Viel E, Eledjam J-J, Jaber S. A prospective study of pain at rest: incidence and characteristics of an unrecognized symptom in surgical and trauma versus medical intensive care unit patients. Anesthesiology. 2007;107(5):858–60. https://doi.org/10.1097/01.anes.0000287211.98642.51.
46. Puntillo KA, Max A, Timsit J-F, et al. Determinants of procedural pain intensity in the intensive care unit. The European® study. Am J Respir Crit Care Med. 2014;189(1):39–47. https://doi.org/10.1164/rccm.201306-1174OC.
47. McCaffery M, Beebe A. Pain: clinical manual for nursing practice. UK ed. St. Louis: Mosby; 1994. https://doi.org/10.7748/ns.9.11.55.s69.
48. Payen JF, Bru O, Bosson JL, et al. Assessing pain in critically ill sedated patients by using a behavioral pain scale. Crit Care Med. 2001;29(12):2258–63.
49. Gélinas C, Fillion L, Puntillo KA, Viens C, Fortier M. Validation of the critical-care pain observation tool in adult patients. Am J Crit Care. 2006;15(4):420–7.
50. Payen J-F, Chanques G, Mantz J, et al. Current practices in sedation and analgesia for mechanically ventilated critically ill patients: a prospective multicenter patient-based study. Anesthesiology. 2007;106(4):687–95.; quiz 891–892. https://doi.org/10.1097/01.anes.0000264747.09017.da.
51. Kamdar BB, Combs MP, Colantuoni E, et al. The association of sleep quality, delirium, and sedation status with daily participation in physical therapy in the ICU. Crit Care. 2016;19(1):261. https://doi.org/10.1186/s13054-016-1433-z.
52. Kamdar BB, Needham DM, Collop NA. Sleep deprivation in critical illness: its role in physical and psychological recovery. J Intensive Care Med. 2012;27(2):97–111. https://doi.org/10.1177/0885066610394322.
53. Khan BA, Fadel WF, Tricker JL, et al. Effectiveness of implementing a wake up and breathe program on sedation and delirium in the ICU. Crit Care Med. 2014;42(12):e791–5. https://doi.org/10.1097/CCM.0000000000000660.
54. Riker RR, Picard JT, Fraser GL. Prospective evaluation of the sedation-agitation scale for adult critically ill patients. Crit Care Med. 1999;27(7):1325–9.
55. Ely EW, Truman B, Shintani A, et al. Monitoring sedation status over time in ICU patients: validity and reliability of the Richmond agitation-sedation scale (RASS). JAMA. 2003;289(22):2983. https://doi.org/10.1001/jama.289.22.2983.
56. Sessler CN, Gosnell MS, Grap MJ, et al. The Richmond agitation–sedation scale: validity and reliability in adult intensive care unit patients. Am J Respir Crit Care Med. 2002;166(10):1338–44. https://doi.org/10.1164/rccm.2107138.
57. Zaal IJ, Devlin JW, Peelen LM, Slooter AJC. A systematic review of risk factors for delirium in the ICU. Crit Care Med. 2015;43(1):40–7. https://doi.org/10.1097/CCM.0000000000000625.
58. Shehabi Y, Howe BD, Bellomo R, et al. Early sedation with dexmedetomidine in critically ill patients. N Engl J Med. 2019; https://doi.org/10.1056/NEJMoa1904710.
59. Shehabi Y, Forbes AB, Arabi Y, et al. The SPICE III study protocol and analysis plan: a randomised trial of early goal directed sedation compared with standard care in mechanically ventilated patients. Crit Care Resusc. 2017;19(4):318–26.
60. Ely EW, Margolin R, Francis J, et al. Evaluation of delirium in critically ill patients: validation of the confusion assessment method for the intensive care unit (CAM-ICU). Crit Care Med. 2001;29(7):1370–9. https://doi.org/10.1097/00003246-200107000-00012.
61. Ely EW, Inouye SK, Bernard GR, et al. Delirium in mechanically ventilated patients: validity and reliability of the confusion assessment method for the intensive care unit (CAM-ICU). JAMA. 2001;286(21):2703–10.
62. Bergeron N, Dubois MJ, Dumont M, Dial S, Skrobik Y. Intensive care delirium screening checklist: evaluation of a new screening tool. Intensive Care Med. 2001;27(5):859–64.
63. Andrews L, Silva SG, Kaplan S, Zimbro K. Delirium monitoring and patient outcomes in a general intensive care unit. Am J Crit Care. 2015;24(1):48–56. https://doi.org/10.4037/ajcc2015740.

64. Bigatello LM, Amirfarzan H, Haghighi AK, et al. Effects of routine monitoring of delirium in a surgical/trauma intensive care unit. J Trauma Acute Care Surg. 2013;74(3):876–83. https://doi.org/10.1097/TA.0b013e31827e1b69.
65. van den Boogaard M, Pickkers P, van der Hoeven H, Roodbol G, van Achterberg T, Schoonhoven L. Implementation of a delirium assessment tool in the ICU can influence haloperidol use. Crit Care. 2009;13(4):R131. https://doi.org/10.1186/cc7991.
66. Reade MC, Eastwood GM, Peck L, Bellomo R, Baldwin I. Routine use of the confusion assessment method for the intensive care unit (CAM-ICU) by bedside nurses may underdiagnose delirium. Crit Care Resusc. 2011;13(4):217–24.
67. Devlin JW, Fong JJ, Schumaker G, O'Connor H, Ruthazer R, Garpestad E. Use of a validated delirium assessment tool improves the ability of physicians to identify delirium in medical intensive care unit patients. Crit Care Med. 2007;35(12):2721–4.. quiz 2725
68. van Eijk MMJ, van Marum RJ, Klijn IAM, de Wit N, Kesecioglu J, Slooter AJC. Comparison of delirium assessment tools in a mixed intensive care unit. Crit Care Med. 2009;37(6):1881–5. https://doi.org/10.1097/CCM.0b013e3181a00118.
69. Spronk PE, Riekerk B, Hofhuis J, Rommes JH. Occurrence of delirium is severely underestimated in the ICU during daily care. Intensive Care Med. 2009;35(7):1276–80. https://doi.org/10.1007/s00134-009-1466-8.
70. Inouye SK, Foreman MD, Mion LC, Katz KH, Cooney LM. Nurses' recognition of delirium and its symptoms: comparison of nurse and researcher ratings. Arch Intern Med. 2001;161(20):2467–73.
71. Engel HJ, Needham DM, Morris PE, Gropper MA. ICU early mobilization. Crit Care Med. 2013;41:S69–80. https://doi.org/10.1097/CCM.0b013e3182a240d5.
72. Needham DM, Korupolu R, Zanni JM, et al. Early physical medicine and rehabilitation for patients with acute respiratory failure: a quality improvement project. Arch Phys Med Rehabil. 2010;91(4):536–42. https://doi.org/10.1016/j.apmr.2010.01.002.
73. Schweickert WD, Pohlman MC, Pohlman AS, et al. Early physical and occupational therapy in mechanically ventilated, critically ill patients: a randomised controlled trial. Lancet. 2009;373(9678):1874–82. https://doi.org/10.1016/S0140-6736(09)60658-9.
74. Brummel NE, Jackson JC, Girard TD, et al. A combined early cognitive and physical rehabilitation program for people who are critically ill: the activity and cognitive therapy in the intensive care unit (ACT-ICU) trial. Phys Ther. 2012;92(12):1580–92. https://doi.org/10.2522/ptj.20110414.
75. Nickels MR, Aitken LM, Walsham J, Barnett AG, McPhail SM. Critical care cycling study (CYCLIST) trial protocol: a randomised controlled trial of usual care plus additional in-bed cycling sessions versus usual care in the critically ill. BMJ Open. 2017;7(10):e017393. https://doi.org/10.1136/bmjopen-2017-017393.
76. Parry SM, Berney S, Warrillow S, et al. Functional electrical stimulation with cycling in the critically ill: a pilot case-matched control study. J Crit Care. 2014;29(4):695.e1–7. https://doi.org/10.1016/j.jcrc.2014.03.017.
77. Fumagalli S, Boncinelli L, Lo Nostro A, et al. Reduced cardiocirculatory complications with unrestrictive visiting policy in an intensive care unit: results from a pilot, randomized trial. Circulation. 2006;113(7):946–52. https://doi.org/10.1161/CIRCULATIONAHA.105.572537.
78. Rosa RG, Tonietto TF, da Silva DB, et al. Effectiveness and safety of an extended ICU visitation model for delirium prevention. Crit Care Med. 2017;45(10):1660–7. https://doi.org/10.1097/CCM.0000000000002588.
79. Munro CL, Cairns P, Ji M, Calero K, Anderson WM, Liang Z. Delirium prevention in critically ill adults through an automated reorientation intervention – a pilot randomized controlled trial. Hear Lung J Acute Crit Care. 2017;46(4):234–8. https://doi.org/10.1016/j.hrtlng.2017.05.002.
80. Partridge JS, Martin FC, Harari D, Dhesi JK. The delirium experience: what is the effect on patients, relatives and staff and what can be done to modify this? Int J Geriatr Psychiatry. 2013;28(8):804–12. https://doi.org/10.1002/gps.3900.

81. Smithburger PL, Korenoski AS, Kane-Gill SL, Alexander SA. Perceptions of family members, nurses, and physicians on involving patients' families in delirium prevention. Crit Care Nurse. 2017;37(6):48–57. https://doi.org/10.4037/ccn2017901.
82. Smithburger PL, Korenoski AS, Alexander SA, Kane-Gill SL. Perceptions of families of intensive care unit patients regarding involvement in delirium-prevention activities: a qualitative study. Crit Care Nurse. 2017;37(6):e1–9. https://doi.org/10.4037/ccn2017485.
83. Rotondi AJ, Chelluri L, Sirio C, et al. Patients' recollections of stressful experiences while receiving prolonged mechanical ventilation in an intensive care unit. Crit Care Med. 2002;30(4):746–52.
84. Freedman NS, Gazendam J, Levan L, Pack AI, Schwab RJ. Abnormal sleep/wake cycles and the effect of environmental noise on sleep disruption in the intensive care unit. Am J Respir Crit Care Med. 2001;163(2):451–7. https://doi.org/10.1164/ajrccm.163.2.9912128.
85. Cooper AB, Thornley KS, Young GB, Slutsky AS, Stewart TE, Hanly PJ. Sleep in critically ill patients requiring mechanical ventilation. Chest. 2000;117(3):809–18.
86. Patel J, Baldwin J, Bunting P, Laha S. The effect of a multicomponent multidisciplinary bundle of interventions on sleep and delirium in medical and surgical intensive care patients. Anaesthesia. 2014;69(6):540–9. https://doi.org/10.1111/anae.12638.
87. Bourne RS, Minelli C, Mills GH, Kandler R. Clinical review: sleep measurement in critical care patients: research and clinical implications. Crit Care. 2007;11(4):226. https://doi.org/10.1186/cc5966.
88. Trompeo AC, Vidi Y, Locane MD, et al. Sleep disturbances in the critically ill patients: role of delirium and sedative agents. Minerva Anestesiol. 2011;77(6):604–12.
89. Van Rompaey B, Elseviers MM, Van Drom W, Fromont V, Jorens PG. The effect of earplugs during the night on the onset of delirium and sleep perception: a randomized controlled trial in intensive care patients. Crit Care. 2012;16(3):R73. https://doi.org/10.1186/cc11330.
90. Maldonado JR. Delirium pathophysiology: an updated hypothesis of the etiology of acute brain failure. Int J Geriatr Psychiatry. 2017:1–30. https://doi.org/10.1002/gps.4823.
91. van de Pol I, van Iterson M, Maaskant J. Effect of nocturnal sound reduction on the incidence of delirium in intensive care unit patients: an interrupted time series analysis. Intensive Crit Care Nurs. 2017;41:18–25. https://doi.org/10.1016/j.iccn.2017.01.008.
92. Litton E, Carnegie V, Elliott R, Webb SAR. The efficacy of earplugs as a sleep hygiene strategy for reducing delirium in the ICU: a systematic review and meta-analysis. Crit Care Med. 2016;44(5):992–9. https://doi.org/10.1097/CCM.0000000000001557.
93. Guo Y, Sun L, Li L, et al. Impact of multicomponent, nonpharmacologic interventions on perioperative cortisol and melatonin levels and postoperative delirium in elderly oral cancer patients. Arch Gerontol Geriatr. 2016;62:112–7. https://doi.org/10.1016/j.archger.2015.10.009.
94. Bryczkowski SB, Lopreiato MC, Yonclas PP, Sacca JJ, Mosenthal AC. Delirium prevention program in the surgical intensive care unit improved the outcomes of older adults. J Surg Res. 2014;190(1):280–8. https://doi.org/10.1016/j.jss.2014.02.044.
95. Kamdar BB, King LM, Collop NA, et al. The effect of a quality improvement intervention on perceived sleep quality and cognition in a medical ICU. Crit Care Med. 2013;41(3):800–9. https://doi.org/10.1097/CCM.0b013e3182746442.
96. Ángeles-Castellanos M, Ramírez-Gonzalez F, Ubaldo-Reyes L, Rodriguez-Mayoral O, Escobar C. Loss of melatonin daily rhythmicity is asociated with delirium development in hospitalized older adults. Sleep Sci. 2016;9(4):285–8. https://doi.org/10.1016/j.slsci.2016.08.001.
97. Dessap AM, Roche-Campo F, Launay J-M, et al. Delirium and circadian rhythm of melatonin during weaning from mechanical ventilation. Chest. 2015;148(5):1231–41. https://doi.org/10.1378/chest.15-0525.
98. Artemiou P, Bily B, Bilecova-Rabajdova M, et al. Melatonin treatment in the prevention of postoperative delirium in cardiac surgery patients. Pol J Cardio-Thorac Surg. 2015;2(2):126–33. https://doi.org/10.5114/kitp.2015.52853.

99. Chen S, Shi L, Liang F, et al. Exogenous melatonin for delirium prevention: a meta-analysis of randomized controlled trials. Mol Neurobiol. 2016;53(6):4046–53. https://doi.org/10.1007/s12035-015-9350-8.
100. Burry L, Scales D, Williamson D, et al. Feasibility of melatonin for prevention of delirium in critically ill patients: a protocol for a multicentre, randomised, placebo-controlled study. BMJ Open. 2017;7(3):e015420. https://doi.org/10.1136/bmjopen-2016-015420.
101. Huang H, Jiang L, Shen L, et al. Impact of oral melatonin on critically ill adult patients with ICU sleep deprivation: study protocol for a randomized controlled trial. Trials. 2014;15(1):327. https://doi.org/10.1186/1745-6215-15-327.
102. Martinez FE, Anstey M, Ford A, et al. Prophylactic melatonin for delirium in intensive care (Pro-MEDIC): study protocol for a randomised controlled trial. Trials. 2017;18(1):4. https://doi.org/10.1186/s13063-016-1751-0.
103. Ono H, Taguchi T, Kido Y, Fujino Y, Doki Y. The usefulness of bright light therapy for patients after oesophagectomy. Intensive Crit Care Nurs. 2011;27(3):158–66. https://doi.org/10.1016/j.iccn.2011.03.003.
104. Simons KS, Laheij RJF, van den Boogaard M, et al. Dynamic light application therapy to reduce the incidence and duration of delirium in intensive-care patients: a randomised controlled trial. Lancet Respir Med. 2016;4(3):194–202. https://doi.org/10.1016/S2213-2600(16)00025-4.
105. Taguchi T, Yano M, Kido Y. Influence of bright light therapy on postoperative patients: a pilot study. Intensive Crit Care Nurs. 2007;23(5):289–97. https://doi.org/10.1016/j.iccn.2007.04.004.
106. Barr J, Fraser GL, Puntillo K, et al. Clinical practice guidelines for the management of pain, agitation, and delirium in adult patients in the intensive care unit: executive summary. Am J Heal Pharm. 2013;70(1):53–8. https://doi.org/10.1097/CCM.0b013e3182783b72.
107. Balas MC, Burke WJ, Gannon D, et al. Implementing the awakening and breathing coordination, delirium monitoring/management, and early exercise/mobility bundle into everyday care: opportunities, challenges, and lessons learned for implementing the ICU pain, agitation, and delirium guidelines. Crit Care Med. 2013;41(9 Suppl 1):S116–27. https://doi.org/10.1097/CCM.0b013e3182a17064.
108. Trogrlić Z, van der Jagt M, Bakker J, et al. A systematic review of implementation strategies for assessment, prevention, and management of ICU delirium and their effect on clinical outcomes. Crit Care. 2015;19(1):157. https://doi.org/10.1186/s13054-015-0886-9.
109. Carrothers KM, Barr J, Spurlock B, Ridgely MS, Damberg CL, Ely EW. Contextual issues influencing implementation and outcomes associated with an integrated approach to managing pain, agitation, and delirium in adult ICUs. Crit Care Med. 2013;41(9 Suppl 1):S128–35. https://doi.org/10.1097/CCM.0b013e3182a2c2b1.
110. Costa DK, Valley TS, Miller MA, et al. ICU team composition and its association with ABCDE implementation in a quality collaborative. J Crit Care. 2018;44:1–6. https://doi.org/10.1016/j.jcrc.2017.09.180.
111. Boehm LM, Dietrich MS, Vasilevskis EE, et al. Perceptions of workload burden and adherence to ABCDE bundle among intensive care providers. Am J Crit Care. 2017;26(4):e38–47. https://doi.org/10.4037/ajcc2017544.

Chapter 14
Treatment Strategies for Delirium

Noll L. Campbell and Babar A. Khan

Key Concepts

1. The lack of evidence for treatment of delirium, outside of critically ill populations, limits the ability to make recommendations in other populations or care environments.
2. Non-pharmacologic approaches are the only universally recommended treatment for delirium.
3. Pharmacologic treatment options have not yet provided sufficient evidence to be recommended in any population or care environment.
4. Reducing potential harm through deprescribing or medication-sparing principles is reasonable.

N. L. Campbell (✉)
Department of Pharmacy Practice, Purdue University College of Pharmacy, West Lafayette, IN, USA

Center for Health Innovation and Implementation Science, Regenstrief Institute, Indianapolis, IN, USA

Indiana University Center for Aging Research, Regenstrief Institute, Indianapolis, IN, USA
e-mail: campbenl@iupui.edu

B. A. Khan
Center for Health Innovation and Implementation Science, Regenstrief Institute, Indianapolis, IN, USA

Indiana University Center for Aging Research, Regenstrief Institute, Indianapolis, IN, USA

Department of Medicine, Indiana University School of Medicine, Indianapolis, IN, USA

C. G. Hughes et al. (eds.), *Delirium*, https://doi.org/10.1007/978-3-030-25751-4_14

Introduction

The last 30 years of delirium research has informed many aspects of delirium treatment; nevertheless this field is currently described more by the gaps in knowledge than by the evidence supporting current recommendations. Most of the literature describing delirium treatment has been derived from heterogeneous populations of critically ill adults, with little or no high-quality research to make recommendations on potential treatments in disparate populations. While the critically ill population represents the majority of participants included in delirium treatment trials, other populations at high risk of delirium such as older adults with and without dementia, those in post-acute care facilities, children, and populations at the end of life have been poorly studied and as such have little or no evidence for which to make clinical recommendations. Similarly, current literature fails to evaluate a diverse battery of treatment approaches (non-pharmacologic and pharmacologic) and clinically relevant delirium-associated outcomes.

The underlying heterogeneity in the etio-pathology of delirium creates a challenge to develop uniform therapeutic interventions efficacious for diverse patient populations. Additionally, the very same heterogeneity afforded by the myriad of etiologies and clinical phenotypes may lead to differential delirium duration and severity, relationship with mortality, and long-term cognitive and psychological sequelae. As such, the heterogeneity of delirium pathology may require a similar degree of heterogeneity in treatment approaches. Taking into consideration the advancements in understanding delirium pathophysiology and focusing on desirable treatment outcomes of delirium duration, severity, downstream mortality, and delirium-associated cognitive impairment, therapeutic interventions are likely to require personalization in both their design and delivery.

In this chapter, we will discuss the current pharmacologic and non-pharmacologic treatment strategies for delirium management focusing on patient populations and treatment approaches that have been studied to date. Because much of the evidence published to date reflects trials conducted in critically ill or surgical populations, recommendations cited herein should be applied only to those populations in which trials were conducted. While in this chapter we review the current literature and where it applies, we also note that the absence of particular treatment approaches reflects the absence of investigation as delirium treatments. For example, melatonin and ketamine have been studied in the prevention of delirium, but there is no study evaluating the treatment of delirium, and as such are not discussed in this chapter. Therefore, recommendations made in this chapter intend to highlight available research with applications for clinical practice and appreciate the existing gaps in delirium treatment.

Non-pharmacologic Approaches to Delirium Treatment

Non-pharmacologic approaches to delirium treatment borrow from delirium prevention literature in both hospitalized and critical care populations and address risk factors for delirium common across different patient populations. The approaches include orientation strategies, supporting and normalizing sleep/wake cycles, and mobility and sensory (visual and auditory) support [1–6]. Studies utilizing non-pharmacologic strategies for delirium prevention have identified variable results, with some showing as much as a 50% reduction in delirium incidence [1, 4–6], while others show no difference [2, 3]. In a study by Inouye and colleagues, although the severity and recurrence rates of delirium were not different between intervention and usual care, there was a significant reduction in the total number of hospital days with delirium (105 vs. 161 days, $p = 0.02$). Among critically ill subjects, a combination of aggressive early physical and occupational therapy provided to patients receiving daily awakening protocols with reduced sedation exposure resulted in a 50% decrease in delirium duration (2 days versus 4 days, $p = 0.03$) [7].

Recently, attention has been focused on the ABCDE bundle (awakening and breathing coordination, delirium monitoring/management, and early exercise and mobility) among critically ill patients. The ABCDE bundle is a promising non-pharmacologic approach to decrease delirium burden in the ICU setting pulling together components that make intuitive sense to reduce delirium burden [8–11]. Implementation of the bundle in the ICU was found to be significantly associated with a lower incidence of delirium (49% vs. 62%, OR 0.55; 95% CI 0.33–0.93) in a before-after study [12]. A newer expanded version of the bundle, the ABCDEF bundle (with "A" modified to assess and manage pain and "F" for family engagement), was evaluated in a larger, multicenter, before-after, cohort study. Improvements in bundle compliance were significantly associated with reduced mortality and more ICU days without coma or delirium [13]. A recent pre-/post-implementation project showed that complete ABCDEF bundle implementation could decrease odds of delirium the next day (AOR 0.60, 95% CI 0.49–0.72). However, complete bundle performance was limited; only 8% of all ICU days reached full adherence, reflecting the challenges of multicomponent interventions in the ICU [14].

Based on the current literature on non-pharmacological treatment of delirium in the ICU setting, the Society of Critical Care Medicine (SCCM) and 2018 Clinical Practice Guidelines for the Prevention and Management of Pain, Agitation/Sedation, Delirium, Immobility, and Sleep Disruption (PADIS) guidelines suggest use of multicomponent non-pharmacologic interventions such as the ABCDEF bundle for delirium management although acknowledging the low quality of evidence [15]. Similarly, the American Geriatrics Society's Clinical Practice Guideline for Postoperative Delirium in Older Adults (published in 2015) recommends that healthcare professionals "consider" multicomponent interventions in older adults diagnosed with postoperative delirium (based on a weak level of evidence available at the time) [16].

Value of Future Research: Non-pharmacologic Approaches

While non-pharmacologic interventions for delirium treatment are suggested, key elements of multicomponent interventions are still needed from rigorous clinical trials to improve application and implementation of such interventions. First, developing consistent definitions and protocols for each element of multicomponent intervention would improve rigor in both comparing results of clinical trials and implementing in clinical practice. Second, understanding which element(s) of multicomponent interventions contribute to the improvements in clinical outcomes could improve efficiency of work force efforts and perhaps improve understanding of mechanisms of disease. Lastly, understanding if and how families can support non-pharmacologic strategies during episodes of delirium would also improve adherence to delirium prevention and treatment strategies.

Pharmacologic Approaches to Delirium Treatment

Although a number of theories exist that explain potential etiologies of delirium [17, 18], the neurotransmitter imbalance hypothesis serves as the primary justification for pharmacologic treatments evaluated to date. Neurotransmitter imbalances may be derived from a number of sources, including hypoxemia, inflammation, endocrine disturbances, and concomitant medications. The neurotransmitter hypothesis initially developed as an explanation for presumed cholinergic deficiency states [19–23] and subsequently expanded to include a state of heightened dopaminergic transmission [24, 25]. In addition to acetylcholine deficiency and dopaminergic excess, the most commonly described neurotransmitter imbalances associated with delirium include norepinephrine and glutamate pathways. Additionally, decreases or increases in serotonin, histamine, and gamma-aminobutyric acid (GABA) may also contribute to neurotransmitter imbalances depending on the population and comorbid medical factors.

In some cases, neurotransmitter imbalances can be aligned with symptom presentations, with cholinergic deficiency explaining symptoms of inattention and dopaminergic imbalance explaining hyperactive states and hallucinations. Dopaminergic effects may be a result of direct dopaminergic activity or by potentiating excitotoxic effects of glutamate [24, 26]. While these theories provide a framework through which to justify treatments, clinical trials have failed to provide a valid treatment effect to date. Potential explanations for treatment failures must include flawed hypotheses; however it is important to note again that the available evidence is drawn from critically ill populations, with heterogeneity in cause of illness and pathophysiologic disease processes. Therefore, recommendations for or against treatment must be made based on results of existing clinical trials and the populations in which they were conducted. Whether unique populations within those trials could benefit from a treatment, or different treatment approaches result in benefit in future trials, remains to be determined. As such, recommendations made by available clinical guidelines [16, 27] state clearly the intent to apply the guidelines only to those patients for which data are included (i.e., guidelines for delirium treatment in *all* critically ill patients published by the Society of Critical Care Medicine).

Failed Pharmacologic Approaches to Delirium Treatment

Antipsychotics

As antagonists at dopaminergic receptors, both typical and atypical antipsychotics have been evaluated as treatments of delirium in critically ill, surgical, and palliative populations [28–33]. While typical (first-generation) antipsychotics are primarily used to reduce hyperactive neurotransmission at dopaminergic receptors (though have lesser affinity for other receptors at higher doses), atypical (second-generation) antipsychotics have a more diverse profile of activity that includes dopaminergic receptors as well as serotonin, histamine, and muscarinic receptors.

Despite evidence from delirium prevention trials suggesting that atypical antipsychotics may prevent delirium in surgical populations, neither typical nor atypical antipsychotics have consistently improved delirium or other clinical outcomes as a treatment approach in critically ill or palliative populations. Five randomized controlled trials have compared either typical or atypical antipsychotics to placebo, and one randomized trial compared a typical antipsychotic as part of a multicomponent pharmacologic intervention with usual care (see Table 14.1). One trial comparing haloperidol to placebo did not show any reduction in the duration of delirium, duration of mechanical ventilation, length of stay in the ICU, or mortality [31]. While one small pilot study comparing quetiapine to placebo did reduce duration of delirium [34], findings from the analysis have been debated [35], and a second pilot trial of quetiapine failed to show differences in delirium severity compared with placebo in hospitalized older adults [36]. Additionally, two larger trials comparing the atypical antipsychotic ziprasidone with haloperidol and placebo also failed to show a difference in the duration of delirium and other important outcomes [28, 29].

Addressing the multicomponent neurotransmitter abnormalities hypothesized to contribute to delirium, Khan and colleagues attempted a multicomponent pharmacological intervention including low-dose haloperidol, along with deprescribing interventions for benzodiazepines and anticholinergic medications in critically ill adults admitted to a mixed medical and surgical ICU. While this trial again found no differences in duration of delirium, it was unique in its assessment of delirium severity and found a small but statistically significant improvement in the intervention group. The impact of this finding on delirium severity and reproducibility from other trials is not yet known. As such, guidelines from both the Society for Critical Care Medicine [27] and the American Geriatrics Society [16] *recommend against the routine use of antipsychotics in the treatment of delirium in all critically ill adults and postoperative older adults.*

Although the randomized trials evaluating antipsychotics in the treatment of delirium were conducted in both medical and surgical patients who were critically ill, each used open-label antipsychotic rescue medication for agitation or hallucinations. Administration of open-label medication particularly in the placebo group may bias the results toward the null hypothesis. Fortunately, and as a result of generally lower doses and short duration of use, tolerability assessments from delirium

Table 14.1 RCTs comparing antipsychotics with placebo or usual care in the treatment of delirium

Author/title	Population	Intervention	Delirium outcome	Secondary outcomes
Girard et al. MIND [28]	Mixed medical and surgical ICU, $n = 102$	Adjusted-dose haloperidol vs. ziprasidone vs. placebo up to 14 days	No difference in delirium duration	No difference in ventilator-free days, LOS, or mortality
Page et al. HOPE-ICU [31]	Mechanically ventilated ICU, n-141	Fixed-dose haloperidol vs. placebo up to 14 days	No difference in delirium duration	No difference in ventilator-free days, LOS, or mortality
Devlin et al. [34]	Mixed medical and surgical ICU, $n = 36$	Adjusted-dose quetiapine vs. placebo up to 10 days	Shorter duration of delirium in quetiapine group (36 h vs. 120 h; $p = 0.006$)	Shorter time to delirium resolution, less agitation. No difference in ICU LOS or mortality
Girard et al. MIND-USA [29]	Mixed medical and surgical ICU, $N = 566$	Adjusted-dose haloperidol vs. ziprasidone vs. placebo up to 14 days	No difference in coma-free days alive without delirium	No differences in duration of mechanical ventilation, length of stay, or mortality
Khan et al. PMD [32]	Mixed medical and surgical ICU, $N = 350$	Fixed-dose haloperidol, deprescribing of benzodiazepines and anticholinergics	No difference in coma-free days alive without delirium	Intervention group had a small but statistically significant reduction in delirium severity; no differences in LOS or mortality
Agar et al. [30]	Inpatient hospice or palliative care $N = 247$	Adjusted-dose risperidone vs. haloperidol vs. placebo	Higher delirium symptoms in treatment arms	More extrapyramidal symptoms and higher rate of mortality in both active treatment groups

treatment trials have not found significant increases in adverse effects, namely, movement-related disorders such as extrapyramidal symptoms and cardiac arrhythmias including QTc prolongation. However, given a lack of benefits in delirium or other clinical outcomes, recommendations to avoid use of antipsychotics in the treatment of delirium are intended to prevent potential adverse events including risk of prolonged use after discharge from the ICU or hospital.

Antipsychotics in the Management of Agitation (Symptoms of Hyperactive Delirium)

While current guidelines recommend against routine use of antipsychotics in the treatment of delirium, some patients experience distressing thoughts, symptoms, or behaviors as a result of delirium. These may include anxiety, hallucinations, delusions, and agitation. As a result, delirious patients may become physically harmful to themselves or others. Such patients may benefit from short-term use of haloperidol or an atypical antipsychotic until these distressing symptoms resolve. When using pharmacologic agents to manage behaviors, the following strategies are recommended based on expert opinion:

1. Initiate at lowest dose possible and titrate as needed.
2. Evaluate efficacy and tolerability continuously, allowing appropriate time for clinical effect based on pharmacokinetic principles and onset of effect.
3. Avoid unnecessary continuation by setting stop date parameters (48-h symptom-free, discharge from acute care, discharge from hospital) to avoid inappropriate continuation.

As many as 30% of patients in whom an antipsychotic for delirium is initiated in the ICU are at risk of continuing these medications unnecessarily after discharge [37–40]. Continued exposure to antipsychotic medications after discharge from the ICU or hospital can result in significant morbidity and financial cost. Additionally, recommendations from the American Geriatrics Society regarding the management of agitation in postoperative older adults include the avoidance of benzodiazepines [16]. The AGS guideline states practitioners may use antipsychotics at the lowest effective dose for the shortest possible duration to treat patients who are severely agitated or distressed and are threatening substantial harm to themselves and/or others. In all cases, treatment with antipsychotics should be employed only if behavioral interventions have failed or are not possible, and ongoing use should be evaluated daily with in-person examination of patients.

Acetylcholinesterase Inhibitors

Responding to the well-recognized cholinergic deficiency theory, cholinesterase inhibitors have been tested in the treatment of delirium in both ICU and hospitalized older adult populations. While two pilot trials identified no differences in the severity or duration of delirium (total sample size of both pilots was 31 participants) [41, 42], two larger randomized, placebo-controlled trials of acetylcholinesterase inhibitors failed to show improvements in delirium outcomes [43, 44]. In fact, one study of adults admitted to the ICU was stopped after only 35% of the planned population was recruited due to longer duration of delirium and higher mortality rates in those randomized to the intervention group [44]. As a result, the American Geriatrics Society [16] recommends against using acetylcholinesterase inhibitors in the treatment of delirium in postoperative older adults, and this recommendation is generally accepted among other populations as well.

Statins

Statins, in addition to decreasing cholesterol synthesis, have complex pleiotropic effects [9]. These pleiotropic effects might prevent or attenuate delirium in critical illness by acting on causative mechanisms including neuroinflammation, blood-brain barrier injury, neuronal apoptosis, ischemia, hemorrhage, and microglia activation [45–47]. Despite evidence from two observational studies suggesting statin users were less likely to experience delirium in the ICU [48, 49], two randomized trials of critically ill adults failed to show improvements in delirium outcomes including incidence and duration of delirium [50, 51]. As such, the SCCM guidelines [27] *recommend against* the routine use of statins as a treatment of delirium, though note that the quality of evidence supporting this recommendation was low.

Unclear Role of Pharmacologic Approaches in Delirium Treatment

Dexmedetomidine

Dexmedetomidine is an alpha-2 receptor agonist with sedative and analgesic properties used as an adjuvant for general surgery and as a sedative in mechanically ventilated populations. Only one randomized trial has evaluated dexmedetomidine as a treatment for delirium particularly in mechanically ventilated adults in whom agitation precludes extubation. This study fell short of its planned sample size due to financial limitations despite screening over 21,000 intubated patients from 15 ICUs [52]. Compared with placebo, the dexmedetomidine group experienced a small but statistically significant increase in ventilator-free hours in the first 7 days after study randomization (17.3 h.; 95% CI, 4.0–33.2) and reduction in delirium duration (24 h; 95% CI 6–41 h); however dexmedetomidine did not influence ICU or hospital LOS, or disposition location at hospital discharge [52]. As with studies of other pharmacologic interventions, patients were allowed to receive open-label dexmedetomidine 48 h after randomization and were also allowed to receive antipsychotics to manage agitation, which may have contaminated the comparator groups, biasing results toward the null hypothesis. Given this single study, the SCCM guideline [27] recommends (based on a low quality of overall evidence) the use of dexmedetomidine in the specific population of mechanically ventilated adults where agitation is precluding weaning/extubation. Whether dexmedetomidine can be used to reduce delirium and other clinically relevant outcomes in patients with delirium but not agitation or in those with delirium and agitation who are not mechanically ventilated has yet to be determined.

Table 14.2 summarizes the applicable guidelines in the acute care of patients at risk of or with delirium. These guidelines represent recommendations generated from expert consensus panels that take into account the quality of evidence as well as the application to routine use of pharmacologic options in all patients. As noted elsewhere in this chapter, these recommendations cite a low quality of evidence, largely driven by the heterogeneity of populations included in clinical trials and delivery of various pharmacologic interventions and protocols.

Table 14.2 Summary of guideline recommendations regarding pharmacologic treatment of delirium in ICU or postoperative populations

	SCCM (2013, 2018) critically ill adults [15, 27]	AGS (2015) postoperative older adults [16]
Antipsychotics First- or second-generation	Recommended against use	Recommended against use
HMG-CoA reductase inhibitors Statins	Recommended against use	Not evaluated
Acetylcholinesterase inhibitors	Not evaluated	Recommend against use
Dexmedetomidine	Unable to make recommendation	Not evaluated

AGS American Geriatrics Society, *SCCM* Society of Critical Care Medicine

Pharmacologic Risk Factor Reduction in Delirium Prevention and Treatment

Medications including benzodiazepines and anticholinergics may be risk factors for delirium and should be discontinued or used sparingly in those with or at risk of delirium. Benzodiazepines are well-recognized to increase the risk of delirium [53–55], while anticholinergics have been associated with cholinergic deficiency delirium in several studies [20]. Deprescribing strategies in those at risk of delirium have not been well developed or studied in ICU populations; available literature includes two studies unable to significantly reduce exposure to benzodiazepines and anticholinergics compared to usual care [32, 33]. Recommendations against the new use of benzodiazepines and anticholinergics in those with delirium are included in both SCCM and AGS guidelines; however no evidence is available to weigh the risks and benefits of deprescribing benzodiazepines or anticholinergics among prevalent users with delirium in any care environment [16, 27].

Despite rigorous evidence that deprescribing classes of medications with adverse cognitive effects improves outcomes in those with delirium, collaboration with transdisciplinary practitioners in the execution of risk factor reduction can improve efficiency of such interventions; however the optimal approach has not been evaluated with rigorous scientific or implementation approaches.

Value in Future Research: Pharmacologic Approaches

Despite failures of current delirium treatment approaches to improve clinical outcomes, many valuable lessons have been learned that will guide next steps toward treatment of delirium. Guidelines qualify current recommendations largely with low or low-to-moderate quality of evidence given the heterogeneity in delirium etiology and monotherapy approaches attempted. The next phase of research in delirium treatments is challenged with both reducing the heterogeneity in trial participants and diversifying approaches tested with a personalized treatment regimen. Further work with promising agents including melatonin, ketamine, valproic acid, and dexmedetomidine is also warranted. Of particular importance to any pharmacologic intervention found effective (and safe) in delirium treatment trials are appropriate system approaches to prevent harm from such treatments, which include study into the appropriate duration and cessation of treatment to prevent unnecessary and prolonged exposure.

Additional considerations to optimally defining and measuring the outcomes important in guiding research and clinical practice in the treatment of delirium are important in order to reduce variability across settings and populations. Currently, there is no systematic approach to the selection and reporting of outcomes and their measures in these studies resulting in reporting of numerous and varied study outcomes and measures. Rigorous consensus processes involving key stakeholders including patients and caregivers are ongoing and will develop standardized definitions of core outcome sets to be used in multiple populations and care settings. Lastly, evaluation of a key outcome of extreme importance among those experiencing delirium, long-term functional and cognitive impairment, has been grossly absent from delirium treatment trials. Whether delirium treatment may impact short-term outcomes may be equally as important as their influence on long-term outcomes among delirium survivors.

Summary

It is important to emphasize, again, that gaps in existing knowledge of delirium treatment are prevalent and compromise the ability to make recommendations for or against delirium treatments in many care environments. As such, most recommendations in available guidelines are made with low quality of evidence and may change as rigorous research becomes available. In critically ill and surgical populations, where delirium is perhaps most prevalent, existing evidence does not support the use of pharmacologic approaches to manage delirium. As noted in other chapters of this text, the final common pathway of delirium pathogenesis, if one exists, is currently unclear and is possibly unique to a population or specific etiology. As such, it is unlikely that a one-size-fits-all treatment approach will be effective. The most important actions that clinicians must employ when treating delirium are the identification and correction of underlying causes, along with supportive non-pharmacologic care and management of emergent behaviors as needed. Future research will undoubtedly provide confirmatory evidence to current recommendations or improve clarity into which populations may receive short-term (acute delirium outcomes) or delayed (reduced risk of chronic cognitive impairment or mortality) benefit from pharmacologic or non-pharmacologic treatments of delirium.

References

1. Colombo R, Corona A, Praga F, et al. A reorientation strategy for reducing delirium in the critically ill. Results of an interventional study. Minerva Anestesiol. 2012;78:1026–33.
2. Foster J, Kelly M. A pilot study to test the feasibility of a nonpharmacologic intervention for the prevention of delirium in the medical intensive care unit. Clin Nurse Spec. 2013;27:231–8.
3. Moon KJ, Lee SM. The effects of a tailored intensive care unit delirium prevention protocol: a randomized controlled trial. Int J Nurs Stud. 2015;52:1423.
4. Hanison J, Conway D. A multifaceted approach to prevention of delirium on intensive care. BMJ Qual Improv Rep 2015;(1)4. https://doi.org/10.1136/bmjquality.u209656.w4000.
5. Rivosecchi RM, Kane-Gill SL, Svec S, Campbell S, Smithburger PL. The implementation of a nonpharmacologic protocol to prevent intensive care delirium. J Crit Care. 2016;31:206–11.
6. Inouye SK, Bogardus STJ, Charpentier PA, et al. A multicomponent intervention to prevent delirium in hospitalized older patients. N Engl J Med. 1999;340:669–76.
7. Schweickert WD, Pohlman MC, Pohlman AS, et al. Early physical and occupational therapy in mechanically ventilated, critically ill patients: a randomised controlled trial. Lancet (London, England). 2009;373:1874–82.
8. Girard TD, Kress JP, Fuchs BD, et al. Efficacy and safety of a paired sedation and ventilator weaning protocol for mechanically ventilated patients in intensive care (awakening and breathing controlled trial): a randomised controlled trial. Lancet. 2008;371:126–34.
9. Kress JP, Pohlman AS, O'Connor M, Hall JB. Daily interruption of sedative infusions in critically ill patients undergoing mechanical ventilation. N Engl J Med. 2000;342:1471–7.
10. Schweickert WD, Pohlman MC, Pohlman AS, et al. Early physical and occupational therapy in mechanically ventilated, critically ill patients: a randomised controlled trial. Lancet. 2009;373:1874–82.
11. Ely EW, Baker AM, Dunagan DP, et al. Effect on the duration of mechanical ventilation of identifying patients capable of breathing spontaneously. N Engl J Med. 1996;335:1864–9.
12. Balas MC, Vasilevskis EE, Olsen KM, et al. Effectiveness and safety of the awakening and breathing coordination, delirium monitoring/management, and early exercise/mobility bundle. Crit Care Med. 2014;42:1024–36.
13. Barnes-Daly MA, Phillips G, Ely EW. Improving hospital survival and reducing brain dysfunction at seven California community hospitals: implementing PAD guidelines via the ABCDEF bundle in 6,064 patients. Crit Care Med. 2017;45:171–8.
14. Pun BT, Balas MC, Barnes-Daly MA, et al. Caring for critically ill patients with the ABCDEF bundle: results of the ICU liberation collaborative in over 15,000 adults. Crit Care Med. 2019;47:3–14.
15. Barr J, Fraser GL, Puntillo K, et al. Clinical practice guidelines for the management of pain, agitation, and delirium in adult patients in the intensive care unit. Crit Care Med. 2013;41:263–306.
16. Adults AGSEPoPDiO. American Geriatrics Society abstracted clinical practice guideline for postoperative delirium in older adults. J Am Geriatr Soc. 2015;63:142–50.
17. Maldonado JR. Pathoetiological model of delirium: a comprehensive understanding of the neurobiology of delirium and an evidence-based approach to prevention and treatment. Crit Care Clin. 2008;24:789–856.
18. Maldonado JR. Neuropathogenesis of delirium: review of current etiologic theories and common pathways. Am J Geriatr Psychiatry. 2013;21:1190–222.
19. Hshieh TT, Fong TG, Marcantonio ER, Inouye SK. Cholinergic deficiency hypothesis in delirium: a synthesis of current evidence. J Gerontol Ser A Biol Med Sci. 2008;63:764–72.
20. Tune LE, Egeli S. Acetylcholine and delirium. Dement Geriatr Cogn Disord. 1999;10:342–4.
21. Flacker JM, Cummings V, Mach JR, Bettin k KDK, Wei J. The association of serum anticholinergic activity with delirium in elderly medical patients. Am J Geriatr Psychiatry. 1998;6:31–41.

22. Itil T, Fink M. Anticholinergic drug-induced delirium: experimental modification, quantitative EEG and behavioral correlations. J Nerv Ment Dis. 1966;143:492–507.
23. Holinger PC, Klawans HL. Reversal of tricyclic-overdosage-induced central anticholinergic syndrome by physostigmine. Am J Psychiatry. 1976;133:1018–23.
24. Trzepacz PT. Is there a final common neural pathway in delirium? Focus on acetylcholine and dopamine. Semin Clin Neuropsychiatry. 2000;5:132–48.
25. van der Mast RC. Pathophysiology of delirium. J Geriatr Psychiatry Neurol. 1998;11:138–45.
26. Graham DG. Catecholamine toxicity: a proposal for the molecular pathogenesis of manganese neurotoxicity and Parkinson's disease. Neurotoxicology. 1984;5:83–95.
27. Devlin JW, Skrobik Y, Gelinas C, et al. Clinical practice guidelines for the prevention and management of pain, agitation/sedation, delirium, immobility, and sleep disruption in adult patients in the ICU. Crit Care Med. 2018;46:e825–73.
28. Girard TD, Pandharipande PP, Carson SS, et al. Feasibility, efficacy, and safety of antipsychotics for intensive care unit delirium: the MIND randomized, placebo-controlled trial. Crit Care Med. 2010;38:428–37.
29. Girard TD, Exline MC, Carson SS, et al. Haloperidol and ziprasidone for treatment of delirium in critical illness. N Engl J Med. 2018;379:2506–16.
30. Agar MR, Lawlor PG, Quinn S, et al. Efficacy of oral risperidone, haloperidol, or placebo for symptoms of delirium among patients in palliative care: a randomized clinical trial. JAMA Intern Med. 2017;177:34–42.
31. Page VJ, Ely EW, Gates S, et al. Effect of intravenous haloperidol on the duration of delirium and coma in critically ill patients (HOPE-ICU): a randomised, double-blind, placebo-controlled trial. Lancet Respir Med. 2013;1:515–23.
32. Khan BA, Perkins AJ, Campbell NL, et al. Pharmacological management of deliruim (PMD) in the intensive care unit: a randomized pragmatic clinical trial. J Am Geriatr Soc. 2019;
33. Campbell NL, Perkins AJ, Khan BA, et al. Deprescribing in the pharmacologic management of delirium (de-PMD): a randomized trial in the intensive care unit. J Am Geriatr Soc. 2019;67:695–702.
34. Devlin JW, Roberts RJ, Fong JJ, et al. Efficacy and safety of quetiapine in critically ill patients with delirium: a prospective, multicenter, randomized, double-blind, placebo-controlled pilot study. Crit Care Med. 2010;38:419–27.
35. Devlin JW, Michaud CJ, Bullard HM, Harris SA, Thomas WL. Quetiapine for intensive care unit delirium: the evidence remains weak. Pharmacotherapy. 2016;36:e12–3.
36. Tahir TA, Eeles E, Karapareddy V, et al. A randomized controlled trial of quetiapine versus placebo in the treatment of delirium. J Psychosom Res. 2010;69:485–90.
37. Jasiak KD, Middleton EA, Camamo JM, Erstad BL, Snyder LS, Huckleberry YC. Evaluation of discontinuation of atypical antipsychotics prescribed for ICU delirium. J Pharm Pract. 2013;26:253–6.
38. Marshall J, Herzig SJ, Howell MD, et al. Antipsychotic utilization in the intensive care unit and in transitions of care. J Crit Care. 2016;33:119–24.
39. Tomichek JE, Stollings JL, Pandharipande PP, Chandrasekhar R, Ely EW, Girard TD. Antipsychotic prescribing patterns during and after critical illness: a prospective cohort study. Crit Care. 2016;20:378.
40. Kram BL, Kram SJ, Brooks KR. Implications of atypical antipsychotic prescribing in the intensive care unit. J Crit Care. 2015;30:814–8.
41. Marcantonio ER, Palihnich K, Appleton P, Davis RB. Pilot randomized trial of donepezil hydrochloride for delirium after hip fracture. J Am Geriatr Soc. 2011;59:S282–8.
42. Overshott R, Vernon M, Morris J, Burns A. Rivastigmine in the treatment of delirium in older people: a pilot study. Int Psychogeriatr. 2010;22:812–8.
43. Liptzin B, Laki A, Garb JL, Fingeroth R, Kushell R. Donepezil in the prevention and treatment of post-surgical deliruim. Am J Geriatr Psychiatry. 2005;13:1100–6.

44. van Eijk MM, Roes KC, Honing ML, et al. Effect of rivastigmine as an adjunct to usual care with haloperidol on duration of delirium and mortality in critically ill patients: a multicentre, double-blind, placebo-controlled randomized trial. Lancet. 2010;376:1829–37.
45. Bu DX, Griffin G, Lichtman H. Mechanisms for the anti-inflammatory effects of statins. Curr Opin Lipidol. 2011;22:165–70.
46. Niessner A, Steiner S, Speidl WS, et al. Simvastatin suppresses endotoxin-induced upregulation of toll-like receptors 4 and 2 in vivo. Atherosclerosis. 2006;189:408–13.
47. Wang H, Lynch JR, Song P, et al. Simvastatin and atorvastatin improve behavioral outcome, reduce hippocampal degeneration, and improve cerebral blood flow after experimental traumatic brain injury. Exp Neurol. 2007;206:59–69.
48. Morandi A, Hughes CG, Thompson JL, et al. Statins and delirium during critical illness: a multicenter, prospective cohort study. Crit Care Med. 2014;42:1899–909.
49. Page VJ, Davis DH, Zhao XB, et al. Statin use and risk of delirium in the critically ill. Am J Respir Crit Care Med. 2014;189:666–73.
50. Page VJ, Casarin A, Ely EW, et al. Evaluation of early administration of simvastatin in the prevention and treatment of delirium in critically ill patients undergoing mechanical ventilation (MoDUS): a randomised, double-blind, placebo-controlled trial. Lancet Respir Med. 2017;5:727–37.
51. Needham DM, Colantuoni E, Dinglas VD, et al. Rosuvastatin versus placebo for delirium in intensive care and subsequent cognitive impairment in patients with sepsis-associated acute respiratory distress syndrome: an ancillary study to a randomised controlled trial. Lancet Respir Med. 2016;4:203–12.
52. Reade MC, Eastwood GM, Bellomo R, et al. Effect of dexmedetomidine added to standard care on ventilator-free time in patients with agitated delirium: a randomized clinical trial. J Am Med Assoc. 2016;315:1460–8.
53. Pandharipande P, Shintani A, Peterson J, et al. Lorazepam is an independent risk factor for transition to delirium in intensive care unit patients. Anesthesiology. 2006;104:21–6.
54. Pandharipande PP, Pun BT, Herr DL, et al. Effect of sedation with dexmedetomidine vs lorazepam on acute brain dysfunction in mechanically ventilated patients: the MENDS randomized controlled trial. JAMA. 2007;298:2644–53.
55. Pandharipande PP, Sanders RD, Girard TD, et al. Effect of dexmedetomidine versus lorazepam on outcome in patients with sepsis: an a priori-designed analysis of the MENDS randomized controlled trial. Crit Care. 2010;14:R38.

Chapter 15
Building a Delirium Network

James L. Rudolph, Elizabeth Archambault, Marianne Shaughnessy, Malaz Boustani, and Karin J. Neufeld

The syndrome of delirium impacts all ages with severe consequences to morbidity and mortality [1, 2]. Yet, much remains unknown about prevention, management, and treatment. Limited understanding of this complex, heterogeneous, and hard-to-identify condition can lead to negativity and hopelessness regarding outcomes and can stunt the progress of both research and patient recovery. Patients, family members, and healthcare providers must all be considered in the approach moving forward. There is significant potential and promise in building a unified network to improve delirium outcomes and research discovery [3]. The purpose of this chapter is to provide tangible guidance for turning the negative emotions associated with delirium into a positive force, by building an informed and passionate network to improve delirium awareness, reduce negative outcomes, and one day eliminate the devastating impact of this syndrome.

J. L. Rudolph (✉) · E. Archambault
Center of Innovation in Long Term Services and Supports, Providence VAMC, Providence, RI, USA
e-mail: James.Rudolph@va.gov

M. Shaughnessy
Office of Geriatrics and Extended Care, Veterans Health Administration, Washington, DC, USA

M. Boustani
Center for Brain Care Innovation, Regenstrief Institute, Indiana University School of Medicine, Indianapolis, IN, USA

K. J. Neufeld
Johns Hopkins University School of Medicine, Baltimore, MD, USA

C. G. Hughes et al. (eds.), *Delirium*, https://doi.org/10.1007/978-3-030-25751-4_15

Delirium Is an Emotional Experience for the Patient, the Family, and the Healthcare Professionals

Delirium is a medical emergency and therefore invokes heightened emotions. Whether the subtype is hypoactive, hyperactive, or mixed, the loved ones of those experiencing an episode of delirium witness the individual in an altered state. The individual is isolated within an inner world, despite having medical professionals and loved ones eager to help them by their side. Unfortunately, these care providers may be perceived as hostile threats, and the individual experiencing delirium is left not only feeling alone but also at grave risk. Both the medical providers and family members may feel helpless as their efforts to calm and comfort are met with resistance and distrust.

Isolation, Fear, and Helplessness

A case of unrecognized delirium was recently reviewed at the annual American Delirium Society (ADS) conference. The patient keenly remembered the disturbing cognitive experiences during the delirium. These experiences were not understood by family and staff, and the patient felt alone, afraid, and helpless to change the course of the disturbing experience.

The nurse had not received training to care for a patient with hyperactive delirium who lashed out verbally and physically in fear and anger. The nurse requested support, but the delirium knowledge gap left her need unmet. This nurse was feeling alone, afraid, and helpless to alter the immediate threats to her safety as well as that of the patient.

In an instant, it seemed that everything had changed for the patient's spouse. She feared for his physical health, but a new terror arose from the behavior of the suddenly unrecognizable individual to whom she had been married for 50 years. Her mind was flooded with questions of what was happening. Would he stay like this for the remainder of his life? How could she care for him if he stayed like this? She found the environment of the hospital, the multitude of treatments, and the medical language to be overwhelming. The wife felt alone, afraid, and helpless to care for her loved one.

The physician focused on the patient's acute medical condition that resulted in the hospitalization. The delirium was an unwanted consequence of the illness. Without evidence or FDA approval of a medication for delirium, the best course of action was to treat the underlying illness. The patient's cognitive condition seemed to be rapidly deteriorating. The nurse was requesting medications to decrease the agitation. The patient's spouse was angry with the physician that more wasn't being done, and the patient yelled obscenities at every opportunity. The physician felt alone, afraid, and helpless to alleviate the condition.

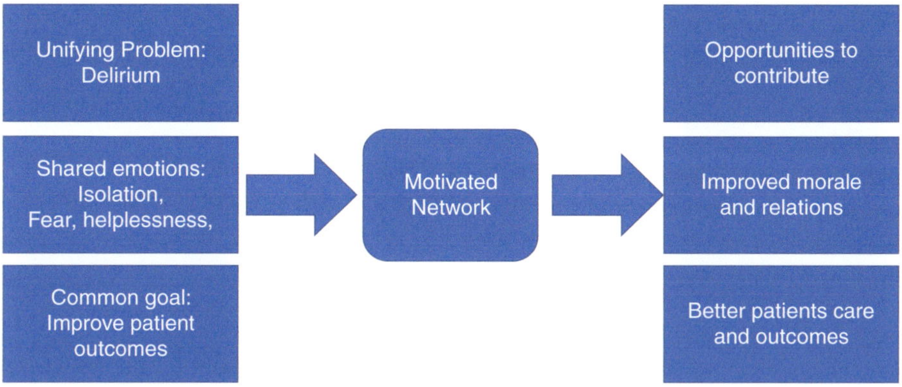

Fig. 15.1 Precursors and potential results of building a delirium network

Delirium: One Common Goal

While these individuals seemed to be entirely at odds with one another, they share the same three emotions – isolation, fear, and helplessness. More significantly, they all shared the singular goal of improvement for the patient. Channeled into this goal for improvement, these emotions can fuel a motivational force to action. A network allows patients, caregivers, nurses, and physicians to share the common bond of the emotions of delirium (Fig. 15.1). Such a network becomes a powerful force for the reduction of both the short- and long-term negative consequences associated with this syndrome and broader dissemination of delirium awareness, knowledge, and best practices.

Addressing the Emotional Experience of Delirium: Together

The first critical step toward improvement is to reduce the isolation associated with delirium. This applies to both the isolation that individuals currently impacted are experiencing and those who are unfamiliar with delirium. There remains a lack of awareness in both the professional and broader community about delirium and its consequences [4–6]. Bringing together people affected by delirium reduces the isolation and allows the emotional experience of delirium to be shared. This mutual experience creates a comfort and bond, which is the essence of the network.

Engaging Highly Motivated People with a Common Bond

Emotions such as fear can fester into anger, which can lead to the breakdown of relationships that are essential to patient-centered care. It is much more feasible to facilitate a network from a place of fear than one of anger which is divisive and alienating. A key strategy to preventing the progression of fear into anger is listening. Hospital environments typically do not lend themselves to extraneous time for nurses and physicians, but the time-consuming task of listening is critical. A sense that there is only one expert in the room impedes listening, if both the providers and the family members believe that those with medical training hold a monopoly on valuable information. The reality is that medical staff are experts on illness and care provision, but the loved one is an expert on the patient's baseline, and the patient is the only expert on what they themselves are feeling. Everyone in the room needs to feel heard, seen, and valued.

A delirium network can leverage the emotions of those affected by delirium by creating an environment in which people who have a common experience listen to and understand one another [7]. If the network provides an outlet for the emotions, there is the opportunity for mutual benefit – energy focused on a constructive outcome, which improves the gaps in delirium knowledge and care. For example, a delirium-focused organization might have an education committee that enables people impacted by delirium to address the knowledge gap by talking to professionals or the public.

Matching People and Opportunity to Advance Delirium Knowledge and Care

While most people who encounter delirium are negatively impacted, their motivations and personal characteristics are individual. The opportunities to advance delirium need to be consistent with this individuality. For example, a family member who observed delirium and doesn't like public speaking is not going to go on a lecture circuit to speak about the experience of delirium. The person and the opportunity need to match.

In building a delirium network, focus should be on the overall mission, some leveraging of available resources, and a bit of luck. The development of Internet-based social networking platforms has brought about unprecedented opportunities to spread information and education at little cost. So, the family member above need not speak in public but could use social media to engage other stakeholders in the discussion.

As evidenced by the case study, strong and uncomfortable emotions are experienced because of delirium. This presents an opportunity to positively channel those emotions by building a motivated network. In establishing a delirium network, care teams should engage in debate and have an honest exchange of ideas. Invitations within the medical center should be extended to key stakeholders impacted by delirium including patient safety committees, falls prevention groups, and occupational safety representation. There may be a snowball effect as these individuals can suggest others who will be important additions to the network. However, some unexpected allies may also surprise you. Once a network is initiated, there will be the potential for ongoing growth. A strategy for keeping individuals engaged is to have a concrete measure of success and to celebrate efforts.

Reconnecting

As the emotional bond of delirium is shared and effort is directed toward positive outlets, a critical component to sustainment of the network is reconnecting with the people who engaged [8]. This reconnection should be simple – expressing gratitude for being a part of the network, invitation to continue to engage, and opportunities for that engagement. The importance of this reconnection cannot be overstated; it is what creates a home for the emotion, effort, and enthusiasm. Put toward a common goal, such as delirium, the sustainability of the network is dependent on this reconnection.

Examples of Delirium Networks

Local Hospital

The Johns Hopkins Delirium Consortium bridges disciplines, departments, and multiple hospitals to increase the free exchange of ideas about delirium [9]. Brought together by their delirium experiences and institutional sponsorship of lunch, multiple disciplines come together and have developed clinical, education, and research collaborations to meet the needs of patients and institutions. Some notable collaborations are the integration of delirium screening in surgery patients and research proposals in the basic mechanisms of delirium.

National Organization

The American Delirium Society (ADS) was built on core fundamentals that engage delirium professionals in the activities of the society [10]. Delirium professionals feel an emotional connection to delirium. They have witnessed firsthand the toll this syndrome takes on the lives of individuals. The American Delirium Society provides opportunities to contribute to advances in care, which keep the individual engaged. Through its annual conferences, the ADS has provided an opportunity for thoughtful engagement, scientific critique, and building a community. ADS leverages the bond of shared delirium experience and contributions to advance clinical care, education, and research. Similar delirium-centered organizations have developed in Europe, Australasia, and now Latin America.

Collaborations Among International Organization

More recently, the world's delirium associations joined together with a common goal to increase delirium awareness. Recognizing that each society was spending a large effort on increasing awareness, iDelirium was formed to coordinate efforts across the globe. The collaboration produced "World Delirium Awareness Day" about which more information can be found at www.idelirium.org. In 2018 and 2019, iDelirium accumulated over 21 million Twitter impressions on a single day during World Delirium Awareness Day. The coordinating task force has grown significantly as the delirium professionals identify an opportunity to direct their emotional energy into creative social media content.

Scientific Networks

The Network for Investigation of Delirium: Unifying Scientists (NIDUS) is a collaborative, multidisciplinary network dedicated to the acceleration of scientific discovery in delirium research, through focused collaboration and creation of sustainable infrastructure to enhance innovative and high-quality research. NIDUS was created in response to a call from the National Institutes on Aging to support a collaborative network to advance scientific research on the causes, mechanisms, outcomes, diagnosis, prevention, and treatment of delirium in older adults.

Summary

Delirium creates an emotional experience in those impacted including patients, families, and healthcare professionals. By bringing together highly motivated people with a common emotional experience, there is an opportunity for mutual understanding and action. Delirium networks provide an opportunity to improve clinical care, education, and research.

References

1. Marcantonio ER. Delirium in hospitalized older adults. N Engl J Med. 2017;377(15):1456–66.
2. Patel AKBM, Traube C. Delirium in pediatric critical care. Pediatr Clin N Am. 2017;64(5):1117.
3. Shaughnessy M, Rudolph JL. Building a Delirium Network. J Am Geriatr Soc. 2011;59(s2):S233–S.
4. Bull MJ, Boaz L, Sjostedt JM. Family caregivers' knowledge of delirium and preferred modalities for receipt of information. J Appl Gerontol: Off J Southern Gerontol Soc. 2016;35(7):744–58.

5. Kales HC, Kamholz BA, Visnic SG, Blow FC. Recorded delirium in a national sample of elderly inpatients: potential implications for recognition. J Geriatr Psychiatry Neurol. 2003;16(1):32–8.
6. Steis MR, Fick DM. Are nurses recognizing delirium? A systematic review. J Gerontol Nurs. 2008;34(9):40–8.
7. Manville B. You need a community, not a network. Harv Bus Rev. 2014. https://hbr.org/product/you-need-a-community-not-a-network/H00ZIT-PDF-ENG?referral=02749. Accessed Aug 26, 2019.
8. Schawbel D. 7 ways to build a strong Netowrk. American Express Open Forum.
9. Neufeld KJ, Joseph Bienvenu O, Rosenberg PB, Mears SC, Lee HB, Kamdar BB, et al. The Johns Hopkins delirium consortium: a model for collaborating across disciplines and departments for delirium prevention and treatment. J Am Geriatr Soc. 2011;59(Suppl 2):S244–8.
10. Rudolph JL, Boustani M, Kamholz B, Shaughnessey M, Shay K. Delirium: a strategic plan to bring an ancient disease into the 21st century. J Am Geriatr Soc. 2011;59(s2):S237–S40.

Index

C. G. Hughes et al. (eds.), *Delirium*, https://doi.org/10.1007/978-3-030-25751-4

MIX
Papier aus verantwortungsvollen Quellen
Paper from responsible sources
FSC® C105338

If you have any concerns about our products,
you can contact us on
ProductSafety@springernature.com

In case Publisher is established outside the EU,
the EU authorized representative is:
Springer Nature Customer Service Center GmbH
Europaplatz 3, 69115 Heidelberg, Germany

Printed by Libri Plureos GmbH
in Hamburg, Germany